Management of Gastrointestinal Cancer

Management of Gastrointestinal Cancer

Edited by

Peter McCulloch
and
Andrew Kingsnorth

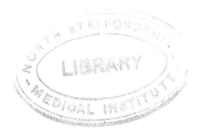

BMJ
Publishing
Group

© BMJ Publishing Group 1996

First published in 1996
by the BMJ Publishing Group, BMA House, Tavistock Square,
London WC1H 9JR

British Library Cataloguing in Publication Data

A catalogue record for this book is available from the
British Library

ISBN 0-7279-1071-X

Typeset by Latimer Trend & Company Ltd, Plymouth
Printed by Craft Print, Singapore

Contents

Contributors

Riccardo A Audisio
Division of General Surgery, European Institute of Oncology, Milan, Italy

John Bancewicz
Reader in Surgery and Consultant Surgeon
University of Manchester Department of Surgery, Hope Hospital, Salford, UK

Stephen R Bloom
Professor of Endocrinology
Royal Postgraduate Medical School, Hammersmith Hospital, London, UK

Han J Bonenkamp
Department of Surgery, Leiden University Hospital, The Netherlands

Peter Boyle
Director
Division of Epidemiology and Biostatistics, European Institute of Oncology, Milan, Italy

Brian Cottier
Consultant in Clinical Oncology and Chief Executive
Clatterbridge Centre for Oncology, Bebington, UK

Martin M Eatock
Registrar in Medical Oncology
Glasgow Royal Infirmary University NHS Trust, Glasgow, UK

Hugh M Gilmour
Senior Lecturer
Department of Pathology, University of Edinburgh, UK

J Hermans
Department of Medical Statistics, Leiden University Hospital, The Netherlands

Nicholas D James
Senior Lecturer in Clinical Oncology
CRC Institute for Cancer Studies, Queen Elizabeth Hospital, Edgbaston, Birmingham, UK

H I Keizer
Department of Oncology, Leiden University Hospital, The Netherlands

David J Kerr
Professor of Clinical Oncology
CRC Institute for Cancer Studies, Queen Elizabeth Hospital, Edgbaston, Birmingham, UK

Andrew Kingsnorth
Professor of Surgery
Plymouth Postgraduate Medical School, Derriford Hospital, Plymouth, UK

A R Kinsella
Senior Lecturer (non-clinical)
Department of Surgery, University of Liverpool, Liverpool, UK

Witold Kmiot
Senior Lecturer in Surgery
Royal Postgraduate Medical School, Hammersmith Hospital, London, UK

Andrew S Krajewski
Senior Lecturer
Department of Pathology, University of Edinburgh, UK

Nicholas R Lemoine
Professor of Molecular Pathology
Imperial Cancer Research Fund Oncology Unit, Royal Postgraduate Medical School, Hammersmith Hospital, London, UK

Peter McCulloch
Senior Lecturer in Surgery
University of Liverpool, UK

Arthur B McKie
Research Fellow
Imperial Cancer Research Fund Oncology Unit, Royal Postgraduate Medical School, Hammersmith Hospital, London, UK

Patrick Maisonneuve
Division of Epidemiology and Biostatistics, European Institute of Oncology, Milan, Italy

Masatoshi Makuuchi
Professor and Chairman
Second Department of Surgery, Faculty of Medicine, University of Tokyo, Tokyo, Japan

Shinichi Miyagawa
Associate Professor
First Department of Surgery, Shinshu University School of Medicine,
Matsumoto, Japan

Derrick F Martin
Consultant Radiologist
Withington Hospital, Manchester, UK

J R G Nash
Reader
Department of Pathology, University of Liverpool, Liverpool, UK

Donal O'Shea
Senior Lecturer in Endocrinology
Royal Postgraduate Medical School, Hammersmith Hospital, London,
UK

Harushi Osugi
Senior Lecturer in Surgery
Second Department of Surgery, Osaka City University Medical School,
Osaka, Japan

Alistair C Parker
Senior Lecturer
Department of Medicine, University of Edinburgh, Edinburgh, UK

David R Peake
Senior Registrar in Clinical Oncology
Clatterbridge Centre for Oncology, Bebington, UK

Mitsuru Sasako
Chief, Gastric Surgery Division
National Cancer Centre Hospital, Tokyo, Japan

I Songun
Department of Surgery, Leiden University Hospital, The Netherlands

Mike Soukop
Consultant Physician and Medical Oncologist
Glasgow Royal Infirmary University NHS Trust, Glasgow, UK

Kenichi Sugihara
Staff Surgeon
Division of Colorectal Surgery, National Cancer Center Hospital, Tsukij,
Tokyo, Japan

Tadatoshi Takayama
Chief, Hepatic Surgery Division
Second Department of Surgery, Tokyo University School of Medicine,
Tokyo, Japan

C J H van de Velde
Professor of Surgery Head of Department of Surgical Oncology and
Chairman
Dutch Gastric Cancer Group, Leiden University Hospital, The
Netherlands

Alison Waghorn
Research Registrar
Royal Postgraduate Medical School, Hammersmith Hospital, London,
UK

Robin C N Williamson
Professor of Surgery
Royal Postgraduate Medical School, London, UK

Preface

What kind of book is this, and why? A preface should tell you these things, and should do so briefly and clearly. This is a practical book on the management of gastrointestinal cancers. It is aimed at busy specialists who need a concise but authoritative reference work, and at higher trainees in all the disciplines which make up the modern integrated cancer care team. It contains descriptions of the currently accepted methods of diagnosis, staging, and treatment in this group of tumours, with critical analysis of their success rate and problems. It focuses on controversial areas in management and puts the arguments for the different views. It tries to integrate the surgical and oncological approaches to each tumour type by putting together a contribution from a surgical and a medical/radiation oncological specialist. It does not dwell in great detail on novel approaches that have yet to find their way into practice, but it does pay special attention to aetiology, palliative care, and the principles behind new approaches to treatment.

Why did we design it this way? Because we perceived that the way in which cancer care is organised is changing fundamentally in many countries. The long term future vision for cancer management clearly involves the formation of interdisciplinary specialist teams, with surgeon, radiotherapist, and oncologist working together much more closely than in the past. There is, therefore, a need for a text that can update clinicians on the contributions of their colleagues to the team, and give a broader understanding of the context of their own contribution to the treatment of the individual patient. When uncertainty arises over the choice of approach, a well referenced authoritative account by an expert in the field can be very useful in deciding what to do. This was one reason for the very practical focus of the text. We hope this approach will be relevant across national boundaries, as the modern care of gastrointestinal tract cancer will not differ in its essentials in all well developed health care systems. The situation in the United Kingdom exemplifies these changes: British cancer services are in a state of upheaval following the recent adoption by the government of a report recommending the restructuring of cancer services along multidisciplinary lines. Those currently in training both here and abroad will inhabit a world in which integrated cancer care is the norm, and to them the suggestion that a text should approach cancer care from the viewpoint of one speciality only will seem bizarre.

The reasons for the publication of a book confined to gastrointestinal cancers are probably well accepted. Firstly, the clinicians (mainly surgeons and gastroenterologists) whose specialist training leads them to an interest in this area form a distinct group. Because of their background it is common for these specialists to have interests or involvement in the management of several forms of gastrointestinal cancer. They will readily appreciate the degree to which the methods used in diagnosis and in surgical and minimally invasive treatment overlap. The differential diagnosis of one form of gastrointestinal tract cancer will often include other forms, and the approach to diagnosis and staging is common to most, if not all, forms. The same can be said of many of the surgical problems posed by these tumours because they arise in large part from operating in the abdominal cavity, and in particular on the digestive tube and associated secretory organs. The prime example is the importance of anastomotic leakage as a complication of surgery in cancers of the pancreas, oesophagus, and rectum. In each case leakage is the most common potentially lethal complication of surgery, and similarities in prevention, diagnosis, and management of this complication reflect the common problems posed by the corrosive effects of enzymatic and digestive secretions together with the infective potential of the gut microflora. A second important unifying factor is the similarity in behaviour of many gastrointestinal tract cancers. These reflect similarities in histogenesis, anatomy, and pathogenesis. When contrasted with tumours of the breast, lung, or central nervous system, the gut cancers have a number of notable common features. The diseases have a marked tendency towards lymphatic and transcoelomic metastasis and relatively rapid progression, with poor five year survival rates. On the other hand, survival after attempted curative treatment does appear to give good prospects of remaining permanently disease free in those patients who do survive five years, in contrast to the situation in tumours such as melanoma, breast cancer, and renal cancer, where metastatic recurrence after many years is relatively common. Anatomy dictates that most bloodborne metastasis from gastrointestinal cancers occurs in the liver, and this has led to a particular interest in the treatment of such metastasis by surgical or regional rather than systemic approaches. Frustratingly, the other common characteristic shared by many of these carcinomas is their relative resistance to radiotherapy and chemotherapy. It is partly this that has led to their remaining for so long the territory of the surgeon alone, but there are signs that surgical predominance in management, already weakened by the widespread acceptance of adjuvant chemotherapy for Dukes's C colon cancer, will continue to decline. To the extent that this reflects improved efficacy of a multimodal approach it should be welcomed.

We have divided some of the chapters into two parts, and have asked the surgeons to deal not only with surgical management, but also with epidemiology, pathogenesis, diagnosis and staging, while the oncologists have been asked to discuss quality of life issues and terminal care as well as adjuvant or definitive non-surgical treatment. This seemed a sensible scheme to us, because there is a certain logic to dealing with aetiological concerns before discussing diagnosis and staging, and surgeons are generally more likely to be directly involved in the latter than are their oncological colleagues. Conversely, oncologists and radiotherapists often have more direct involvement in palliative care than surgeons, although the circumstances of each case will determine which speciality is principally involved. Oncologists and surgeons have different perspectives, and each can discuss most authoritatively those aspects of cancer management that they themselves feel fall within their ambit. Where perspectives differ sufficiently to cause controversy or disagreement it is the job of the editors to attempt to harmonise views, or, if this is not possible, to allow a balanced presentation of the different arguments while avoiding contradiction or repetition. We feel that this approach has worked well, and would point in particular to the long chapter on hepatobiliary cancers. This is a joint production from five main authors in three different disciplines. Such a cooperative was necessary to cover the range of the subject material, including, as it does, tumours as different as bile duct carcinoma and colorectal liver metastasis, and the variety of therapeutic approaches now available, from alcohol injection to endoscopic retrograde cholepan-creatography interventions to radical surgery. Each subsection was written independently by an authority in the field, and the contributions were then blended into a coherent whole.

A unique feature of this book is the large Japanese contribution to a text principally aimed at a non-Japanese readership. We hope this will increase the international appeal of the book. The Japanese provide an independent perspective on cancer care, which will be novel to many readers, and we feel that the cross fertilisation of ideas that has resulted from this collaboration may help clinicians in many countries in re-examining the concepts on which they base their practice. The British approach to cancer care is very much moulded by working within the constraints of a "socialised" health care system. This has many advantages for the overall standard of health care but places restrictions on the activity of the clinician, to which many become so inured that they cease to notice them. This partly explains the British tradition of conservatism and scepticism in the adoption of new treatments. This is not to denigrate the British approach, which is widely praised by thoughtful clinicians from many other countries, alarmed by the harm and waste that can be caused by incautious enthusiasm unhampered by a sufficiency of rational scepticism. The commonplace contrast is the American viewpoint, but this too is hugely influenced by the economics of the health system in the USA. The unsustainability of the American approach since the 1960s, even for the world's largest economy, has become clear in recent years. Given this fact, we feel that it is not always helpful to clinicians in other countries to be advised on management by colleagues working in a system that still has a natural tendency to regard cost as no object and new technology as an end in itself. The Japanese offer another alternative view, from which we can learn much. Unlike clinicians in Britain and America, Japanese cancer specialists have not been particularly influenced by the sea change in thinking about the metastatic behaviour of tumours that has resulted from advances in breast cancer research and treatment. The refutation of the Halsted and Handley "centripetal" model of metastasis—from localised growth to lymph nodes to bloodstream in the case of breast cancer—has resulted in widespread application of the "alternative" paradigm known as "biologic predeterminism", in relation not only to breast cancer but also to many other tumours whose observed natural history is very different. The main implication of this theory—namely, that surgery has no role beyond excision of visible primary tumour—has, we feel, been damaging to the technical development of Western cancer surgery. The fact that the Japanese have never accepted this implication in practice has given them (and through them, us) a unique opportunity to study the value of radical surgery empirically. The increasing number of European surgeons visiting Japan are uniformly impressed by the technical excellence of their surgery and the safety of even superradical procedures in Japanese hands. Japanese surgeons are undoubtedly blessed with an extraordinarily slim fit population whose low incidence of atherosclerotic heart disease greatly benefits them. None the less, those of us who have become regular visitors are convinced that Japanese diligence in meticulous haemostasis and anatomical dissection play no small part in their success. The Japanese remain somewhat reluctant to embrace the methodology of the controlled clinical trial, for lack of which much of their reported success in cancer surgery remains subjudice in the rest of the world. While convinced that we in the West are right to continue urging the Japanese to carry out randomised controlled trials, we feel that the West should not ignore the strengths of the Japanese approach to clinical research. This is essentially conducted as a rolling complete audit cycle, with regular re-evaluation of the current practice and agreement on changes to be made for the period until the next evaluation. The impressive feature of the Japanese version of audit is the meticulous cooperative data collection in huge numbers of patients. The oft quoted example of the National Cancer Centre database on gastric cancer in Tokyo is illustrative, containing the records of over 5000 consecutive cases. The completeness and accuracy of the data collection in this and other Japanese series is such that a missing data rate of 1% would be regarded as a disaster by those who use and run the system, a level of performance to which few outside Japan can currently aspire. Attention to detail can never substitute for randomisation as a means of eliminating bias, but it does allow us to measure influences we suspect with great precision. We should remember that in Popperian terms the randomised controlled trial is only one of a large number of possible tools available for testing hypotheses, and that its use is relatively rare in most branches of science other than medicine. The success of the Japanese approach in technical developments throughout industry should give us pause for thought, as in many ways the process of modern cancer treatment can be described more accurately as a technical than as a scientific exercise. All of which is simply to say that the Japanese surgical authors in this text are not only superb technicians, whose expertise should be respected, but also clear and logical thinkers whose understanding of the diseases with which they deal is profound.

The value of textbooks to the group for whom we are writing can be legitimately challenged. Experienced clinicians and senior trainees will be well aware of the main management options and the important factors that will guide these in most cases. They will also be more critical of ex cathedra statements advising on the best course in controversial areas than more junior trainees because they will be familiar with the uncertainties of the process of clinical research by which treatment gradually evolves. Even the most experienced and knowledgeable clinician sometimes needs to refresh his or her memory, however, and we hope that our balanced approach will make the broad picture of treatment options more coherent for the reader coming to the text for a perspective on a clinical problem. Both practising clinicians and higher trainees need help from time to time in sorting out the evidence and the various arguments in acknowledged areas of controversy. We hope that by providing detailed, adequately referenced discussion of these areas we can give this.

This kind of book on management can rapidly become outdated, and we are as vulnerable to this process as anyone. The speed of progress is not so great in established practice as it is in the research field, however, as a review of major management changes since the 1980s will indicate. This is principally because clinical trials are necessarily a slow business, a fact which is unlikely to change. In common with the rest of the scientific and technical publishing world, we hope to be in a position to take advantage of the ever accelerating advances in computerised information media in the future. Whether paper texts survive into the twenty first century or whether they are replaced by interactive CD-ROM type programs remains to be seen. We are ready to change with the times, but the promises of the paperless office of 10 years ago ring a little hollow to those of us now regularly deluged with a torrent of mail merged, word processed paper, which would have been impossible without the devices that were supposed to have the reverse effect.

We have consistently attempted to bring out certain themes and topics that are of general importance to those dealing with gut cancer. The background to the diseases is one of these: the epidemiological aspects of this are given a separate chapter by Peter Boyle and colleagues, as well as sections at the beginning of each organ based chapter. The pathophysiology of disease is not considered in exhaustive detail, but chapters on the molecular biology of gastrointestinal tract cancer, cell biology, and metastases give an overview of the similarities in the molecular background of many of these tumours, as well as some of the differences. Quality of life and palliative care nowadays receive more consideration in management discussions than heretofore, and rightly so. We have specifically asked each contributor to consider these issues as they affect the management of the particular tumour they are writing about. We have not discouraged our authors from looking to the future. Some, like Nicholas James and David Kerr, have responded by sketching the outline of what may form the basis of treatments in the twenty first century, based on principles completely different from those in use today. Others have been more modest in their speculations. We hope this view of the future from the viewpoint of experts deeply involved in the development of the field will prove stimulating. As to accuracy, we shall have to wait and see. We hope you find this book informative, sensible, useful, and stimulating.

Finally, we should not forget to thank those who have helped to make the book possible, particularly Mary Banks of the BMJ Publishing Group, Maureen Crowley and Yvonne Cross at the Department of Surgery in Liverpool, all the contributors to the chapters and of course the wives and families of the two editors. Thank you all, and bonne chance.

Peter McCulloch
Andrew Kingsnorth

1: Epidemiology

PETER BOYLE, PATRICK MAISONNEUVE, and
RICCARDO A AUDISIO

The gastrointestinal tract is a common and important site for cancer in men and women throughout the world. It is, however, very difficult to make broad epidemiological statements about cancer of the gastrointestinal tract because there is a variety of different types of cancer in this category, some of which dominate in some parts of the world (for example, stomach cancer in the former Soviet Union and colorectal cancer in western Europe) and are rarer in others. As is the case when considering treatment and pathological aspects of these diseases, it is essential to consider the epidemiology of the various sites of cancer separately, and the different types of cancer which can be seen within one site. In what follows, all rates quoted are average, annual age-adjusted rates per 100,000 person years, adjusted to the world standard population.

Cancer of the oesophagus

Perhaps more than any other form of cancer, oesophageal cancer is characterised by an enormous range in occurrence throughout the world with incidence rates as high as 195·3 in females and 165·3 in males in northern Gonbad in the Caspian region of Iran[1] and mortality rates of 211·2 in males and 136·5 in females recorded in Linxian county in China.[2] These rates are in marked contrast to those from Cluj county in Romania where reported incidence rates were 1·2 in males and 0·2 in females around the early 1980s.[3]

The highest risk areas of the world include the so-called *Asian oesophageal cancer belt* that stretches from the Caspian littoral in northern Iran, through the southern Republics of the (former) USSR, to eastern China.[4] Moderately high rates are observed in south-east Africa, parts of eastern South America and certain areas of western Europe, such as France and Switzerland. The pattern of oesophageal cancer in men in the European Union is dominated by the aggregation of départements in north-west France with similar and high rates of oesophageal cancer mortality. In sharp contrast is the situation

1

in women where the highest rates are found in the counties of Scotland and Ireland.[5]

The highest male incidence rate reported is from the département of Calvados in France (26·5 per 100 000) and with two other French départements in the highest ten: Somme (19·3) and Bas Rhin (18·7).[6] Other population groups with high rates include Porto Alegre in Brazil, Afro-American populations in the United States and Bermuda, and Chinese

TABLE 1.1—*Ten highest and ten lowest incidence rates of oesophageal cancer in men and women around 1985 (ICD-9 150)*

Male			Female		
Area	Cases	Rate*	Area	Cases	Rate*
Highest					
France, Calvados	466	26·5	India, Bangalore	384	8·8
Brazil, Porto Alegre	108	25·9	India, Bombay	901	8·4
Bermuda: black	18	24·9	China, Tianjin	671	8·0
US, Connecticut: black	100	19·5	Canada, NWT and Yukon	5	7·0
France, Somme	126	19·3	Brazil, Porto Alegre	44	6·9
France, Bas Rhin	480	18·7	China, Shanghai	1 477	6·4
Hong Kong	2 391	18·1	India, Madras	352	6·3
US, Atlanta: black	141	17·4	India, Ahmedabad	217	5·6
China, Tianjin	1 294	16·6	Kyrgyzstan	212	5·5
US, Detroit: black	336	15·9	UK, East Scotland	126	4·9
Lowest					
Algeria, Setif	15	1·4	Czech., Boh. and Morav.	263	0·5
Mali, Bamako	6	1·3	US, Hawaii: Japanese	7	0·4
Israel: born Afr. Asia	38	1·3	Spain, Zaragoza	12	0·4
US, Hawaii: Chinese	3	1·2	Romania, County Cluj	10	0·4
Singapore: Malay	5	1·2	Poland, Warsaw Rural	10	0·4
Israel: non-Jews	8	1·1	Hungary, Vas	4	0·3
Peru, Trujillo	5	1·0	Spain, Granada	7	0·3
The Gambia	5	1·0	Italy, Ragusa	3	0·2
US, Los Angeles: Filipino	2	0·6	US, Los Angeles: Japanese	1	0·1
Israel: born Israel	4	0·6	Israel: non-Jews	0	

* Per 100 000 population.

communities (Table 1.1). For women, there are four states of India among the highest ten regions, as well as two Chinese communities, Kyrgyzstan and the east of Scotland (Table 1.1). Even the highest incidence rates in women are substantially lower than the highest recorded in men.[7]

Striking differences in occurrence have been demonstrated, more than for any other site, over small geographic areas in northern Iran, in the Transkei, and in Brittany in France.[8-10] Differences are also seen between ethnic groups residing in the same area with, for example, the incidence rates in Afro–Americans (13·9 in all SEER areas) being threefold higher than those in the white population (4·0), and rates for the Chinese in Singapore being double those in Indians and 10 times greater than those in Malays in the same population. Even within different dialect groups in the Chinese of Singapore, marked variations have been reported,[11] the highest levels being seen in Teochew males (27·0). The same pattern is seen in females, albeit at lower levels of incidence. A slow but significant decrease in incidence has been observed.

A decline in mortality rates has been noted in the youngest age groups in Linxian county, the highest incidence area of the People's Republic of China, presumably in relation to an improvement of nutritional standards.[2] However, rates have doubled in the Afro–American population in the United States over the past 30 years.[12] A considerable increase was also observed in the Transkei in the 1960s, this cancer having been practically unknown before 1930.[9]

Temporal trends in mortality

There are mortality data available at national levels from over 100 countries for a varying period of time within the World Health Organisation (WHO) Mortality database. Rather than assemble all available information, we have taken nine representative countries of Europe, east (Czechoslovakia and Poland) and west (Germany, United Kingdom, Denmark, and Italy), North America (Canada) and Asia (Japan and Australia).[13] Unfortunately, mortality data are unavailable from many populations where the levels and temporal pattern of gastrointestinal cancer may be of great interest: this includes most countries of Africa and Asia.

In Canada both the truncated and overall age adjusted mortality rates have been increasing in males since 1955. The rates in females, however, remain stable during the period. Consequent birth cohort examination shows an increase in rates in successive birth cohorts born after 1900. In females the mortality rates remain stable in successive birth cohorts for age groups over 50. For those at ages below 50, the rates have been decreasing in recent birth cohorts.

In Japan there is no overall tendency in either truncated or overall age adjusted mortality rates in males since 1955. In females the truncated rates have been decreasing during the entire study period. The overall age adjusted mortality rates, however, remained unchanged until 1970 and then decreased. Birth cohort examination shows relatively stable rates in successive birth cohorts in males for age groups over 40. For those with ages below 40, the rates have been decreasing. In females, a rapid decrease in rates in successive birth cohorts born after 1890 has been observed.

In former Czechoslovakia both the truncated and overall age adjusted mortality rates in males underwent a slight decrease until 1970, and have been increasing since. A 4·5-fold increase was observed in truncated rates between 1970 and 1988. In females the mortality rates have been stable since 1955. Examination by birth cohort shows a consistent decrease until around the 1920 cohort. For those born after this, the rates have been increasing rapidly in successive birth cohorts. In females no systematic change in rates has been observed in successive birth cohorts.

In Poland a slight decrease was observed for both truncated and overall age adjusted mortality rates in males between 1962 and 1978; however the rates have since been increasing, particularly the truncated rates. In females both the truncated and overall age adjusted mortality rates have been decreasing during the entire study period. Birth cohort examination shows a decrease in rates in males for cohorts born before 1920. For cohorts born thereafter, the rates have been increasing in successive birth cohorts except for the age group 30–34, which shows an unstable rate. In females the mortality rates have been decreasing in successive birth cohorts for almost all the age groups examined.

In Germany the truncated rates in males remained stable until 1972. Recently, however, they have been increasing. The overall age adjusted mortality rates in males in fact showed a slight decrease between 1955 and 1975 but then started to increase. In females no remarkable time trend was observed for either truncated or overall age adjusted mortality rates, although a slight increase in truncated rates is noticeable since 1980. Birth cohort examination shows a decline in rates in successive birth cohorts born around 1910 and a rapid increase in rates for cohorts born after this. In females most of the age groups showed a decrease in rates in successive birth cohorts except for age groups between 40 and 59 in which an increase in rates has been observed for recent birth cohorts.

In the United Kingdom both the truncated and overall age adjusted mortality rates have been increasing in males since 1955, and there is no sign of a levelling off. In females a slight but steady increase was observed for overall age adjusted mortality rates since 1955. For truncated rates, however, a slight increase was observed only for the period 1955–75; the rates have been stable ever since. Birth cohort examination shows a consistent increase in rates in successive birth cohorts born after 1910 in males. In females the rates have been increasing in successive birth cohorts for age groups over 50. For other age groups, the rates have been either stable or decreasing.

In Denmark both the truncated and overall age adjusted mortality rates did not show a clear time trend in males until 1975, when an increase was observed. In females although the overall age adjusted mortality rates have remained stable, the truncated rates showed a slight increase during the study period. Examination by birth cohorts shows an increase in rates for cohorts born after 1895 in males. In females an increase in rates in successive birth cohorts was observed only for age groups between 45 and 54. For other age groups the rates are either stable or decreasing.

In Italy the truncated rates have been increasing in males since 1955. The overall age adjusted mortality rates, however, increased until 1975 and have remained stable ever since. In females both the truncated and overall age adjusted mortality rates have been stable since 1955. Birth cohort examination shows the mortality rates in males have been stable in successive birth cohorts except for the age groups between 40 and 59 where the rates have been increasing in successive birth cohorts. In females the rates are similar in all birth cohorts and in all age groups examined.

Aetiology

The most important risk factors for cancer of the oesophagus in developed countries are cigarette smoking and alcohol consumption.[14 15] The highest rates of oesophageal cancer in Europe are to be found in France[5 16] and findings from a series of studies conducted in the north west of this country have led to the estimation that 85% of all oesophageal cancers could be attributable to the joint effects of cigarette smoking and alcohol consumption. The associations between cigarette smoking, alcohol consumption, and oesophageal cancer are difficult to treat separately, largely because of the correlation in the two exposures and their mutual association with risk of cancer of the oesophagus. The risk of oesophageal cancer has also been shown to be increased among non-smokers by the consumption of alcohol, and among non-drinkers of alcohol by smoking.[17]

Studies from France[18] and Italy[19] have reported a strong association with tobacco smoking and relative risks of between 5 and 10 for heavy smokers. As is the case for cancer of the oral cavity, the association was found to be particularly strong for pipes and cigars and, among cigarette smokers, for high tar/dark tobacco cigarettes.[20]

A high prevalence of alcoholism among patients with oesophageal cancer and an apparent association between the disease and employment in the production and distribution of alcoholic beverages have been noted since the early nineteenth century.[21] In more modern times a prospective study of Danish brewery workers showed a twofold increased risk of oesophageal cancer over that expected.[22] The role of alcohol consumption was most clearly demonstrated in the French département of Ille-et-Vilaine where the risk rose steadily with dose of alcohol consumed.[18 23] There is good support for this association from ecological data.[24]

The relative risks for alcohol and tobacco tend to combine in a multiplicative manner: the relative risk in individuals who consumed more than 120/g/day of alcohol and more than 30/g/day of tobacco was 149 compared with non- or moderate drinkers and smokers.[18 23] Although this magnitude of risk should be extremely worrisome for people exposed to high levels of both risk factors, it offers important prospects for prevention because elimination of either of these risk factors could lead to substantial reductions in the overall risk. All forms of tobacco smoking, including pipes and cigars, are associated with the increased risk of oesophageal cancer but the risk is apparently less strong for the newer filter, lower tar cigarettes than for the older, high tar ones. Likewise various types of alcoholic beverages including spirits, wine, and beer, are related to oesophageal cancer risk. Although it is the combined effect of these two exposures that gives rise to these large risks, each of these factors is an independent carcinogen for the oesophageal epithelium.[17]

In addition to alcohol and tobacco, several other factors have been demonstrated to be involved in the aetiology of oesophageal cancer. Neither alcohol nor tobacco is substantially involved in the aetiology in high incidence areas of some developing countries, such as Iran[25] and China. Several potential determinants related to dietary intake have been identified, including thermal irritation or contamination of foodstuffs, but generalised dietary deficiencies are probably a major contributing factor to the carcinogenic process.[26] Diet in these high risk areas is poor in vitamins A and C and several other micronutrients and, more generally, fruits and vegetables;[27] these factors may also be related to oesophageal cancer risk in developed countries. Further, studies conducted in Africa as well as northern Italy have suggested an association between oesophageal cancer risk and increased consumption of maize,[26] which has been recognised as capable of inducing deficiencies of several micronutrients (thiamine, riboflavin, and particularly niacin) and, in severe cases, pellagra, a disease that entails widespread inflammation of the upper digestive tract mucosa. The risk of oesophageal cancer is also increased among individuals with Barrett's oesophagus.[28]

Cancer of the stomach

Stomach cancer remains numerically the second most common form of cancer in the world, accounting for around 10% of all cancers, with an estimated 755 000 new cases a year for both sexes combined.[29] Overall rates in men are approximately double those in females.

Remarkable in both men and women, the six highest incidence rates are reported from cancer registries of Japan (Table 1.2). In men the highest rate is in Yamagata (93·3 per 100 000), with the highest incidence rate outside a Japanese population being considerably less and reported from St Petersburg (52·8). In women the highest rate, also reported from Yamagata (42·9 per 100 000), is substantially lower than the incidence rate recorded in men in the same population. Low incidence rates are reported

TABLE 1.2—*Ten highest and ten lowest incidence rates of stomach cancer in men and women around 1985 (ICD-9 151)*

Male			Female		
Area	Cases	Rate*	Area	Cases	Rate*
Highest					
Japan, Yamagata	3 457	93·3	Japan, Yamagata	2 052	42·9
Japan, Hiroshima	2 048	85·8	Japan, Hiroshina	1174	38·9
Japan, Miyagi	5 563	85·4	Japan, Saga	898	36·9
Japan, Saga	1 487	81·7	Japan, Miyagi	2 987	36·7
Japan, Nagasaki	1 035	79·0	Japan, Osaka	9 622	32·7
Japan, Osaka	16 694	73·6	Japan, Nagasaki	553	31·7
Russia, St Petersburg	6 071	52·8	Peru, Trujillo	132	26·5
China, Shanghai	10 213	51·7	Russia, St Petersburg	6 647	25·4
China, Qidong	1 206	49·8	Portugal, V N de Gaia	183	23·9
Portugal, V N de Gaia	239	47·8	US, Los Angeles: Korean	52	22·9
Lowest					
US, Iowa	669	6·5	Canada, PEI	27	3·3
Singapore: Malay	34	6·4	US, Utah	144	3·2
US, Utah	234	6·3	Israel: non-Jews	28	3·0
US, Atlanta: white	189	5·9	US, Iowa	434	2·7
Bermuda: white and other	8	5·7	Thailand, Khon Kaen	27	2·5
Thailand, Khon Kaen	47	5·0	US, Atlanta: white	128	2·5
Kuwait: Kuwaitis	26	4·2	Kuwait: Kuwaitis	13	2·0
US, Los Angeles: Filipino	16	4·0	India, Ahmedabad	70	1·5
The Gambia	22	3·9	The Gambia	7	1·51
India, Ahmedabad	100	2·1	Bermuda: white and other	0	

* Per 100 000 population.

from a disparate group of communities. It is surprising to consider the difference in the incidence rate in men in Japan and to contrast this with the incidence rate reported in men in various white or predominantly white populations of the United States, such as Iowa (6·5 per 100 000), Utah (6·3), and Atlanta (5·9) (see Table 1.2).

The highest recorded incidence rates in men are those from the Far East with very high rates in males in Japan and in the former Soviet Union.[30] Fairly high rates have also been reported from parts of China, Latin America, and central and eastern Europe. In western Europe age standardised incidence rates are generally lower. Rates in northern Italy (40·2 in Florence) are substantially higher than in Ragusa in Sicily (16·1), a differential confirmed in studies of southern Italian migrants to the north of the country.[31] In Africa, areas of high frequency have been reported in certain mountainous regions in Rwanda, south-west Uganda, and Tanzania, around Mount Kilimanjaro. Relatively low levels are recorded in white population groups in the United States.

There are marked variations by socioeconomic status, with a twofold difference in cumulative mortality rates between the highest and lowest socioeconomic groups seen in England and Wales.[32] Low rates are none the less observed in India (around 10) and in the Philippines, being even lower in Filipinos in California and in Hawaii.

The risk of stomach cancer changes slowly in populations moving from high risk to low risk communities, and incidence rates in American Japanese, although about one-third of those in Japan, are none the less about twice those in the white population. Declines in risk with increasing duration of residence have been observed for at least some European populations migrating to Australia.[33]

The most remarkable feature in the epidemiology of stomach cancer is the universal declining trend for both sexes, which is characterised by falling more quickly in western than in central and eastern Europe.[34] Paradoxically, the decline in mortality in the high incidence area of Japan has been more marked than elsewhere.[35] Decreasing trends in Norway and Japan appear to be due to the disappearance of the "intestinal" type of this cancer (the variant more subject to international variation), the "diffuse" type being more constant.

Temporal trends in mortality

The truncated and overall age adjusted mortality rates of stomach cancer have been decreasing throughout the time period examined in men and women, in successive birth cohorts, in the United Kingdom, Australia, Canada, Italy, Germany, Denmark and even in those countries where the rates are higher, Poland, Czechoslovakia and Japan.

Despite the widespread decreases in the occurrence of stomach cancer, tumours in the sub-site cardia are reported to be increasing in frequency in both the United States[36] and Europe.[37 38] Although this may be the result of greater precision in the registration of tumour site with the increased use of, for example, endoscopy, it is noteworthy that at the same time there has been an increase in the incidence of adenocarcinoma of the oesophagus, even in populations where the incidence of squamous cell tumours at this site is declining.[39]

Aetiology

Cancer of the stomach was the leading cause of cancer death on a global scale up to the early 1980s; only recently has it been overtaken by the tobacco induced, lung cancer epidemic. There are still areas of the world, notably China and Japan, but also eastern European countries and northern

Italy, where gastric cancer rates are notably high. The substantial declines in gastric cancer observed over recent years in developed countries,[40] but also observed in some developing areas, have occurred earlier in upper social classes and in women[41] and are still continuing in all areas, with little evidence of an end to declines in the rate of gastric cancer even in the young. There is no adequate explanation of the determinants of the declines; however, there is now consistent evidence from descriptive as well as analytical epidemiology that a more affluent diet and improved methods of food preservation, including specifically refrigeration, are to some extent linked to these favourable trends, although the effects appear after a considerable time lag. Together with studies of migrants showing that the changes in stomach cancer mortality occur later than those of mortality due to colorectal (or breast) neoplasms, these observations underline the importance of diet early in life as being relevant in gastric carcinogenesis.

Further, several studies have found that a diet rich in fresh fruit and vegetables[42 43] and, specifically, allium[44 45] is protective, while some traditional starchy foods tend to be positively associated with risk, although it is not known whether they simply represent some indicator of a less affluent diet. This could perhaps explain, at least in part, some of the associations identified with nutrients, particularly the elevated risk for starches. *A posteriori* scores based on optimal combination of high and low risk foods lead to ranges of variation of risk in the order of 5- to 10-fold,[46 47] which could partially explain the geographical differences in gastric cancer rates. The evidence in relation to a possible association with salt and nitrates/nitrites is less clear, as is that related to protection by specific micronutrients, in particular antioxidants such as β-carotene or ascorbic acid.[48]

Intervention with β-carotene, vitamin E, and selenium has been shown to reduce the mortality and incidence of cancer of all forms and particularly stomach cancer in Linxian county,[49] where the rates of oesophageal cancer and stomach cancer are extremely high.[2] This is the first intervention study to show a significantly decreased mortality rate in the intervention group as compared with the placebo group. The study was based on five years follow up of approximately 30 000 people resident in Linxian county, China. The results confirm the importance of micronutrients in the determination of stomach cancer risk and could lead to the development of intervention strategies in other regions of the world where this form of cancer is unusually frequent.

The identification of *Helicobacter pylori* (formerly called *Campylobacter pylori*) in chronic inflammatory conditions of the stomach has stimulated interest in its potential role in gastric carcinogenesis.[50 51] *H. pylori* has been linked to chronic atrophic gastritis,[52] an established precursor of the intestinal type of gastric carcinoma (the type which is decreasing in Western countries).[53] It has been suggested that current evidence supports the conclusion that as many as 60% of gastric adenocarcinomas are attributable to infection with *H. pylori*. Spontaneous cures of *H. pylori* infection have not been documented and it is likely that juvenile infections might persist throughout life.

Apart from the mainly dietary factors and those relating to infection, the risk of stomach cancer has been reported as being raised among atomic bomb survivors,[54] especially for those individuals exposed under the age of 20,[55] and among persons treated for ankylosing spondylitis.[56]

Cancer of the colon and rectum

Colorectal cancer is one of the most important forms of cancer worldwide. The disease is most frequent in developed countries, and particularly so in North America, Australia, New Zealand, and parts of Europe. The diseases of colon and rectal cancer appear to be distinct, but unfortunately there are recognised difficulties in distinguishing colon and rectal cancer in mortality statistics for a variety of reasons.[57] Wherever possible, the distinction between colon and rectum will be preserved but it should be borne in mind at all times that there are recognised difficulties in the recording of this distinction, as well as that with other subdivisions of colorectal cancer.

Colon cancer is a disease of economically *developed* countries, frequently affecting both sexes almost equally. Before 60 years of age, the disease is slightly more common in females, whereas it is more frequent in males thereafter.[58][59] In men, 9 of the 10 highest incidence rates of colon cancer are recorded in population groups in the United States, with the 10th highest in neighbouring Canada (Table 1.3). It is of potentially considerable significance that these high rates are to be found in a variety of population groups including Japanese in Hawaii (37·2) and Los Angeles (33·1), white populations in Connecticut (35·9) and Iowa (32·6) and black populations in Alameda (35·7) and Los Angeles (33·6). In men the lowest incidence rates are found in a variety of population groups in the developing countries, with the lowest rate reported in The Gambia (0·67 per 100 000). In women the group of highest incidence rates includes population groups in North America, with the lowest rates recorded in a similar group of populations as in men (see Table 1.3). In each sex, a number of low rate regions are found in India.

Ethnic and racial differences in colon cancer as well as studies on migrants suggest that environmental factors play a major role in the aetiology of the disease. In Israel male Jews born in Europe or America are at higher risk for colon cancer than those born in Africa or Asia, and a change in risk in the offspring of Japanese migrants to the United States, foreseen by Haenszel

TABLE 1.3—*Ten highest and ten lowest incidence rates of colon cancer in men and women around 1985 (ICD-9 153)*

Male			Female		
Area	Cases	Rate*	Area	Cases	Rate*
Highest					
US, Hawaii: Japanese	414	37·2	Bermuda: black	31	34·4
US, Connecticut: white	3 749	35·9	Canada, Newfoundland	499	30·7
US, Alameda: black	187	35·8	New Zealand: non-Maori	3 398	30·5
US, NYS (less City)	11 860	33·7	US, New Orleans: black	330	30·3
US, Los Angeles: black	708	33·6	US, Bay Area: black	388	29·6
US, Detroit: black	756	33·5	US, Alameda: black	206	29·5
US, Los Angeles: Japanese	110	33·1	US, Los Angeles: Japanese	120	28·9
US, New York City	7 958	32·9	US, Los Angeles: black	857	28·8
US, Iowa	3 419	32·6	US, Iowa	4 343	28·3
Canada, Newfoundland	473	32·5	US, Detroit: black	802	26·6
Lowest					
Peru, Trujillo	17	3·6	Poland, Nowy Sacz	43	3·7
India, Bombay	428	3·2	Kuwait: Kuwaitis	22	3·4
Mali, Bamako	12	2·9	India, Bombay	284	2·6
India, Bangalore	123	2·3	China, Qidong	70	2·2
China, Qidong	52	2·0	Mali, Bamako	8	1·8
Kuwait: Kuwaitis	13	1·9	India, Bangalore	81	1·8
India, Ahmedabad	91	1·8	India, Madras	79	1·5
India, Madras	94	1·5	India, Ahmedabad	42	1·0
Algeria, Setif	12	1·0	Algeria, Setif	10	0·9
The Gambia	3	0·7	The Gambia	0	

* Per 100 000 population.

and Kurihara[62] has now taken place, the incidence rates approaching or surpassing those in white members of the same population and being three or four times higher than among Japanese in Japan.

In general, incidence rates of colon cancer are rising slowly, in particular in areas formerly at low risk; left-sided tumours have shown larger increases.[58] More complex patterns are seen in high risk countries. While mortality rates are increasing in black Americans of both sexes, in the white population the increase is confined to older males and rates are decreasing in females. In the United States incidence is rising slowly in females. Increasing rates are observed in the Nordic countries while in England and Wales mortality rates are declining in all age groups in both sexes.

Although somewhat less frequent than colon cancer, rectal cancer shows many of the features of colon cancer in geographic distribution. In contrast to colon cancer, rectal cancer is more common in males, with a sex ratio of 3:4. Little difference exists in the incidence rates between the western countries of North America, Europe, and Australia, with rates in the range

15–20 for males and 8–12 for females. In contrast mortality rates in the United States are among the lowest in developed countries, with large declines in mortality rates seen in black and white populations for both sexes and very little change in incidence. This is believed to be artefactual as half the patients diagnosed with rectal cancer have their deaths certified to colon cancer.[61] Elsewhere time trends are not consistent, with rising rates in Japan and declining rates in Denmark and England and Wales.

The highest incidence rate of rectal cancer in men is found in Bohemia and Moravia in the Czech Republic (22·9 per 100 000). There is little geographic pattern to the highest rate regions, which contain a diversity of populations in the United States, Hungary, Italy, France, Australia, Canada,

TABLE 1.4—*Ten highest and ten lowest incidence rates of rectal cancer in men and women around 1985 (ICD-9 154)*

Male			Female		
Area	Cases	Rate*	Area	Cases	Rate*
Highest					
Czech., Boh. and Morav.	7 496	22·9	Israel: born Eur. Amer.	1 114	16·1
US, Los Angeles: Japanese	70	21·4	Israel: all Jews	1 519	13·6
Hungary, Vas	205	20·5	New Zealand: non-Maori	1 374	12·3
New Zealand: non-Maori	1 815	20·4	Hungary, Vas	161	12·0
US, Hawaii: Japanese	216	20·3	US, Hawaii: Chinese	30	11·8
Italy, Trieste	111	20·1	Canada, Brit. Col.	1 339	11·7
France, Bas Rhin	558	20·0	Canada, Quebec	2 776	11·7
Australian Cap. Terr.	88	19·9	Czech., Boh. and Morav.	5 546	11·7
Canada, Quebec	3 501	19·4	Canada, New Brunswick	236	11·7
Israel: born Eur. Amer.	1 259	19·0	US, Alameda: white	383	11·4
Lowest					
India, Bangalore	161	3·0	India, Bangalore	125	2·7
Thailand, Khon Kaen	27	2·8	India, Bombay	273	2·5
Mali, Bamako	12	2·6	Bermuda: white and other	5	2·5
Paraguay, Asuncion	27	2·5	India, Ahmedabad	104	2·5
Peru, Trujillo	12	2·5	India, Madras	112	1·9
India, Madras	140	2·4	Thailand, Khon Kaen	16	1·5
Kuwait: Kuwaitis	17	2·4	Algeria, Setif	17	1·3
Kuwait: non-Kuwaitis	28	1·3	Mali, Bamako	6	1·2
Algeria, Setif	11	1·0	Kuwait: Kuwaitis	10	1·1
The Gambia	5	0·7	The Gambia	3	0·6

* Per 100 000 population.

and Israel (Table 1.4). An unexpected feature of these data is the high incidence rates found in Japanese men in Los Angeles (21·4) and Hawaii (20·3). In women, the highest rates are lower than those in men and there is a variety of population groups among the highest incidence rates. For each sex, there is a variety of population groups from the developing world among the regions with the lowest rates (see Table 1.4).

Unlike colon cancer, mortality from rectal cancer did not rise much in Japanese migrants to the United States.[62] Polish migrants have shown an increased risk for both sites.[63]

Temporal trends in mortality

The major problem in separately comparing death rates from colon and rectal cancer between populations is the problem of attribution of "vaguely" defined cancers on the death certificate. The root of the problem was that any death ascribed by the certifying physician as "cancer of the large intestine" was given the three digit code for colon; it could, of course, have been a rectal cancer. For this and several other reasons, it is preferable to investigate mortality from colon and rectal cancer together as a single entity; however, there is a recognised loss of information that could be available if mortality data were of a higher quality.

In those western populations considered, the mortality rates of colorectal cancer are generally stable (for example, in Canada) or changing slowly (for example, United Kingdom and Germany). In contrast mortality rates are increasing noticeably in Japan and in Poland and Czechoslovakia.

For comparison purposes incidence data from colon and rectal cancer have been combined (Table 1.5): this serves to illustrate more clearly the impact of colorectal cancer on communities worldwide. For colorectal cancer the highest incidence rates in men are reported from Japanese communities in Los Angeles (54·5) and Hawaii (57·4) and the highest rates are dominated by populations in North America. The lowest rates are found in various developing countries with the range between the lowest rate (1·3 in The Gambia) and the highest (57·4 in Hawaiian Japanese) being considerable. Similar patterns and differences exist in women (see Table 1.5).

Aetiology

Colorectal cancer is currently estimated to be the third most common form of cancer occurring worldwide, with an estimated 678 000 new cases diagnosed in 1980.[29] High incidence rates are found in western Europe and North America, intermediate rates in eastern Europe, and the lowest rates in sub-Saharan Africa.[58] Few specific risk factors of a non-dietary origin have been established for colorectal cancer; inflammatory bowel diseases and familial polyposis syndromes produce a high risk of colorectal cancer in affected individuals but account for only a small proportion of the overall incidence. Colorectal cancer aetiology is becoming better understood, with major genetic and environmental components being

TABLE 1.5—*Ten highest and ten lowest incidence rates of colorectal cancer in men and women around 1985 (ICD-9 153–154)*

Male			Female		
Area	Cases	Rate*	Area	Cases	Rate*
Highest					
US, Hawaii: Japanese	630	57·5	New Zealand: non-Maori	4 772	42·8
US, Los Angeles: Japanese	180	54·5	Bermuda: black	38	42·0
US, Connecticut: white	5 473	53·1	Canada, Newfoundland	642	39·9
Italy, Trieste	286	51·5	US, Los Angeles: Japanese	166	39·5
New Zealand: non-Maori	4 602	51·3	US, Alameda: black	274	39·3
US, NYS (less City)	17 596	50·5	US, Bay Area: black	511	39·1
US, Detroit: white	4 596	48·8	US, New Orleans, black	417	38·1
US, New York City	11 433	48·0	US, Los Angeles: black	1 110	37·5
US, Iowa	4 951	47·9	US, Iowa	5 626	37·3
US, Bay Area: white	4 089	47·9	US, Detroit: black	1 086	36·5
Lowest					
Kuwait: non-Kuwaitis	86	7·3	Israel: non-Jews	65	7·5
India, Ahmedabad	297	6·4	Thailand, Khon Kaen	57	5·7
India, Bombay	843	6·4	India, Bombay	557	5·1
Peru, Trujillo	29	6·0	Kuwait: Kuwaitis	32	4·5
Mali, Bamako	24	5·4	India, Bangalore	206	4·5
India, Bangalore	284	5·3	India, Ahmedabad	146	3·5
Kuwait: Kuwaitis	30	4·3	India, Madras	191	3·4
India, Madras	234	3·9	Mali, Bamako	14	3·0
Algeria, Setif	23	2·0	Algeria, Setif	27	2·3
The Gambia	8	1·3	The Gambia	3	0·7

* Per 100 000 population.

identified, and offers the best possibility at present to explore the interactions between both sets of aetiological factors on the development of this disease. At the same time advances in knowledge indicate that the prevention of colorectal cancer may be becoming a realistic possibility.[64]

There appears to be strong evidence from epidemiological studies that males with high levels of occupational or recreational physical activity appear to be at a lower risk of colon cancer.[65] Such evidence comes from follow up studies of cohorts who are physically active or who have physically demanding jobs as well as case–control studies that have assessed physical activity by, for example, measurement of resting heart rate, or by questionnaire. The association remains, even after control for potentially confounding factors such as diet and body mass index. The reason for such an inverse association has not been identified but has been postulated as being the effect of exercise on bowel transit time,[66] the immune system,[67] or serum cholesterol and bile acid metabolism.[68] The same consistent results have not been reported on studies in women, but one possible explanation is that the smaller variation in, for example, occupational activity among women may make such an association more difficult to detect.

It has been a fairly consistent finding in studies that have examined the issue that energy intake is higher in patients with colorectal cancer than it is in comparison groups: the mechanism is, however, complex.[69] Physically active individuals are likely to consume more energy but recent studies suggest that physical activity reduces colorectal cancer risk.[70 71 72] The available data, however, show no consistent association between obesity and colorectal cancer risk (although analysis and interpretation of this factor is difficult in retrospective studies where weight loss may be a sign of the disease). This positive effect of energy does not therefore appear to be merely the result of overeating, and may reflect differences in metabolic efficiency. (If the possibility that the association with energy intake is a methodological artefact is excluded, as it seems unlikely that such a consistent finding would emerge from such a variety of study designs in a diversity of population groups, it would imply that individuals who utilise energy more efficiently may be at a lower risk of colorectal cancer.)

There appears to be consistent evidence from epidemiological studies that intake of dietary fat is positively related to colorectal cancer risk: this evidence is obtained from ecological studies, animal experiments, and case–control and cohort studies, although there have been few methodologically sound analytical studies performed in humans. Many of these studies have failed to demonstrate that the observed association with fat intake is independent of energy intake. Willett *et al* published the results obtained from the United States Nurses Health study (a prospective design) involving follow up of 88 751 women aged 34–59 who were without cancer or inflammatory bowel diseases at recruitment.[73] After adjustment for total energy intake, consumption of animal fat was found to be associated with increased colon cancer risk. The trend in risk was highly significant ($p = 0.01$) with the relative risk in the highest compared with the lowest quintile being 1·89 (95% CI (1·13–3·15)). No association was found with vegetable fat. The relative risk of colon cancer in women who ate beef, pork, or lamb as a main dish every day was 2·49 (95% CI (1·24–5·03)), compared with those women reporting consumption less than once a month. The authors interpreted their data as providing evidence for the hypothesis that a high intake of animal fat increases the risk of colon cancer, and they support existing recommendations to substitute fish and chicken for meats high in fat.[68]

This study provides the best epidemiological evidence to date identifying increased meat consumption as a risk factor for colon cancer independently of its contribution to fat intake and total energy intake. There is laboratory evidence that strongly suggests that cooked meats may be carcinogenic, particularly with regard to aminoimidazoazarenes (AIAs) that are produced when meats are cooked.[74][75] As well as being highly mutagenic in bacterial assays, there is now evidence that AIAs are mammalian carcinogens; feeding experiments in mice have produced tumours in various anatomical sites.[76] The situation is not, however, entirely straightforward – for example, it has been shown that anticarcinogenic compounds are produced in fried ground beef;[77] thus in the same food there is the potential for mixtures of potentially carcinogenic and anticarcinogenic substances.

Whittemore *et al* performed a case–control study of Chinese in North America and China thus ingeniously utilising the large difference in risk of colorectal cancer that exists between the two continents.[72] Colorectal cancer risk in both continents was increased with increasing intake of total energy, specifically saturated fat; however, no relationship was found with other sources of energy in the diet. Colon cancer risk was elevated among men employed in sedentary occupations and, in both continents and in both sexes, the risks for cancer of the colon and rectum increased with increased time spent sitting; the association between colorectal cancer risk and saturated fat was stronger among the sedentary than the active. Risk among sedentary Chinese Americans of either sex increased more than fourfold from the lowest to the highest category of saturated fat intake. Among migrants to North America, risk increased with increasing years spent in North America. Attributable risk calculations suggest that, if these associations are causal, saturated fat intakes exceeding 10 g/day, particularly in combination with physical inactivity, could account for 60% of colorectal cancer incidence among Chinese American men and 40% among Chinese American women.[72]

The specific fatty acids in the diet may also be important: animal experiments suggest that linoleic acid (an n–6 polyunsaturated fatty acid) promotes colorectal carcinogenesis[78][79] and that a low fat diet rich in eicopentaenoic acid (an n–3 polyunsaturated fatty acid) has an inhibitory effect on colon cancer;[80] however, there have been no epidemiological studies conducted to date regarding n–3 and n–6 fatty acids and colorectal cancer risk.

The original hypothesis of the protective effect of dietary fibre was based on a clinical/pathological observation and a hypothesised mechanism whereby increasing intake of dietary fibre increases faecal bulk and reduces transit time; more recent thinking suggests that this mechanism may not be as relevant to colorectal carcinogenesis as previously thought.[81] The term "fibre" encompasses many components, each of which has specific physiological functions. The most common classification is into insoluble, non-degradable constituents (mainly present in cereal fibre) and soluble, degradable constituents like pectin and plant gums, which are mainly present in fruits and vegetables. Epidemiological studies have reported differences in the effect of these components. For example, Tuyns et al[82] and Kune et al[83] found a protective effect for total dietary fibre intake in case–control studies, and the same effect was found in one prospective study[84]. However, a large number of studies could find no such protective effect.[73] The large majority of studies in humans have found no protective effect of fibre from cereals but have found a protective effect of fibre from vegetable and, perhaps, fruit sources.[73] This could conceivably reflect an association with other components of fruits and vegetables, with "fibre" intake acting merely as an indicator of consumption.

Although calcium has been proposed as potentially having a modifying role in colorectal carcinogenesis,[85] little supporting evidence is forthcoming from epidemiological studies. These studies in humans are of limited value because of questionable study design or the inadequacy of the estimation of diet. A number of studies have reported positive associations with alcohol consumption but it remains to be proven whether the putative association is with alcohol per se and not with the energy contribution of alcohol. There is some experimental evidence that vitamin E and selenium may be protective against colon tumours[77] and there is support for the hypothesis that vitamin A and/or its precursor β-carotene are also protective.[72] Lactobacilli, found in some dairy products, may have a favourable effect on the intestine.[86] Twelve case–control studies of sufficient quality have addressed the issue of coffee consumption and the risk of colorectal cancer and 11 of these have indicated inverse (protective) associations. No association has been found with tea drinking or caffeine intake from any sources considered.

In summary, dietary factors are the most important life style determinants of colorectal cancer risk. Methodological problems in nutritional epidemiology prevent a completely unequivocal interpretation of the available data, although the situation is becoming very much clearer. Our interpretation is that an effect of saturated fat appears to exist independently of energy intake and that vegetable fibre, directly or indirectly, appears to be protective, as does coffee consumption. Meat intake may also increase risk but whether this is independent of its fat content or its contribution to energy is currently unclear: if independent, the risk could be related to mutagenic products formed in the cooking process. Intake of cereal fibre appears to be protective against the formation of colorectal polyps, although it does not appear to have a role in the later stages of the carcinogenic process involving transformation of the adenomatous polyp into the carcinoma.

Arguably more is known about the genetics of colorectal cancer than any other common form of the disease. There are a number of clinical syndromes that predispose to colorectal cancer: the majority are inherited as autosomal dominant genes (on average, a carrier of this mutation passes on the mutation to half of the offspring). Offspring have a high chance of developing colorectal cancer. These syndromes include those which predispose to large numbers of polyps (for example, familial adenomatous polyposis (FAP)), those which predispose to adenomatous polyps with high malignant potential (for example, hereditary non-polyposis colorectal cancer (HNPCC)), and those syndromes associated non-adenomatous polyps) with an increased risk less than that associated with adenomatous polyps (for example, Peutz–Jeghers syndrome). Apart from these syndromes, epidemiological studies provide evidence that other weaker genetic factors are also involved in the pathogenesis of colorectal cancer.[87] Virtually all studies conducted indicate that families of colorectal cancer cases are more likely to have a history of colorectal cancer than families of "controls": the increased risk of cancer in relatives is between 2 and 4 when compared with the general population.[88]

It is obvious that colorectal cancer is increasingly understood and prospects for prevention are becoming apparent[64]: this could be a great success for epidemiology.

Cancer of the liver

Epidemiological study of liver cancer is hampered not only by underdiagnosis of this disease but also by the potential misclassification of primary and secondary neoplasms. Thus death certification and even incidence registration statistics may be seriously flawed and are difficult to interpret. Liver cancer is, however, extremely common in the Far East and some areas of subequatorial Africa. Worldwide it is the eighth most common cancer, with an estimated number of 250 000 new cases diagnosed in 1980. With reference to methodological problems in analytical epidemiology, cohort studies risk missing cases, and both cohort and case–control studies could include a proportion of patients who have secondary cancer.

Liver cancer is particularly common in males in East and South East Asia and sub-Saharan Africa.[91] In North America, only the Inuit (Eskimos) and the populations of Asian origin show high rates, reaching values above 30. The disease is more common in men than in women and this difference is particularly marked in regions of the world with high levels of this form of cancer.

The situation regarding the geographical distribution of primary liver cancer is completely different from that of colorectal cancer. The highest rates are found in populations in South East Asia and Africa (Table 1.6). The highest incidence rate in each sex is reported from Khon Kaen in Thailand, the rates being 90·0 per 100 000 in men although much lower in women (38·3). In men, extremely high rates are reported also from Qidong in China (89·9 per 100 000). The third highest rate is about half

TABLE 1.6—*Ten highest and ten lowest incidence rates of primary liver cancer in men and women around 1985 (ICD-9 155)*

Male			Female		
Area	Cases	Rate*	Area	Cases	Rate*
Highest					
Thailand, Khon Kaen	861	90·0	Thailand, Khon Kaen	365	38·3
China, Qidong	2 381	89·9	China, Qidong	693	24·5
Mali, Bamako	258	47·9	Mali, Bamako	98	21·5
Japan, Osaka	9 466	41·5	The Gambia	65	12·1
Hong Kong	5 274	39·3	China, Shanghai	2 423	10·8
Japan, Nagasaki	511	38·8	Thailand, Chiang Mai	224	10·5
Japan, Saga	681	38·2	Japan, Osaka	2 793	9·7
The Gambia	248	36·0	Hong Kong	1 471	9·7
China, Shanghai	6 146	30·6	Japan, Saga	259	9·6
Japan, Hiroshima	672	28·2	China, Tianjin	750	8·7
Lowest					
Canada, PEI	6	1·5	France, Tarn	11	0·6
UK, Trent	256	1·5	Canada, Mar. Provs.	35	0·5
Netherlands, Eindhoven	33	1·4	Canada, Newfoundland	7	0·5
UK, Oxford	112	1·4	Australia, Western	22	0·5
Australia, South	59	1·3	France, Isere	17	0·4
Canada, Newfoundland	18	1·3	Australia, Tasmania	7	0·4
Paraguay, Asuncion	12	1·1	Netherland, Eindhoven	11	0·4
Ireland, Southern	14	1·1	Israel: born Israel	6	0·4
Netherlands, Maastricht	13	0·8	Canada, PEI	1	0·1
Bermuda: white and other	0		Canada, NWT and Yukon	0	

* Per 100 000 population.

these two highest values and is reported from Bamako in Mali (47·9). In women the highest rates are found in similar population groups and the lowest rates in each sex generally are reported from developed countries (Table 1.6). The difference in levels between men and women in the high rate regions of the world and the variation between high and low rates internationally are of considerable significance and have not yet been adequately exploited in the investigation of risk factors.

In China primary liver cancer has a predominantly coastal distribution with incidence rates recorded in Shanghai of the same order as those reported from Hong Kong and Singapore. Within Singapore, unlike other cancer sites, such as nasopharynx, lung, and oesophagus, the incidence in Hokkien, Teochew, Cantonese, Hainanese, and Hakka is very similar. The incidence in Singapore born Chinese is very close to that of the foreign born. In contrast, migrant Chinese in California exhibit much lower rates, although these are substantially greater than among white populations residing in the same city. Koreans in Los Angeles have levels of incidence comparable to those in Chinese. Incidence in Japanese resident in California is much lower than in Japan. Intermediate incidence levels are found in Rizal province in the Philippines; those in the Malay population of Singapore are at much the same level. In contrast to Indians in Singapore, rates within India are uniformly much lower.

Rates of liver cancer are low in South America, Australia, and New Zealand for white populations, whereas rates for the Melanesian and Polynesian inhabitants, although unstable as a result of being based on relatively small numbers of cases, appear similar to those seen in Asians. Rates in Europe are also generally low, in the range 1–3, but there is a tendency for rates in southern Europe to be higher. The highest rates in southern Europe are found in Italy, although previously the highest rate was seen in Geneva, Switzerland perhaps a reflection of the high autopsy rate.[92]

In adults, a large majority of liver cancers are hepatocellular carcinomas, cholangiocarcinomas being rare by contrast except in parts of South East Asia and around the shore of Lake Baikal in Siberia, in association with liver flukes (for example, *Clonorchis sinensis, Opisthorchis viverrini*).[93] Most childhood liver cancers are hepatoblastomas, rare tumours showing little worldwide variation.[94]

Temporal trends in mortality

Mortality data are usually unreliable, being distorted not only by unrecognised secondary neoplasms but also by change in rubric content between (ICD) revisions. There is also the difficulty that in many countries for many years the data on primary liver cancer were not presented individually. Examination of mortality trends does not give a readily interpretable pattern although there is a general increase reported in most countries' data. It is difficult to avoid concluding that there are causes of variation present in the mortality data for primary liver cancer over and above those expected through changes brought about by changes in the distribution of exposure factors.

Aetiology

Patterns of hepatocellular cancer are generally related to the prevalence of chronic carriers of hepatitis B surface antigen (HBsAg) in the population.[95] Several epidemiological studies and laboratory investigations have established that there is a strong and specific association between infection with hepatitis B virus (HBV) and hepatocellular carcinoma.[96] The association is restricted to chronically active forms of HBV infection which are characterised by the presence in serum of HBsAg, commonly referred to as "carrier status". The association is strong: in a cohort study from Taiwan based on 22 707 subjects, of which 3454 were HBsAg positive, the relative risk for hepatocellular carcinoma was found to be 104 (95% CI

(51–212)) and the calculated attributable risk was 93·9%.[96 97] The relative risk is, however, about one order of magnitude smaller (approximately 10) in studies conducted in Europe,[98 99] or the United States.[100] This is possibly related to some cofactor (for example, poorer diet in East Asia), but a different duration of exposure to the virus, which in the Far East is usually transmitted perinatally but in Europe and North America is contracted late in life, can by itself explain such a substantial difference. This hypothesis has recently found epidemiological support from a study conducted in Greece, which demonstrated a tendency for cases of hepatocellular carcinoma to have a higher birth order.[101] There does not appear to be an association with the presence of hepatitis B antibodies alone, so that past exposure is not a risk factor.[102] With reference to implications for prevention, perinatal immunisation against hepatitis B could probably be the single most effective resource against cancer worldwide after the elimination of tobacco smoking.

An increased frequency of primary liver cancer has been observed among individuals with a high alcohol intake in a number of studies, although this is not a universal finding.[15] Of four published cohort studies, two found an increased risk with increasing consumption of alcoholic beverages, while in a further study, elevated risk was restricted to a subgroup. An overview of published studies of alcoholics shows a general tendency for alcoholics to have a 50% excess of liver cancer over non-alcoholics. These risks, however, may well be underestimated because alcohol-induced liver damage may result in reduction or cessation of alcohol before the diagnosis of liver cancer.

Part of the excess liver cancer risk in alcoholics can be attributable to dietary deficiencies, because it has been shown that a diet poor in vitamin A and other (micro)nutrients is related to an increased risk of hepatocellular carcinoma.[199] In tropical areas of Africa and Asia aflatoxin, a product of metabolism of *Aspergillus flavus* which contaminates foods, and particularly cereals, has been related to an elevated risk of primary liver cancer, with a positive interaction with HBV and alcohol. The risk of primary liver cancer has been found to be greatly elevated among subjects exposed to more than one factor.[103]

Use of combined oral contraceptives substantially increases the risk of liver carcinoma, and these are effective in the process of hepato-carcinogenesis in rodents. An association between long term oral contraceptive use and hepatocellular carcinoma has been observed in five of five studies conducted in developed countries (although not in a sixth based mainly on developing countries).[104] Primary liver cancer is, however, extremely rare in young women in Western countries, and the public health impact of such an association is small (unless such an association persists when the same generation of women become older).

21

Some studies have demonstrated an association between tobacco smoking and liver cancer,[105] particularly in hepatitis B negative subjects.[106] Although this is aetiologically plausible because many carcinogens in tobacco are metabolised by the liver, direct epidemiological evidence is largely inconsistent and difficult to interpret.

Patients injected for diagnostic purposes with Thorotrast (a colloidal preparation of thorium–232) had a very high frequency of cholangio-cellular carcinoma:[107] this procedure is now obsolete. Thorotrast was deposited in phagocytic cells in very high concentration, especially in the liver, and in consequence nearby cells were intensely irradiated with α-particles.

The rare subtype of liver cancer, angiosarcoma, has been shown to have been caused by exposure to vinyl chloride monomer.[108]

Cancer of the gall bladder and extrahepatic bile ducts

Over two thirds of these rare cancers arise in the gall bladder. This form of cancer has the unusual feature of being one of the very few cancers in an organ of similar function in men and women that exhibits a higher occurrence rate (about double) in women than it does in men. Mortality data have seldom been published on gall bladder cancer on its own, and those data available cover too short a time and have too few cases to make any useful interpretation of trends possible.

The highest rates (17·6) have been observed in the Alaskan native female population[109] and in Bolivia (14·6) by Rios-Dalenz et al.[110] In the American Indian population of New Mexico incidence rates in the early 1980s were 13·2 in females and 10·8 in males.[3] Hispanic populations in the United States have rates that are intermediate between those in American Indians and white populations.

Just as was the case when stomach cancer was considered, the highest incidence rates in men are from the six population based registries in Japan (see Table 1.7). The lowest rates are generally from population groups in the developed countries or the Indian subcontinent. In women, by contrast, the highest incidence rates include regions of South America, as well as Japanese groups (see Table 1.7). The pattern of high rates in Japan cannot yet be explained.

Mortality in the former Federal Republic of Germany shows an unusual regional pattern in both sexes, with elevated rates, which are much higher than elsewhere in western Europe, down the centre of the country.[111] In central and eastern Europe, there is a grouping of high rates in Poland, Hungary, and the former Czechoslovakia.[112]

TABLE 1.7—*Ten highest and ten lowest incidence rates of gall bladder and bile duct cancer in men and women around 1985 (ICD-9 156)*

Male			Female		
Area	Cases	Rate*	Area	Cases	Rate*
Highest					
Japan, Nagasaki	104	8·0	Peru, Trujillo	63	12·9
Japan, Yamagata	276	7·4	Colombia, Cali	222	9·8
Japan, Miyagi	467	7·2	Hungary, Vas	126	9·2
Japan, Saga	126	6·5	Ecuador, Quito	81	8·7
Japan, Osaka	1 323	6·0	Poland, Warsaw City	756	8·7
Japan, Hiroshima	118	5·1	Japan, Yamagata	434	7·9
US, Los Angeles: Korean	8	5·0	Algeria, Setif	82	7·4
Ecuador, Quito	39	4·9	Japan, Nagasaki	138	7·3
US, Los Angeles: Chinese	18	4·9	Czech., Boh. and Morav.	3 747	7·2
Czech., Boh. and Morav.	1 605	4·8	Japan, Miyagi	626	7·1
Lowest					
Kyrgyzstan	23	0·8	Romania, County Cluj	26	0·9
Romania, County Cluj	16	0·8	Singapore: Malay	6	0·9
US, Hawaii: white	5	0·6	UK, North Scotland	9	0·9
UK, North Scotland	5	0·6	India, Ahmedabad	19	0·5
Bermuda: white and other	1	0·6	India, Madras	27	0·5
India, Madras	28	0·5	India, Bangalore	21	0·5
India, Bangalore	21	0·4	China, Qidong	12	0·4
India, Ahmedabad	16	0·4	Mali, Bamako	0	
Mali, Bamako	0		Bermuda: white and other	0	
The Gambia	0		The Gambia	0	

* Per 100 000 population.

Aetiology of gall bladder cancer

There are few epidemiological studies of gall bladder cancer, a rare but lethal gastrointestinal tumour. The disease is more common in the ageing, in women and in certain racial groups such as native American Indians. The roles of gall stones,[113][114] and obesity[115] appear to be important in the aetiology of gall bladder cancer, but, there has been a recognised lack of a large study of this cancer to investigate better these and other hypotheses.

After adjusting for potential confounding factors (age, sex, centre, years of schooling, alcohol consumption, and cigarette smoking history), a history of gall bladder symptoms was found to be the major risk factor associated with this form of cancer (OR = 4·4, 95% CI (2·6–7·5)).[116] This association was present even in subjects where symptoms predate the cancer for as long as 20 years (OR = 6·2, 95% CI (2·8–13·4)). Other variables found to be associated with gall bladder cancer risk included an elevated body mass index, high total energy intake, high carbohydrate intake (which persisted after adjustment for total energy intake), and chronic diarrhoea. All of these risk factors have been previously associated with gallstone disease. Increased intake of a number of dietary items was shown to be protective: vitamins B_6 (pyridoxine), C, and E, and dietary fibre. Alcohol consumption and lifetime cigarette smoking history do not appear to be associated with the risk of gall bladder cancer in this study.[116]

The findings are all consistent with a major role for gall stones in the aetiology of gall bladder cancer.

Aetiology of bile duct cancer

Epidemiological studies of this form of cancer are very few and many of those conducted to date have failed to separate cancers of the gall bladder, ampulla of Vater, and the extrahepatic bile duct and are published as a grouping of "biliary tract cancer".

There have been a number of case reports proposing to demonstrate an association between bile duct cancer and a history of inflammatory bowel disease, choledochal cyst, primary sclerosing cholangitis, and several other conditions. The strongest reported association appears to be with ulcerative colitis,[117] although it is still difficult to infer causality with this or any other similar association. The best evidence comes from a small case–control study (67 cases) that, based on six cases of ulcerative colitis among cases of bile duct cancer, demonstrated a relative risk of 3·6 (95% CI (1·1–19·1)). Results from studies investigating the association between bile duct cancer risk and gallstones have been inconsistent. Although one study found an excess of bile duct cancer in a cohort of persons who had experienced a cholecystectomy,[118] this result contradicted an earlier null study.[119]

A recent collaborative study (CC Hsieh et al, submitted for publication), based on 95 cases and 1697 controls, demonstrated positive associations with bile duct cancer risk and lifetime cigarette smoking, a positive history of gall bladder symptoms, and a high total energy intake. High intake of dietary fibre and vitamin E were found to be associated with decreased risk. Alcohol and tea consumption, obesity, diabetes, gastric ulcer, and oral contraceptive use did not appear to be associated with the risk of extrahepatic bile duct cancer in this study.

Cancer of the pancreas

In attempting to review the epidemiology of pancreatic cancer it is essential at all times to be aware of problems of misdiagnosis, particularly underdiagnosis, of this lethal disease which can potentially hinder both descriptive and analytical epidemiological studies.[120]

Pancreatic cancer is infrequent on a world basis, accounting for some 3% of all cancers in developed countries. Given the very poor survival, this site is now a major component of cancer mortality.[121] The disease is slightly more frequent in males, the sex-ratio tending to increase in high risk populations.

Seven of the highest ten reported incidence rates in men are among black populations in North America and Bermuda (see Table 1.8). In

TABLE 1.8—*Ten highest and ten lowest incidence rates of pancreas cancer in men and women around 1985. (ICD-9 157)*

Male			Female		
Area	Cases	Rate*	Area	Cases	Rate*
Highest					
US, Alameda: black	71	13·7	US, Alameda: black	81	11·9
US, Bay Area: black	133	13·5	US, Bay Area: black	149	11·6
Bermuda: black	9	13·1	US, Detroit: black	310	10·5
US, Atlanta: black	107	13·1	New Zealand: Maori	33	9·8
US, Detroit: black	277	12·5	US, New Orleans: black	114	9·7
US, New Orleans: black	90	11·9	US, Los Angeles: Japanese	39	8·7
US, Los Angeles: black	245	11·7	US, Hawaii: Hawaiian	27	7·8
Czech., Boh. and Morav.	3 792	11·7	US, Los Angeles: black	239	7·7
Latvia	781	11·2	US, Connecticut: black	50	7·3
New Zealand: Maori	36	11·0	US, Hawaii: Chinese	18	7·2
Lowest					
Thailand, Chiang Mai	45	2·44	France, Tarn	38	1·4
Bermuda: white and other	3	2·41	Singapore: Indian	3	1·4
France, Martinique	19	2·34	Algeria, Setif	14	1·1
Mali, Bamako	10	2·21	Bermuda: white and other	2	1·0
Algeria, Setif	22	2·04	India, Bangalore	32	0·7
Thailand, Khon Kaen	14	1·44	India, Madras	39	0·7
India, Madras	72	1·15	Thailand, Khon Kaen	7	0·7
India, Bangalore	52	1·00	Mali, Bamako	1	0·4
India, Ahmedabad	30	0·69	India, Ahmedabad	10	0·2
The Gambia	2	0·41	The Gambia	0	

* Per 100 000 population.

women, the ten highest rates are found in nine populations of the United States and among the Maori population of New Zealand. Low rate regions in each sex include India, registries in Africa, and populations in South East Asia (see Table 1.8).

Temporal trends in mortality

An increasing trend in mortality and incidence is seen practically everywhere for both sexes, which could be partly due, at least in some areas, to improvement in diagnosis. The increase has been particularly rapid in black compared with white males in whom incidence now seems to be levelling out. A parallelism between the age specific time trends in mortality from pancreas and lung cancers has been pointed out, in England and Wales, whereas such similarities are less obvious in the United States and in Scandinavia.

Aetiology of pancreas cancer

Pancreatic cancer is consistently reported to occur more frequently in men than in women, in black compared with white populations and in urban compared with rural population groups. In some countries, mortality rates continue to rise whereas in others declining levels of disease can be seen among members of younger birth cohorts.[120] Although some of the patterns observed can be explained by variation in pancreatic cancer risk factors, many cannot.

Analytical studies based on patients with pancreatic cancer consistently demonstrate that cigarette smoking increases the risk of pancreatic cancer.[14] All studies published since this IARC working party evaluation reported an association between cigarette smoking and an elevated risk of pancreatic cancer.[120] There is clear and consistent evidence linking an increased risk of pancreatic cancer with cigarette smoking.[20] A dose–response relationship was found with increasing pancreatic cancer risk and lifetime reported cigarette consumption and the risk is found to reduce among smokers to a level compatible with lifelong non-smokers 15 years after quitting.[122]

Although it has been speculated that there was a positive association with coffee consumption,[123] the overall evidence available does not support this relationship.[122 124] There is no convincing evidence linking alcohol consumption to an increased risk of pancreatic cancer.[125] A recent positive association between pancreatic risk and beer consumption suggested by one study[126] was not found in an overview of three other case–control studies.[127]

Ionising radiation is possibly related to pancreatic cancer. The risk was found to be elevated in a cohort of patients with ankylosing spondylitis who were treated with radiation[56] and in women treated by radiotherapy for cancer of the cervix:[128] however, apparent increases reported earlier among atomic bomb survivors[129] and in workers in the nuclear industry[130] were not confirmed by later observations based on a longer period of follow up.[54 131] The associations between pancreatic cancer risk and a number of other factors including occupational exposures and require clarification and verification.[114]

It appears likely that in coming years dietary factors will emerge as influential in determining pancreatic cancer risk.[132-137] The SEARCH study[137] found positive associations between intake of carbohydrates and cholesterol and inverse associations with dietary fibre and vitamin C. These associations were generally consistent among the five centres who undertook the study, and the consistency, strength and specificity appear to suggest underlying causal relationships.[137]

Some aspects of medical history have been associated with pancreatic cancer risk. It has recently been demonstrated that patients with chronic pancreatitis have an increased risk of developing pancreatic cancer: the risk was 8·5 ten years after the initial diagnosis of chronic pancreatitis.[114] In particular, besides pancreatitis, there is some evidence that diabetes and cholecystectomy may be associated with elevated pancreatic cancer risk, while allergies may represent an indication of reduced risk.[120]

Discussion

The aim of epidemiological study of cancer is to improve knowledge of the aetiopathogenesis of the disease in question with the single aim of increasing prospects for prevention. Aetiological proscription and prescription could serve to reduce the risk of the development of many of the gastrointestinal cancers currently seen, as follows.

- *Oesophageal cancer* risk would decline with decreasing cigarette consumption, decreasing alcohol consumption and increasing consumption of fruits and vegetables.
- *Stomach cancer* risk would be reduced by increased consumption of fruits and vegetables and probably decreased consumption of salt preserved and mouldy foods and reduced cigarette consumption.
- *Colorectal cancer* risk could be reduced by increased consumption of fruits and vegetables and reduced intake of dietary fat, especially saturated fat.
- *Gall bladder cancer* risk may be reduced by better control of gall stones.
- *Pancreatic cancer* risk could be reduced by reducing cigarette smoking and may also be reduced by increased consumption of fruits and vegetables.

However, in the case of gastrointestinal cancers, there is some suggestive evidence emerging that **chemoprevention** could possibly lead to reduced risk of some of these cancers[49] and that potentially **population screening** may have an important role to play in reducing the risk of colorectal cancer.

It is worthwhile considering the rapid changes in knowledge of colorectal cancer that have taken place since the early 1980s.[78] The natural history and the role of several risk factors in the aetiology of colorectal cancer are becoming more clearly understood[87 138 139] and the genetic events involved in colorectal cancer susceptibility are being uncovered with increasing frequency.[140 141] Knowledge of life style risk factors is also becoming clearer. Risk of colorectal cancer appears to be increased by increasing consumption of fat, protein and meat and to be reduced by increased consumption of fruits and vegetables.[142] Thus there are prospects for primary prevention although it is difficult to know how to bring about successfully such large scale alterations to the diets of large proportions of populations. The large bowel is not generally considered as a site where the risk of cancer is linked to cigarette smoking,[14] although it has been recently suggested that it may be an independent risk factor, which may be specifically associated with the early stages of colorectal carcinogenesis[143 144] although this is still controversial. There is also, however, interesting evidence suggesting that specific chemopreventive strategies could prove useful in the prevention of colorectal cancer.

Chemoprevention received a major boost recently with the demonstration that supplementation of the diet of 30 000 Chinese residents of Linxian county with vitamin E, β-carotene and selenium led to a reduction (after five years of use) in total mortality, total cancer incidence, and mortality and incidence of cancer of the stomach.[49] Antioxidants have long been leading candidates for chemoprevention and the findings regarding the protective effect of fruits and vegetables in colorectal cancer are consistent with this possibility. Unusually, there are limited data available from randomised trials. Although not a study hypothesis and not statistically significant, there was a reduced number of cases of colorectal cancer found among Finnish smokers randomised to α-tocopherol (68 cases, 80 per 10 000 person years) when compared with placebo (81 cases, 96 per 10 000 person years):[145] the approximate relative risk appears to be 0·87. A randomised controlled trial of β-carotene and vitamins C and E, involving 864 patients randomised to one of four treatment arms who underwent colonoscopy for polyp identification after one year and four years, reported no evidence that either β-carotene or vitamins C and E, reduced the incidence of adenomas.[146] Although antioxidants are obvious candidates for use as chemopreventive agents in trials and they may have protective effects against other cancers and other diseases, potentially including cardiovascular disease, their potential in colorectal cancer prevention is not proven at the present time. This is surely an area where more research is needed to identify effective chemopreventive agents and where large trials are necessary to prove their effectiveness.

Non-steroidal anti-inflammatory drugs (NSAIDS) have recently been identified as potential protective agents against colorectal cancer and adenomatous polyps. Initial anecdotal reports noting regression of adenomas in patients with familial adenomatous polyps have been followed by substantial epidemiological studies. There is a general level of agreement in the finding of a protective effect from such studies. There are randomised trials of familial adenomatous polyps demonstrating the regression of adenomas by NSAIDS: for example, complete regression of rectal polyps in six of nine patients taking sulindac and partial regression in three others: in the placebo group, polyps increased in five, remained unchanged in two and decreased in the remaining two.[147] In laboratory rodents, piroxicam, sulindac, and aspirin have all been shown to reduce the frequency of development of colorectal neoplasia.[148] The mechanism of any effect remains obscure, as does the dose required, and it is disappointing that the randomised intervention trial of low dose aspirin in United States physicians was null, although this may represent a situation where the dose given was too low or the period of use too short to achieve the protective effect;[149] however, there is a very good case for a controlled trial of NSAID, probably using aspirin, in the prevention of colorectal cancer.[150]

Colorectal cancer is not uniformly fatal, although there are large differences in survival according to stage of disease. In advanced colorectal cancer in which curative resection is possible, five year survival in Dukes's B is 45% which drops to 30% in Dukes's C.[151] Five year survival in resected Dukes's A is around 80% and survival after simple resection of an adenomatous pedunculated polyp containing carcinoma in situ (or severe dysplasia) or intramucosal carcinoma is generally close to 100%. It is estimated that there are, however, still 394 000 deaths from colorectal cancer worldwide annually.[121]

The large differences in survival between early and late stage disease clearly indicate the advantage in detecting colorectal cancer at an early stage. The simplest advice is to ensure that any change in bowel habits or unexpected presence of blood in the stool should be investigated. Faecal occult blood testing (FOBT) is aimed at the detection of early asymptomatic cancer and is based on the assumption that such cancers will bleed and that small quantities of blood lost in the stool may be detected chemically or immunologically. A significant reduction in colorectal cancer mortality with annual testing using guaiac has been reported.[152] The cumulative annual mortality rate in the group screened annually was 5·88 per 1000 compared with 8·83 in the control group and 8·33 in the group screened biennially. The results are of considerable importance but it is difficult to ignore the observation that 38% of those screened annually and 28% of those screened biennially underwent at least one colonoscopy during the study period, although it is somewhat reassuring that the incidence of colorectal cancer was so similar in the three groups (23, 23 and 26 per 1000 for those screened annually, those screened biennially, and those in the control group respectively). The authors considered that the likely effect of colonoscopy, in removing polyps, had not yet affected the incidence and mortality from colorectal cancer. These findings are important confirmation that guaiac screening may be effective against colorectal cancer, and confirmatory findings from other trials are eagerly awaited. There are both advantages and disadvantages to FOBT. On the one hand it is low cost, although the investigation of false positives (around 1–3%) certainly increases the cost, and it "examines" the entire colon and rectum. On the other hand, it is characterised by a low sensitivity (with around 40% of cancers and 80% of adenomas missed by the test[153 154]) and by detecting colorectal cancers at the later stages in the natural history at which lesions bleed, which leads to a short lead time and the requirement for frequent testing. Rehydration of the slides resulted in increased positivity but also an increased number of colonoscopies and a decreased specificity of the test. The costs must be weighed against the benefits before public health policy on this topic is formulated.[152]

Until a randomised controlled trial is undertaken and reported, the efficacy of flexible sigmoidoscopy as a screening test for preventing death from colorectal cancer will remain unproven; however, there is now a good deal of evidence supporting infrequent sigmoidoscopy as an effective screening modality for colorectal cancer. Impressive reductions in rectal cancer and cancer of the proximal colon have been reported from demonstration studies: 85% reduction in 21 000 subjects undergoing "clearing" proctosigmoidoscopy followed by annual proctosigmoidoscopy with removal of all lesions detected;[155] 70% reduction in risk of colorectal cancer for 10 years after sigmoidoscopy;[156] 80% reduction in incidence after examination mostly performed by flexible sigmoidoscopy;[157] and an 85% reduction of rectal cancers achieved by the removal of adenomas.[158] Although the initial examination may be expensive, there is an advantage that polyps may be removed at the time of the initial procedure and no follow up visits will be required. Use of a 65 cm flexible sigmoidoscope appears to be the most effective proposition at present because this avoids the more complicated colonoscopy and yet still covers the region of the large bowel where two-thirds of cancers arise.

Prospects for prevention of colorectal cancer death are much brighter than even in the early 1980s.[78] Large randomised trials of screening with flexible sigmoidoscopy are very important and there is a strong case for chemoprevention trials using aspirin (or another NSAID) and antioxidants (vitamin E, β-carotene, vitamin C). Successful outcomes to these trials could see strategies to prevent the majority of colorectal cancer deaths available to the general population by the early 2000s.

Coupled with developments in genetics, and even treatment,[159] colorectal cancer may emerge as the first *major* neoplasm that turns out to be preventable[160] allying successful treatment with successful prevention strategies using prescription (screening and chemoprevention) rather than proscription.[64] It should be a model for other forms of gastrointestinal cancer.

It is a pleasure to acknowledge that this work was supported by the Italian Association for Cancer Research (*Associazone Italiana per la Ricerca sul Cancro*).

References

1 Day NE, Munoz N. Esophagus. In: Scottenfeld D, Fraumeni JF, eds. *Cancer Epidemiology and Prevention.* Philadelphia: WB Saunders, 1982:596–622.

2 Lu JB, Yang WX, Liu JM, *et al.* Trends in morbidity and mortality for esophageal cancer in Linxian county, 1959–1983. *Int J Cancer* 1985;**36**:643–5.

3 Muir CS, Waterhouse J, Mack T, *et al.* Cancer incidence in five continents, *IARC Sci Pub* 1987:88.

4 Kmet J, Mahboubi E. Esophageal cancer in the Caspian littoral of Iran: initial studies. *Science* 1972;**175**:846–53.

5 Smans M, Boyle P, Muir CS, eds. Cancer mortality atlas of EEC. *IARC Sci Publ* 1993; **107**.

6 Parkin DM, Muir CS, Whelan S, *et al,* eds: *Cancer incidence in five continents, Vol VI, IARC Sci Publ* 1992;**120**.

7 Jensen OM, Estève J, Møller H, *et al.* Cancer in the European Community and member states. *Eur J Cancer* 1990;**26**:1167–256.

8 Mahboubi E, Kmet J, Cook PJ, *et al.* Oesophageal cancer studies in the Caspian littoral of Iran – the Caspian cancer registry. *Br J Cancer* 1973;**28**:197–208.

9 Rose E. Esophageal cancer in the Transkei, 1955–1969. *J Natl Cancer Inst* 1973;**51**: 7–16.

10 Tuyns AJ, Massé G. Cancer of the oesophagus in Brittany. An incidence study in Ille-et-Vilaine. *Int J Epidemiol* 1975;**4**:55–59.

11 Lee HP, Day NE, Shanmugaratnam K, eds. Trends in cancer incidence in Singapore 1968–1982. *IARC Sci Publ* 1988;**91**.

12 Blot WJ, Fraumeni JF. Trends in esophageal cancer mortality among US blacks and whites. *Am J Public Health* 1987;**77**:296–8.

13 Boyle P, La Vecchia C, Maisonneuve P, *et al.* Cancer epidemiology and prevention. Pp 199–273. In: Veronesi U, Peckham MJ and Pinedo R (eds). *Oxford Textbook of Oncology.* Oxford: Oxford University Press, 1995.

14 IARC. Tobacco smoking. *Monogr Eval Carcinog Risks Hum* 1986;**38**.

15 IARC. Alcohol drinking. *Monogr Eval Carcinog Risks Hum* 1988;**44**.

16 Levi F, La Vecchia C, Lucchini F, *et al.* Cancer incidence and mortality in Europe, 1983–87. *Soz Präventivmed* 1993; suppl **3**:S155–229.

17 La Vecchia C, Negri E. The role of alcohol in oesophageal cancer in non-smokers and of tobacco in non-drinkers. *Int J Cancer* 1989;**43**:784–5.

18 To come

19 La Vecchia C, Bidoli E, Barra S, *et al.* Type of cigarettes and cancers of the upper digestive and respiratory tract. *Cancer Causes Control* 1990;**1**:69–74.

20 La Vecchia C, Boyle P, Franceschi S, *et al.* Smoking and cancer with emphasis on Europe. *Eur J Cancer* 1991.

21 Clemmesen J. *Statistical studies in malignant neoplasms. I Review and results.* Copenhagen: Munksgaard, 1965.

22 Jensen OM. Cancer morbidity and causes of death among Danish brewery workers. *Int J Cancer* 1979;**23**:454–63.

23 Tuyns AJ, Pequinot G, Jensen OM. Le cancer de l'oesophage en Ille-et-Vilaine en fonction des niveaux de consommation d'alcool et de tabac. Des risques qui se multiplient. *Bull Cancer* 1977;**64**:45–60.

24 Moller H, Boyle P, Maisonneuve P, *et al.* Changing mortality from oesophageal cancer in males in Denmark and other European countries in relation to changing levels of alcohol consumption. *Cancer Causes Control* 1990;**1**:181–8.

25 Cook-Mozaffari PJ, Azordegan F, Day NE, *et al.* Oesophageal cancer studies in the Caspian littoral of Iran: results of a case-control study. *Br J Cancer* 1979;**39**:203–309.

26 Franceschi S, Bidoli E, Baron A, *et al.* Maize and risk of cancers of the oral cavity, pharynx and oesophagus. *J Natl Cancer Inst* 1990;**82**:1407–11.

27 Iran-IARC study group. Esophageal cancer studies in the Caspian littoral of Iran: results of population studies. A prodrome. *J Natl Cancer Inst* 1977;**59**:1127–38.

28 Levi F, Ollyo JB, La Vecchia C, *et al*. The consumption of tobacco, alcohol, and the risk of adenocarcinoma in Barrett's oesophagus. *Int J Cancer* 1990;**45**:852–4.

29 Parkin DM, Pisani P, Ferlay J. Estimates of the worldwide incidence of eighteen major cancers in 1985. *Int J Cancer* 1993;**55**:594–606.

30 Napalkov NP, Tserkovy GF, Merabishuili VM, *et al*, eds: Cancer incidence in the USSR (supplement to *Cancer incidence in five continents*, vol III). *IARC Sci Pub* 1983;**48**.

31 Vigotti MA, Cislaghi C, Balzi D, *et al*. Cancer mortality in migrant populations within Italy. *Tumori* 1988;**74**:107–28.

32 Logan WPD. Cancer mortality by occupation and social class 1851–1971. *IARC Sci Publ*, 1982;**3b**:31.

33 McMichael AJ, McCall MG, Hartstorne JM, *et al*. Pattern of gastro-intestinal cancer in European migrants to Australia. The role of dietary change. *Int J Cancer* 1980;**25**:431–7.

34 Boyle P, Maisonneuve P, Levi F, *et al*. Cancer patterns in central and eastern Europe: comparison with the rest of Europe. In: Bodmer W, Zaridze DG, eds. *Cancer prevention in central and eastern Europe*. Geneva: *International Union Against Cancer (UICC)*, 1993.

35 Tominaga S. Decreasing trend of stomach cancer in Japan. *Jpn J Cancer Res* 1987;**78**: 1–10.

36 Blot WJ, Devesa SS, Kneller RW, *et al*. Rising incidence of adenocarcinoma of the esophagus and gastric cardia. *JAMA* 1991;**265**:1287–9.

37 Powell J, McConkey CC. Increasing incidence of adenocarcinoma of the gastric cardia and adjacent sites. *Br J Cancer* 1990;**62**:440–3.

38 Levi F, La Vecchia C. Adenocarcinoma of the esophagus in Switzerland. *JAMA* 1991; **265**:2960.

39 Zheng T, Taylor Mayne S, Holford TR, *et al*. Time-trend and age-period-cohort effects on incidence of esophageal cancer in Connecticut 1935–89. *Cancer Causes Control* 1992; **3**:481–92.

40 Howson CP, Hiyama T, Wynder EL. The decline in gastric cancer: epidemiology of an unplanned triumph. *Epidemiol Rev* 1986;**8**:1–27.

41 Decarli A, La Vecchia C, Cislaghi C, *et al*. Descriptive epidemiology of gastric cancer in Italy. *Cancer* 1986;**58**:2560–9.

42 Risch HA, Jain M, Choi NW, *et al*. Dietary factors and the incidence of cancer of the stomach. *Am J Epidemiol* 1985;**122**:947–59.

43 You WC, Blot WJ, Chang YS, *et al*. Diet and high risk of stomach cancer in Shandong, China. *Cancer Res* 1988;**48**:3518–35.

44 Buiatti E, Palli D, Decarli A, *et al*. A case-control study of gastric cancer and diet in Italy. *Int J Cancer* 1989;**44**:611–16.

45 You WC, Blot WJ, Chang YS, *et al*. Allium vegetables and reduced risk of stomach cancer. *J Natl Cancer Inst* 1989;**81**:162–64.

46 Trichopoulos D, Ouranos G, Day NE, *et al*. Diet and cancer of the stomach: a case-control study in Greece. *Int J Cancer* 1985;**36**:291–97.

47 La Vecchia C, Negri E, Decarli A, *et al*. A case-control study of diet and gastric cancer in northern Italy. *Int J Cancer* 1987;**40**:484–9.

48 Buiatti E, Palli D, Decarli A, *et al*. A case-control study of gastric cancer and diet in Italy. II Association with nutrients. *Int J Cancer* 1990;**45**:896–901.

49 Blot WJ, Li J-Y, Taylor P, *et al*. Nutrition intervention trials in Linxian, China: supplementation with specific vitamin/mineral combinations, cancer incidence, and disease-specific mortality in the general population. *J Natl Cancer Inst* 1993;**85**:1483–92.

50 Parsonnet J, Friedman GD, Vandersteen DP, *et al*. Helicobacter pylori infection and the risk of gastric carcinoma. *N Engl J Med* 1991;**71**:1127–31.

51 Nomura A, Stemmerman G, Chyou P-H, *et al*. Helicobacter pylori infection and gastric carcinoma among Japanese Americans in Hawaii. *N Engl J Med* 1991;**325**:1132–6.

52 Blaser MJ. *Helicobacter pylori* and the pathogenesis of gastroduodenal inflammation. *J Infect Dis* 1990;**161**:626–33.

53 Muñoz N, Connelly R. Time trends of intestinal and diffuse types of gastric cancer in the United States. *Int J Cancer* 1971;**81**:58–64.

54 Shimizu Y, Kato H, Schull WJ, *et al*. Life span study report 11, Part 1: comparison of risk coefficients for site specific cancer mortality based on the DS86 and T65DR shielded

kerma and organ doses. Radiation Effects Research Foundation, Hiroshima, Japan, 1987. (*Radiation Effects Research Foundation technical report 12–87*).

55 Preston DL, Kato H, Kopecky KJ, *et al.* Life span study report 10, Part 1: cancer mortality among A-bomb survivors in Hiroshima and Nagasaki, 1950–1982. Hiroshima Radiation Effects Research Foundation: 1986. (*Radiation Effects Research Foundation technical report 1-86*).

56 Smith PG, Doll R. Mortality among patients with ankylosing spondylitis after a single treatment course with x-rays. *BMJ* 1982;**284**:449–54.

57 Boyle P. Relative value of incidence and mortality data in cancer research. *Recent Results Cancer Res* 1989;**114**:41–63.

58 Boyle P, Zaridze DG, Smans M. Descriptive epidemiology of colorectal cancer. *Int J Cancer* 1985;**36**:9–18.

59 Haenszel N, Correa P. Cancer of the colon and rectum and adenomatous polyps. A review of epidemiologic findings. *Cancer* 1971;**28**:14–24.

60 Percy C, Stanek E, Gloeckler L. Accuracy of cancer death certificates and its effect on cancer mortality statistics. *Am J Public Health* 1981;**71**:242–250.

61 Sondik E, Young JL, Horm JW, *et al*, eds. 1985 annual cancer statistics review. Bethesda: National Cancer Institute, 1986. (*NIH Publication 86-2789*).

62 Haenszel W, Kurihara M. Studies of Japanese migrants I. Mortality from cancer and other diseases among Japanese in the United States. *J Natl Cancer Inst* 1968;**40**:43–68.

63 Staszewski J. Migrant studies in alimentary tract cancer. *Recent Results Cancer Res* 1972;**39**:85–97.

64 Boyle P. Progress in preventing death from colorectal cancer. *Brit J Cancer* 1995;**72**:528–30.

65 Shepard RJ. Exercise in the prevention and treatment of cancer – an update. *Sports Med* 1993;**15**:258–80.

66 Holdstock DJ, Misiewicz JJ, Smith T, *et al.* Propulsion (mass movements) in the human colon and its relationship to meals and somatic activity. Gut; 1970;**11**:91–9.

67 Simon HB. The immunology of exercise. *JAMA* 1984;**252**:2735–38.

68 Bartram HP, Wynder EL. Physical activity and colon cancer risk? Physiological consideration. *Am J Gastroenterol* 1989;**84**:109–12.

69 Willett WC. The search for the causes of breast and colon cancer. *Nature* 1989;**338**:389–94.

70 Vena JE, Graham S, Zielezny M, *et al.* Occupational exercise and risk of cancer. *Am J Clin Nutr* 1987;**45**:318–27.

71 Slattery ML, Schumacher ML, Smith KR, *et al.* Physical activity, diet and role of colon cancer in Utah. *Am J Epidemiol* 1988;**128**:989–99.

72 Whittemore AS, Wu-Williams AH, Lee M, *et al.* Diet, physical activity and colorectal cancer among Chinese in North America and China. *J Natl Cancer Inst* 1990;**82**:915–26.

73 Willett WC, Stampfer MJ, Colditz GA, *et al.* Relation of meat, fat, and fiber intake to the risk of colon cancer in a prospective study among women. *N Engl J Med* 1990;**323**:1664–72.

74 Sugimura T. Past, present and future of mutagens in cooked foods. *Environ Health Perspect* 1986;**67**:5–10.

75 Felton JS, Knize MG, Shen NH, *et al.* Identification of the mutagens in cooked beef. *Environ Health Perspect* 1986;**67**:17–24.

76 Schiffman MH, Felton JS. Re: fried foods and the risk of colon cancer. *Am J Epidemiol* 1990;**131**:376–8.

77 Ha WI, Grim NK, Periza MW. Anticarcinogenics from fried ground beef: heat-altered derivatives of linoleic acid. *Carcinogenesis* 1987;**8**:1881–7.

78 Zaridze DG. Environmental etiology of large-bowel cancer. *J Natl Cancer Inst* 1983;**70**:389–400.

79 Sakaguchi M, Hiramatsu Y, Takada H, *et al.* Effect of dietary unsaturated and saturated fats on azoxymethane-induced colon carcinogenesis in rats. *Cancer Res* 1984;**44**:1472–77.

80 Minoura YT, Takata T, Sakaguchi M, *et al.* Effect of dietary eicopentaenoic acid on azoxymethane induced colon carcinogenesis in rats. *Cancer Res* 1988;**46**:4790–4.

81 Kritchevsky D. Diet, nutrition and cancer: the role of fibre. *Cancer* 1986;**58**:1830–6.

82 Tuyns AJ, Haeltermann M, Kaaks R. Colorectal cancer and the intake of nutrients: oligosaccharides are a risk factor, fats are not. A case-control study in Belgium. *Nutr Cancer* 1987;**10**:181–96.

83 Kune S, Kune GA, Watson LF. Case-control study of dietary aetiological factors: the Melbourne colorectal cancer study. *Nutr Cancer* 1987;**9**:21–42.

84 Heilbrun LK, Hankin JH, Nomura AMY, *et al.* Colon cancer and dietary fat, phosphorous and calcium in Hawaiian–Japanese men. *Am J Clin Nutr* 1986;**43**:306–9.

85 Newmark HL, Wargovich MJ, Bruce WR. Colon cancer and dietary fat, phosphate and calcium: a hypothesis. *J Natl Cancer Inst* 1984;**72**:1323–5.

86 Goldin BR, Gorbach SL. The effect of milk and lactobacillus feeding on human intestinal bacterial enzyme activity. *Am J Clin Nutr* 1984;**39**:756–61.

87 Sorenson AW, Slattery ML, Ford MH. Calcium and colon cancer: a review. *Nutr Cancer* 1988;**11**:135–45.

88 Longnecker MP, Orza MJ, Adams ME, *et al.* A meta-analysis of alcoholic beverage consumption in relation to risk of colorectal cancer. *Cancer Causes Control* 1990;**1**:59–68.

89 Bishop DT, Hall NR. The genetics of colorectal cancer. *Eur J Cancer* 1994;**30**:1946–56.

90 Bishop DT, Thomas HJW. The genetics of colorectal cancer. *Cancer Surv* 1990;**9**: 585–604.

91 Kennaway EL. Cancer of the liver in the negro in Africa and America. *Cancer Res* 1944; **4**:571–7.

92 Tuyns AJ, Obradovic M. Unexpected high incidence of primary liver cancer in Geneva, Switzerland. *J Natl Cancer Inst* 1975;**54**:61–64.

93 Srivatanakul S, Sontipong P, Chotiwan P, *et al.* Liver cancer in Thailand: temporal and geographic variations. *J Gastroenterol Hepatol* 1988;**3**:413–20.

94 Parkin DM, Stiller CA, Bieber CA, *et al*, eds. International incidence of childhood cancer. *IARC Sci Publ* 1988;**87**.

95 Szmuness W. Hepatocellular carcinoma and the hepatitis B virus: evidence for a causal association. *Prog Med Virol* 1978;**24**:40–69.

96 Beasley RP, Lin C, Hwang LY, *et al.* Hepatocellular carcinoma and hepatitis B virus. A prospective study of 22·07 men in Taiwan. *Lancet* 1981;**ii**:1129–33.

97 Beasley RP. Hepatitis B virus. The major etiology of hepatocellular carcinoma. *Cancer* 1988;**61**:1942–56.

98 Trichopoulos D, Day NE, Kaklamani E, *et al.* Hepatitis B virus, tobacco smoking and ethanol consumption in the etiology of hepatocellular carcinoma. *Int J Cancer* 1987;**39**: 45–49.

99 La Vecchia C, Negri E, Decarli A, *et al.* Risk factors for hepatocellular carcinoma in Northern Italy. *Int J Cancer* 1988;**42**:872–6.

100 Yu MC, Mark T, Hanisch R, *et al.* Hepatitis, alcohol consumption, cigarette smoking, and hepatocellular carcinoma in Los Angeles. *Int J Cancer* 1987;**39**:45–49.

101 Hsieh CC, Tzonou A, Zavitsanos X, *et al.* Age at first establishment of chronic hepatitis B virus infection and hepatocellular cancer risk. A birth order study. *Am J Epidemiol* 1992;**136**:115–21.

102 Muñoz N, Bosch FX. Epidemiology of hepatocellular carcinoma. In: Okuda K, Ishak KG, eds. *Neoplasms of the liver.* Tokyo: Springer, 1987.

103 Bulatao-Jayme J, Almero EM, Castro MCA, *et al.* A case-control study of primary liver cancer risk from aflatoxin exposure. *Int J Epidemiol* 1982;**11**:112–19.

104 Rosenberg L. The risk of liver neoplasia in relation to combined oral contraceptive use. *Contraception* 1991;**43**:643–52.

105 Hsing AW, McLaughlin JK, Hrubec Z, *et al.* Cigarette smoking and liver cancer among US veterans. *Cancer Causes Control* 1990;**1**:217–21.

106 Trichopoulos D, MacMahon B, Sparros L, *et al.* Smoking and hepatitis B-negative primary hepatocellular carcinoma. *J Natl Cancer Inst* 1980;**65**:111–14.

107 Van Kaick G, Muth H, Kal A, *et al.* Results of the German thorotrast study. In: Boice JD, Fraumeni JF, eds. *Radiation carcinogenesis: epidemiology and biological significance.* New York: Raven Press, 1984.

108 *IARC.* An updating of IARC Monographs 1-42. 1987;Suppl 7.

109 Boss LP, Lanier AP, Dohan PH, *et al.* Cancers of the gallbladder and biliary tract in Alaskan natives, 1970–79. *J Natl Cancer Inst* 1982;**169**:1005–7.

110 Rios-Dalenz J, Correa P, Haenszel W. Morbidity from cancer in La Paz, Bolivia. *Int J Cancer* 1981;**28**:307–14.

111 Becker N, Frentzel-Beyme R, Wagner S. *Atlas of cancer mortality in the Federal Republic of Germany.* 2nd ed. Berlin: Springer, 1984.

112 Zatonski W, Smans M, Tyczynski J, *et al.* Cancer mortality atlas of central and eastern Europe. *IARC Sci Publ* 1996.

113 Diehl AK. Gallstone size and the risk of gallbladder cancer. *JAMA* 1983;**250**: 2323–6.

114 Lowenfels AB, Cavallini G, Ammann RW. Pancreatitis and the risk of pancreatic cancer. *N Engl J Med* 1993;**328**:1433–7.

115 Lew EA, Garfinkel L. Variations in mortality by weight among 750 000 men and women. *J Chron Dis* 1979;**32**:563–76.

116 Zatonski W, Lowenfels AB, Boyle P, *et al.* Epidemiological aspects of gallbladder cancer: a case-control study of the SEARCH programme of the IARC. *J Natl Cancer Inst* (in press).

117 Mir-Madjlessi SH, Farmer RG, Sivak MV. Bile duct carcinoma in patients with ulcerative colitis. Relationship to sclerosing cholangitis: report of six cases and review of the literature. *Dig Dis Sci* 1987;**32**:145–54.

118 Caygill CP, Hill MJ, Hall CN, *et al.* Increased risk of cancer at multiple sites after surgery for peptic ulceration. *Gut* 1987;**28**:924–8.

119 Heilbrun LK, Nomura A, Stemmerman GN. Gastrectomy and cancer of the gallbladder or urinary tract [letter]. *Lancet* 1974;**i**:511.

120 Boyle P, Hsieh Cc, Maisonneuve P, *et al.* Epidemiology of pancreas cancer (1988). *Int J Pancreatol* 1989;**5**:327–46.

121 Pisani P, Parkin DM, Ferlay J. Estimates of the worldwide mortality rate from 18 major cancers in 1985. Implications for prevention and projections of future burden. *Int J Cancer* 1993;**55**:891–903.

122 Boyle P, Maisonneuve P, Bueno de Mesquita B, *et al.* Cigarette smoking and pancreas cancer risk: a case-control study of the SEARCH programme of the IARC. *Int J Cancer* (in press).

123 MacMahon B, Yen S, Trichopoulos D, *et al.* Coffee and cancer of the pancreas. *N Engl J Med* 1981;**304**:630–3.

124 IARC. Coffee, tea, mate, methylxanthines (caffeine, theophylline, theobromine) and methylglyoxal. *Monogr Eval Carcinog Rishs Hum* 1991;**51**.

125 Velema J, Walker AM, Gold E. Alcohol and pancreatic cancer. Insufficient epidemiologic evidence for a causal relationship. *Epidemiol Rev* 1986;**8**:28–41.

126 Cuzick J, Babiker AG. Pancreatic cancer, alcohol, diabetes mellitus and gallbladder disease. *Int J Cancer* 1989;**43**:415–21.

127 Bouchardy C, Clavel F, La Vecchia C, *et al.* Alcohol, beer and cancer of the pancreas. *Int J Cancer* 1990;**45**:842–6.

128 Boice JD, *et al.* Cancer risk following radiation treatment for cervical cancer. An international collaboration among cancer registries. *J Natl Cancer Inst* 1985;**74**:955–75.

129 Kato H and Schull WJ. Studies of A-bomb survivors. 7. Mortality, 1950–1978. Part I. Cancer mortality. *Radiat Res* 1982;**90**:395–432.

130 Gilbert ES, Marks S. An analysis of the mortality of workers in a nuclear facility. *Radiat Res* 1979;**79**:122–48.

131 Tolley HD, Marks S, Buchanan JA, Gilbert ES. A further update of the analysis of mortality of workers in a nuclear facility. *Radiat Res* 1983;**95**:211–13.

132 Howe GR, Jain M, Miller AB. Dietary factors and risk of pancreatic cancer: results of a Canadian population-based case-control study. *Int J Cancer* 1990;**45**:604–8.

133 Bueno de Mesquita HB, Moerman CJ, Runia S, *et al.* Are energy and energy-providing nutrients related to carcinoma of the exocrine pancreas? *Int J Cancer* 1990;**46**:435–44.

134 Ghadirian P, Simard A, Baillargeon J, *et al.* Nutritional factors and pancreatic cancer in the francophone community in Montreal, Canada. *Int J Cancer* 1991;**47**:1–6.

135 Baghurst PA, McMichael AJ, Slavotnik AH, *et al.* A case-control study of diet and pancreas cancer. *Am J Epidemiol.* 1991;**134**:167–79.

136 Zatonski W, Przewozniak K, Howe GR, Maisonneuve P, Walker AM, Boyle P. Nutritional factors and pancreatic cancer: a case-control study from south-west Poland. *Int J Cancer* 1991;**48**:390–4.

137 Howe GR, Ghadirian P, Bueno de Mesquita B, *et al.* Nutrient intake and pancreatic cancer: a collaborative, case-control study within the SEARCH programme. *N Engl J Med* (in press).

138 Fearon ER, Vogelstein B. A genetic model for colorectal tumorigenesis. *Cell* 1990;**61**: 759–67.

139 Morotomi M, Guillem J, LoGerfo P, *et al.* Production of diacylglycerol, an activator of protein kinase C, by human intestinal microflora. *Cancer Res* 1990;**50**:3595–9.

140 Bodmer WF, Balley CJ, Bodmer J, *et al.* Localization of the gene for familial adenomatous polyposis on chromosome 5. *Nature* 1987;**328**:614–8.

141 Hall NR, Murday VA, Chapman P, *et al.* Genetic linkage in Muir-Torre syndrome to the same chromosomal region as cancer family syndrome. *Eur J Cancer* 1994;**30**:180–2.

142 Potter JD, Slattery ML, Bostwick RM, *et al.* Colon cancer: a review of the epidemiology. *Epidemiol Rev* 1993;**15**:499–545.

143 Giovannucci E, Rimm EB, Strampfer MJ, *et al.* A prospective study of cigarette smoking and risk of colorectal adenoma and colorectal cancer in US men. *J Natl Cancer Inst* 1994;**86**:183–91.

144 Giovannucci E, Colditz GA, Strampfer MJ, *et al.* A prospective study of cigarette smoking and risk of colorectal adenoma and colorectal cancer in US women. *J Natl Cancer Inst* 1994;**86**:192–9.

145 The alpha-tocopherol, beta-carotene cancer prevention study group. The effect of vitamin E and beta carotene on the incidence of lung cancer and other cancers in male workers. *N Engl J Med* 1994;**330**:1029–35.

146 Greenberg ER, Baron JA, Tosteson TD, *et al.* A clinical trial of antioxidant vitamins to prevent colorectal cancer, *New Engl J Med* 1994;**331**:141–7.

147 Labayle D, Fischer D, Viel R, *et al.* Sulindac causes regression of rectal polyps in familial adenomatous polyposis. *Gastroenterology* 1991;**101**:307–11.

148 Skinner SA, Penny AG, O'Brien PE. Sulindac inhibits the rate of growth and appearance of colon tumours in rats. *Arch Surg* 1991;**126**:1094–96.

149 Gann PH, Manson J, Glynn RJ, *et al.* Low-dose aspirin and incidence of colorectal tumours in a randomised trial. *J Natl Cancer Inst* 1993;**85**:1220–4.

150 Farmer KC, Goulston K, Macrae F. Aspirin and non-steroidal anti-inflammatory drugs in the chemoprevention of colorectal cancer. *Med J Austr* 1993;**159**:649–50.

151 Morson BC. *Gastrointestinal Pathology.* Oxford: Blackwell Scientific, 1979.

152 Mandel JS, Bond JH, Church TR, *et al.* Reducing mortality from colorectal cancer by screening for fecal occult blood. *N Engl J Med* 1993;**328**:1365–71.

153 Rosen P, Ron E, Fireman Z, *et al.* The relative value of fecal occult blood tests and flexible sigmoidoscopy in screening for large bowel neoplasia. *Cancer* 1987;**60**:2553–58.

154 Allison J, Feldman R, Tekawa I. Hemoccult screening in detecting colorectal neoplasm. *Ann Intern Med* 1990;**112**:328–33.

155 Gilbertson VA, Nelms JM. The prevention of invasive cancer of the rectum. *Cancer* 1978;**41**:1137–9.

156 Selby JV, Friedman GD, Quesenbery CJ, *et al.* A case-control study of screening sigmoidoscopy and mortality from colorectal cancer. *N Engl J Med* 1992;**326**:653–57.

157 Newcomb PA, Norfleet RG, Storer BE, *et al.* Screening sigmoidoscopy and colorectal cancer mortality. *J Natl Cancer Inst* 1992;**84**:1572–5.

158 Atkin WS, Morson BC, Cuzick J. Long-term risk of colorectal cancer after excision of rectosigmoid adenomas. *N Engl J Med* 1992;**326**:658–62.

159 Cunningham D, Findlay M. The chemotherapy of colon cancer can no longer be ignored. *Eur J Cancer* 1993;**29**:2077–9.

160 Greenberg R, Baron J. Prospects for preventing colorectal cancer death. *J Natl Cancer Inst* 1993;**85**:1182–4.

2: Biology of metastasis

A R KINSELLA and PETER McCULLOCH

Current understanding of metastasis biology

Like the progression to localised malignancy (see Chapter 4), metastasis is a genetically controlled multistep process. It involves (a) the detachment of cells from neighbouring tumour or normal cells, (b) their invasion into the surrounding tissue, (c) intravasation into the lymphatics and blood capillaries, (d) attachment of the endothelium of the vessels of the target organ, (e) extravasation into the surrounding tissue, and (f) the establishment of metastases at distant secondary sites. This process is called the "metastatic cascade" and involves the expression by the tumour cell of a number of properties not normally found in the cell types from which it originates. Metastatic spread was originally believed to occur first to the lymph nodes, and only once this "barrier" had been breached would tumour cells enter the bloodstream. The modern concept of metastasis is more sophisticated and allows that lymphatic and bloodborne spread can occur independently (see below). Metastatic cells establish themselves at secondary sites which tend to be specific for the tumour of origin, and one of the challenges for research in this field is to explain these patterns of organ specificity. The complexity of the metastatic process, and the steps that must be accomplished to complete it, suggest the participation of a variety of different proteins. The involvement of matrix degrading proteases, receptors for endothelial cells, matrix binding proteins, motility factors and their receptors, growth factors, and immunological recognition molecules have all been postulated, and some of the genes involved in these processes have been very elegantly reviewed by Ponta et al.[1] It has long been believed that tumour cells acquire their metastatic properties by mutation and selection and that the rare cell that has assembled all these properties will metastasise, but it is equally possible that the metastatic process may involve coregulation of many genes, which would reduce the complexity of this process substantially. The evidence to resolve this debate is not yet available. For the most part, it seems that quantitative not qualitative changes in gene expression are important in governing metatastic behaviour. The genes governing the metastatic process can be divided into *controlling* genes, such as oncogenes, transcriptional and translational genes, and genes involved in signal transduction, and *phenotypic* genes, for example, the structural genes such as the E cadherins and integrins described below. Rather than attempt to discuss in detail all of the mechanisms thought to be implicated in the linked processes of invasion and metastasis, this chapter will review specific areas in which the evidence suggests that the processes studied are particularly important in the metastatic cascade, while briefly mentioning others.

Role of adhesion molecules

The orderly structure of differentiated material is maintained by structures known as adhesion plaques (adherens junctions), desmosomes, and tight junctions, which mediate cell–cell adhesion between neighbouring cells. It has been known for a long time that the scattering of cells in invasive carcinomas is due to the loss of integrity of the adherens junctions, often due to the loss of function of E cadherin. This transmembrane glycoprotein has an extracellular domain that mediates specific homophilic interactions with the extracellular domains of other E cadherin molecules on neighbouring epithelial cells. The cytoplasmic domain of the molecule links to the cytoplasmic protein β catenin, which links in turn through α catenin to α actinin and the actin cytoskeleton.[2] Studies in vitro using two invasion assay systems have suggested that E cadherin has a causal role to play in colorectal tumour cell invasion. In both a collagen gel and a "matrigel" assay system, all colorectal carcinoma cell lines that failed to express E cadherin invaded the artificial membrane.[3] Addition of anti-E cadherin antibody to a cell line expressing E cadherin function rendered it invasive, while the introduction of an E cadherin cDNA into an invasive colorectal carcinoma cell line that was negative for E cadherin expression rendered it non-invasive.[3] The evidence from clinical studies is less clear. Loss of E cadherin expression has been correlated with advanced disease in a variety of tumour systems, including diffuse gastric carcinoma,[4] and a trend towards reduced E cadherin expression in more advanced colorectal carcinomas has been reported,[5 6] but no statistically significant correlation between reduced E cadherin expression and disease spread was observed in the latter studies. Expression of E cadherin has been observed in colorectal carcinomas that went on to metastasise, and in colorectal hepatic metastases.[5]

It is becoming increasingly obvious from recent studies that understanding of the role of E cadherin in the dissemination of disease must include a discussion of E cadherin functionality and of the role of abnormalities in the other components of the E cadherin complex. E cadherin expression can occur in the absence of E cadherin functionality:

E cadherin function is influenced by mutations in the intracellular or extracellular domains of the E cadherin molecule, as reported for gastric carcinomas[7] and gastric carcinoma cell lines,[8] and by mutations in the β catenin molecule for gastric carcinomas.[9 10] Expression of a non-functional E cadherin molecule has also been reported in the absence of α catenin expression in a lung carcinoma cell line[11] and in a colorectal carcinoma cell line.[12] The role of α catenin expression in the regulation of cell–cell adhesion has been highlighted in gastric carcinoma,[13] oesophageal carcinoma,[14] and colorectal carcinoma (Kinsella et al, unpublished data). These data suggest that functionally normal E cadherin, α catenin, and β catenin may have an important role to play as metastasis suppressor genes in tumours of the gastrointestinal tract. Other intercellular couplings mediated by the desmosomes may also have a role to play in malignant progression. Desmosome expression has been reported to be downregulated in transitional cell carcinomas and squamous cell carcinomas of the head and neck, but not in colorectal carcinomas.

A functional role for homophilic intercellular adhesion in neoplastic cells has been proposed for the α_4-β_1 integrin, one of the fibronectin receptors.[15] The integrins are α-β heterodimeric transmembrane proteins comprising at least 13 different α chains and eight different β chains and, along with the cadherins, comprise the main adhesion molecules expressed by normal and transformed epithelial cells.[16 17] They are critical for the maintenance of cell differentiation in vitro and probably in vivo. The integrins, like E cadherin, are transmembrane glycoproteins, the cytoplasmic domains of which also interact with cytoplasmic proteins such as α actinin or talin.[16 18] The majority of integrins are receptors for extracellular matrix proteins such as collagens (α_1-β_1, α_2-β_1, α_3-β_1), fibronectin (α_3-β_1, α_4-β_1, α_5-β_1), or laminin (α_3-β_1, α_6-β_1).[18] Other integrins mediate heterotypic interactions with members of the immunoglobulin supergene family such as the intercellular adhesion module ICAM-1 and the vascular cell adhesion molecule V-CAM.[16] In colorectal carcinoma cell lines E cadherin and β_1 integrins have been reported to mediate the cell–cell and cell–collagen interactions required for the maintenance of their glandular differentiation.[19] Adhesion of colon carcinoma cells to collagen matrix and their morphological and cellular differentiation are inhibited by monoclonal antibodies recognising α_2-β_1 integrin.[20] Similarly migration and collagen gel contraction are inhibited by blocking monoclonal antibodies to α_2-β_1 integrin receptor.[18] There is growing evidence that α_2-β_1 integrin is required in the metastatic pathway of transformed cells[21] and that its regulation might be influenced by growth factors produced both by the neoplastic cells and the adjacent stromal cell compartment. Transforming growth factor (TGF) α has been shown to upregulate the expression of α_2-β_1 and α_3-β_1 integrin and downregulate the fibronectin receptor and α_6 integrin chain. These effects are accompanied by increased adhesion to collagen and enhanced α_2-β_1 integrin mediated morphological differentiation in three dimensional collagen gels. Adhesion to a collagen substratum has been shown to inhibit the mitogenic effects of TGFα in responsive colon carcinoma cell lines.[20] The mechanisms of this differential response to TGFα are not understood and may involve phosphorylation of growth factor receptor tyrosine kinases or other cellular components.[22-24] A number of growth factors such as TGFβ,[25] fibroblast growth factor, and interleukin (IL) 4 have been shown to regulate the expression and function of integrins[18] as well as other adhesion receptors.[26] In the light of such evidence it has been proposed[20] that the inappropriate expression of growth factors seen in malignant cells whose cell matrix adhesion receptors are no longer functioning normally may be part of the mechanism by which normal tissue architecture and growth control are lost. Integrins may require interaction with other adhesion molecules in the regulation of the differentiation and motility of both normal and transformed cells. For example, E cadherin mediated cell–cell interactions are critical for α_2-β_1 mediated differentiation in colorectal tumour cells. Thus metastasis appears to be governed in part by qualitative and quantitative alterations in the adhesive interactions mediated by the cadherins, integrins, and other adhesion molecules.[27] Loss of expression and/or function of any of these molecules would allow colorectal cells to dedifferentiate and lose their cohesive properties and therefore facilitate invasion and metastatis.

Consistent with this, qualitative and quantitative changes in integrin expression have been documented in carcinomas of the colon,[27] stomach,[28] and pancreas.[29] In colorectal cancer, for example, two studies have clearly shown that α_2-β_1 is consistently lost or decreased in moderately and poorly differentiated colorectal tumours.[27 30] A decrease in α_2 integrin expression and loss of normal basolateral localisation has been observed in preinvasive adenomatous lesions and correlated with a cellular atypia and glandular derangement.[30] No significant correlation between reduced α_2 expression and the extent of local invasion and metastatic deposits were found. There is no evidence in vivo to support the role played by α_2-β_1 integrin in invasion and metastasis in colorectal cancer. Reduced α_2 expression has been found in gastric and pancreatic cancers associated with a poorly differentiated morphology.

As we can see from the outline of the metastatic cascade, for migration to occur the "metastasising" tumour cell needs to make new contacts with matrix components, possibly stromal cells and certainly with endothelial cells. CD44, a pleiomorphic receptor for hyaluronan, fibronectin, collagen, laminin, and possibly other ligands, has been identified as a metastasis associated antigen.[31] CD44 undergoes extensive alternative splicing and post-translational modification, rendering the definition of its molecular function rather complex. Using standard immunohistochemical techniques and antibodies recognising all CD44 isoforms, CD44 expression has been analysed on frozen sections of benign gastric mucosa (normal, gastritis, intestinal metaplasia), autologous primary tumours, and metastatic lesions from various locations. The results have been correlated with a panel of conventional risk factors for gastric carcinoma and with tumour recurrence and survival.[32] These data indicate that expression of CF44 on gastric mucosa is restricted to a distinct glandular area and is probably induced as a consequence of cytokine expression by infiltrating leucocytes. Inflammatory cytokines specifically upregulate variant isoforms, especially those containing exons v6 and v9. CD44 expression was, however, detected in only 49% of primary gastric carcinomas and a good correlation was found between total CD44 and CD44 v9 expression in the same tumours, suggesting that CD44 variant analysis may not be useful in defining malignancy or premalignancy in gastric lesions. CD44 and CD44 v9 expression were, however, more common in advanced gastric carcinomas with metastases at the time of surgery than in metastasis-free carcinomas. No correlation was found with other prognostic factors, such as T (tumour) stage, N (node) stage, grade, or lymphatic invasion, nor with leucocyte infiltrate. Since mediation of leucocyte infiltration is thought to be one of the main physiological roles of CD44, this suggests that CD44 expression has a different activation pathway in benign and malignant gastric tissues, Mayer *et al* showed that curatively resected patients with CD44 and CD44 v9 positive primary carcinomas showed more frequent tumour relapse and tumour induced mortality and had a shorter survival time than patients with CD44S and CD44 v9 negative primary tumours.[32] In colorectal carcinogenesis, expression of CD44 exon v5 is an early tumour marker because it is detectable on small dysplastic polyps but not on normal colonic epithelium.[33] In contrast, exon v6 expression is correlated with disease progression and reduced survival.[34] Reverse transcription-Polymerase Chain Reaction (rt-PCR) has revealed the presence of larger splice variants in colorectal tumour progression. It seems likely that tumours expressing CD44 v6 gain a selective advantage during tumour progression and metastasis formation. These clear patterns of expression in premalignant and malignant colonic lesions suggest possible diagnostic and therapeutic applications for CD44. It is important to appreciate that surface and transmembrane molecules, such as E cadherin, integrins, and CD44, not only interact with other cells and components of the extracellular matrix but also send growth regulatory signals. Ligand and growth factor binding has been reported to lead to enhanced phosphorylation, and activation of several genes has been found following activation of either integrins or CD44.

Role of proteolytic enzymes

An essential step in the metastatic process is "invasion" and it is becoming increasingly obvious, from both experimental systems and clinical trials, that matrix metalloproteinase enzymes may have a key role to play in this process. The first evidence for this was obtained from studies with tissue specific inhibitors of metalloproteinases (TIMPs). Addition of TIMP1 to in vitro invasion assays or experimental metastases assays results in inhibition of invasion and metastasis.[35 36] TIMP1 has been shown to be a negative regulator of metastasis in a gastric carcinoma cell line.[37] Another molecule implicated in this process of invasion is the plasminogen activator urokinase, which plays a role in degradation of basement membrane laminin.[38-40] Collagenase IV and cathepsin D are other proteolytic enzymes for which laboratory studies have supported an important role in invasion and metastasis. In the case of cathepsin D there is evidence, from clinical studies, of an association between poor prognosis and expression of the molecule in the primary tumour. Another enzyme system that appears to be important in bloodborne metastasis is the complex series of proteinases that make up the coagulation system. Animal studies have supported a critical role for coagulation in determining the success of circulating tumour cells in seeding as new deposits.[41] There is easily detectable stage related activation of the coagulation system in most types of human cancer.[42]

Other metastasis associated genes

Interpretation of the role of the metastasis suppressor genes discussed so far is straightforward, and functional loss of their protein products, due to either reduced expression or mutation, can easily be understood as having a possible role in the dissemination of tumour cells. Such a clear understanding of the role of another metastasis gene, NM23, is still lacking. The protein encoded by the NM23 gene is located in the cytoplasm and carries a nucleoside diphosphate kinase activity. Its expression is inversely correlated with metastic potential in some rodent tumour systems,[43] where it was first identified, as well as in human infiltrating ductal breast[44] and hepatocellular carcinomas.[45] Metastasis suppressor activity has been confirmed in two experimental systems.[46 47] NM23 expression inversely correlates with poor prognosis in gastric carcinoma but not in colon carcinoma where mutations have been found. Allelic loss of NM23 has been reported in one out of nine cases of colonic adenocarcinoma with a homozygous deletion in the lymph node metastasis from this tumour.[48] Genetic alterations in the NM23 gene have been demonstrated in 50% of metastatic colon tumours with no changes seen in the non-metastatic neoplasm, suggesting that mutations in the NM23 gene play a role in metastasis of colonic tumours.[49] Furthermore, changes in the NM23H1 have been shown to have a possible prognostic significance in colorectal carcinoma.[50] It has been postulated that NM23 may be responsible for inhibiting cell migration in response to defined growth factors, and therefore NM23, like the cadherins and integrins, may have a key role to play in the early stages of the metastatic process.

Several other intracellular proteins that are specifically expressed in metastasising tumour cells, and for which a causal role in the metastatic process is very likely, have recently been recognised: these include MTS1 and TIAM1. MTS1 is highly homologous to the rat calcium binding protein P9KA, and TIAM (T lymphoma invasion and metastasis) belongs to the family of GDP-GTP G proteins related to rho.[51 52] There are also a whole series of motility factors whose role may be influential. These may be classified as: (a) factors that stimulate cancer cell motility invasion—for example, the autocrine motility factors; (b) factors that stimulate both growth and motility—for example, hepatocyte growth factor or scatter factor, epidermal growth factor, and IL1, IL3, and IL6;[53-55] and (c) factors that stimulate motility but inhibit growth—for example, TGFβ and the interferons. Of all these the most important are probably hepatocyte growth factor and the autocrine motility factors.

In conclusion, the process of metastasis is very complex and involves a series of changes that must coincide within a single cell. All the changes described above are permissive for metastasis, but what determines the specificity of those cells that metastisise to the lymph nodes and those that metastisise directly to the liver? In the case of colorectal cancer this remains to be determined but there is considerable evidence of a role for carbohydrate mediated cell adhesion.[56-58] Many questions of considerable clinical interest have still to be answered: for example, what determines the differences in the patterns of metastatic spread between colorectal and gastric malignancies? The interface between the laboratory scientist and the clinician dealing with cancer is vital in ensuring that such questions are identified as important and addressed using the appropriate expertise.

Clinical patterns of metastatic disease

If we consider all of the malignant tumours that arise within the gastrointestinal tract, they present an extremely heterogeneous group with respect to cell of origin, prognosis and metastatic behaviour. If, however, we concentrate on the group of adenocarcinomas that arise from the epithelium of the gut or the associated digestive organs, interesting patterns and parallels begin to become apparent in the natural history and metastatic behaviour of this group of tumours. Histologically, the tumours share certain basic characteristics, such as the tendency to glandular differentiation and mucin production and a marked tendency towards lymphatic invasion.

There are striking similarities in the growth patterns of the adenocarcinomas affecting the oesophagus, stomach, and colon, where initial tumour growth is usually followed by ulceration of the tumour and spread through the thickness of the gut wall to involve the serosal surface. In view of their anatomical arrangement, gastrointestinal tumours share the potential for metastasis to liver via the portal vein, but their actual tendency to do so varies from organ to organ. The tumours share a generally poor prognosis, as well as a capacity for transcoelomic metastasis and spread to local and regional lymph nodes. It is perhaps worth noting that the time scale within which recurrence tends to occur after initial treatment is particularly constant in this group of tumours, most recurrent disease occurring within the first two years. The relative rarity of recurrence more than five years after definitive treatment contrasts with a number of other types of carcinoma, particularly renal and breast cancers and melanoma. All of these are noted for their tendency to produce distant, presumably bloodborne metastases at an interval of many years after resection of the primary tumour. As a group they also differ strikingly from the gastrointestinal cancers by the unpredictability of their growth rate, apparently undergoing growth spurts and periods of quiescence, which are not characteristic of the gastrointestinal tumours. These have a tendency to relentless local and regional growth, together with continuous growth of nodal metastases once these are established. The studies of Fisher et al. established clearly that nodal metastases could be left in situ during the surgical treatment of breast cancer without significantly affecting ultimate prognosis.[59] There is no directly analogous study for any form of gastrointestinal cancer, but extrapolation from numerous studies, each providing part of the same evidence, strongly suggests that this is not the case in these tumours. By contrast, the evidence we have suggests that tumours of the stomach, oesophagus, colon, pancreas, and biliary tract, once established in the lymphatic system, continue to grow rapidly and relentlessly, often causing death by their local effects. It is very difficult to dissect out the exact reasons for this contrast but there are clearly two aspects to it. The first is the different biology of the tumours themselves, which clearly possess different properties with respect to their potential for metastasis by the various routes. The second is the anatomy of the regional lymphatics involved, which make continuing nodal growth in the axilla a much less dangerous phenomenon than growth of a similar extent in nodes adjacent to the great vessels and other vital structures deep within the abdomen. The intra-abdominal gastrointestinal carcinomas share a propensity for metastasis to the peritoneal surfaces. The extent to which this is due to special biological properties of this group of tumour, as opposed to anatomical opportunism, is not clear. The frequency of metastasis by lymphatic, transcoelomic, and haematogenous spread does differ somewhat between the various gastrointestinal tumours. Colorectal cancer appears to have the highest propensity for bloodborne metastasis to the liver, frequently appearing as multiple liver metastases with no evidence of other intra-abdominal disease after apparently curative surgery. Liver metastases in gastric cancer, by contrast, are rarely found either in primary or recurrent disease without evidence of massive local spread and nodal disease at the same time.[60]

Why do these carcinomas share these particular properties, and why do they exhibit these differences? The most probable explanation for the similarities is that the tumours arise from very similar differentiated epithelia, and that they may be exposed to similar carcinogenic influences. This being the case it is not surprising that the resultant malignant tumours appear to share so many properties. By extrapolation of this line of reasoning, one might suggest that the critical gene mutations in the malignant cells might be similar in the various types of gastrointestinal cancer, but here the argument does not appear particularly strong. There are certainly genes, such as p53, c-erb2, c-met, and the BCL2 gene, that have a wide distribution amongst all the carcinomas in this group. There are, however, equally striking differences in the background of the different carcinomas. The extremely high incidence of k-ras abnormalities in pancreatic cancer, which is not mirrored by any other gastrointestinal tumour, springs to mind here. Presumably the critical oncogene disturbances leading to specific metastatic behaviours, such as transcoelomic spread, are common to the tumour types that have been identified as sharing this property. Until the genetic background of the various gastrointestinal tumours has been worked out in considerably more detail, comments about the genetic background to the similarities noted between the cancer types will remain a matter of speculation.

It is interesting to note that the metastatic behaviour of the group of gastrointestinal adenocarcinomas does not fit particularly well into either of the paradigms usually used to understand human cancer metastasis. The outdated Halsted paradigm assumed, on the basis of postmortem studies, that spread of carcinoma was centripetal—that is, from the primary tumour to the lymph nodes and only thereafter to the bloodstream.[61] The practical consequence of this was the belief that a radical en bloc resection of tumour and draining nodes should have a high likelihood of success in producing cure unless distant metastasis could be shown to have already occurred. The alternative paradigm, which arose following the discrediting of the basis for the Halsted paradigm, was that of biological predeterminism.[62] This took an opposite view, assuming that cancer was usually a systemic disease from the outset, because metastases were assumed to have formed at a microscopic level long before the primary tumour became clinically detectable, in those tumours that were biologically capable

45

of ever producing metastases. The practical consequence of this paradigm was a belief that surgery should be limited to excision of the primary tumour and obvious gross local disease, and had an extremely limited role to play other than in the prevention of symptoms from these local deposits. Both theories are frustratingly difficult to test but the evidence of common surgical experience could be said to argue for a middle course that does not accept either paradigm in its entirety. It seems clear that in the case of gastric cancer, for example, the disease does remain localised to the primary site and lymph nodes in many cases, and that hepatic and distant metastases do not later become evident if a curative resection is performed. It is a tautology that the curability of cancers declines steadily as the stage increases, and in the main this reflects the growing probability of distant metastatic disease. It seems clear from this that there are many cases in which the point at which fatal metastasis is initiated is somewhere within the clinically detectable course of the growth of the tumour between stages I and IV. If this were not so, we would expect a stage I (early) gastric carcinoma to have a very gloomy prognosis because of the likelihood of recurrent distant disease after local resection. Experience from mass screening programmes and observational studies suggests that carcinoma in situ is a rarely observed event within the gastrointestinal tract, even the early gastric cancer being a form of invasive disease. The corollary is that the doubtful significance of many in situ lesions, picked up for instance in the breast during screening programmes, is not reflected in the case of gastrointestinal tract tumours. Some data are available from observational studies suggesting that the rate of progression from early to advanced gastric cancer is relatively slow but that none the less the vast majority of early cancers will eventually invade and metastasise given time, which may be as much as eight years. The place of high risk legions such as Barrett's oesophagus, intestinal metaplasia in the stomach, and dysplasia in the colon is more difficult to evaluate. To date it has not been possible to identify any oncogene marker or other prognostic factor that can help us to estimate which of the large number of cases of epithelial abnormality not amounting to cancer will go on to malignant change.

The clinical implications of the facts outlined above about gastrointestinal carcinomas have to be looked at in the context of the uncertainty surrounding the metastatic process. A strong case can be made for an aggressive approach to locoregional excision, in view of the propensity for these tumours to spread via the lymph nodes and on to the local peritoneum. The fact that, unlike breast cancer, this group of tumours does spread in a locoregional fashion without distant metastasis on fairly frequent occasions adds further encouragement. It remains to be determined whether new adjuvant chemotherapy or changes in surgical technique can reduce the risks of local or distant spread of gastrointestinal tumours at the time of surgery, but this is certainly a potential implication of the known metastatic properties described above. For instance, local concentrations of tumour necrosis factor are known to make a major difference to the ability of tumour cells to invade the peritoneum,[63] and other cytokines found in surgical wounds have major stimulatory effect on shed cancer cells. The reports of metastasis to port sites after laparoscopic colectomy have raised a series of interesting questions about the potential effects of surgery (conventional or minimal access) on the process of cancer spread, either locally or systemically. Since surgery is likely to remain one of the mainstays of treatment for this group of tumours for the foreseeable future, this area of study deserves our attention as one in which an increase in theoretical knowledge might well bring early practical benefits for the patient undergoing surgery for gastrointestinal cancer.

References

1 Ponta H, Hofmann M, Herrlich P. Recent advances in the genetics of metastasis. *Eur J Cancer* 1994;**30A**:1995–2001.

2 Knudsen KA, Soler AP, Johnson KR, *et al*. Interaction of alpha actinin with the cadherin catenin cell–cell adhesion complex via alpha-catenin. *J Cell Biol* 1995;**130**:67–77.

3 Kinsella AR, Lepts GC, Hill CL, *et al*. Reduced E-cadherin expression correlates with increased invasiveness in colorectal carcinoma cell lines. *Clin Exp Metastasis* 1994;**12**: 335–42.

4 Shimoyama Y, Hirohashi S. Expression of E- and P-cadherin in gastric carcinoma. *Cancer Res* 1991;**51**:2185–92.

5 Kinsella AR, Green B, Lepts GC, *et al*. The role of the cell–cell adhesion molecule E-cadherin in large bowel tumour cell invasion and metastasis. *Br J Cancer* 1993;**67**:904–9.

6 Gagliardi G, Kandemir O, Liu D, *et al*. Changes in E-cadherin immunoreactivity in the adenoma–carcinoma sequence of the large bowel. *Virchows Arch* 1995;**426**:149–54.

7 Becker KF, Atkinson MJ, Reich U, *et al*. E-cadherin gene mutations provide clues to diffuse type gastric carcinomas. *Cancer Res* 1994;**54**:3845–52.

8 Oda T, Kanai Y, Oyama T, *et al*. E-cadherin gene mutations in human gastric carcinoma cell lines. *Proc Natl Acad Sci USA* 1994;**91**:1858–62.

9 Oyama T, Kanai Y, Ochiai A, *et al*. A truncated β-catenin disrupts the interaction between E-cadherin and α-catenin: a cause of loss of intercellular adhesiveness in human cancer cell lines. *Cancer Res* 1994;**54**:6282–7.

10 Kawanishi J, Kato J, Sasali K, *et al*. Loss of E-cadherin dependent cell–cell adhesion due to mutation of the β-catenin gene in a human cancer cell-line NSC-39. *Mol Cell Biol* 1995;**15**:1175–81.

11 Shimoyama Y, Nagafuchi A, Fujita S, *et al*. Cadherin dysfunction in a human cancer cell line: possible involvement of α-catenin expression in reduced cell–cell-adhesiveness. *Cancer Res* 1991;**52**:5770–4.

12 Breen E, Clarke A, Steel G, *et al*. Poorly differentiated colon carcinoma lines deficient in α-catenin expression express high levels of surface E-cadherin but lack Ca^{2+} dependent cell–cell adhesion. *Cell Adhes Commun* 1993;**1**:239–50.

13 Matsui S, Striozaki H, Inoue M, *et al*. Immunohistochemical evaluation of α-catenin expression in human gastric cancer. *Virchows Arch* 1994;**424**:375–81.

14 Kadowaki T, Shiozaki H, Inoue M, *et al*. E-cadherin α-catenin expression in human esophageal carcinoma. *Cancer Res* 1994;**54**:291–6.

15 Guan J-L, Hynes RO. Lymphoid cells recognise alternatively spliced segment of fibronectin via the integrin receptor α4β. *Cell* 1990;**60**:53–61.

16 Hynes RO. Integrins: versatility, modulation and signalling in cell adhesion. *Cell* 1992; **69**:11–25.

17 Takeichi M. Cadherin cell adhesion receptors as a morphogenetic regulator. *Science* 1991; **251**:1451–3.

18 Pignatelli M, Stamp G. Integrins in tumour development and spread. *Cancer Surv* 1995; **24**:113–127.

19 Pignatelli M, Liu D, Nasim MM, *et al*. Morphoregulatory activities of E-cadherin and β_1 integrins in colorectal tumour cells. *Br J Cancer* 1992;**66**:629–34.

20 Liu D, Gagliardi G, Nasim MM, *et al*. TGF-α can act as a morphogen and/or mitogen in a colon carcinoma cell line. *Int J Cancer* 1994;**56**:603–8.

21 Albeda SM. Biology of disease: role of integrins and other cell adhesion molecules in tumour progression and metastasis. *Lab Invest* 1993;**68**:4–17.

22 Zachary I, Rozengurt E. Focal adhesion kinase (p125[FAK]) a point of convergence in the action of neuropeptides, integrins and oncogenes. *Cell* 1992;**71**:891–4.

23 Juliano RL, Haskill S. Signal transduction from the extracellular matrix. *J Cell Biol* 1993; **120**:577–85.

24 Lin Y-C, Grinnell F. Decreased level of PDGF-stimulated receptor autophosphenylation site mutation of the epidermal growth factor receptor: analysis of kinase activity and endocytosis. *J Biol Chem* 1993;**266**:8355–62.

25 Pignatelli M, Bodmer WF. Integrin-receptor mediated differentiation and growth inhibition are enhanced by TGF-β in colorectal tumour cells grown in collagen gel. *Int J Cancer* 1989;**44**:518–23.

26 Nathan C, Sporn M. Cytokines in context. *J Cell Biol* 1991;**113**:981–6.

27 Nigam AK, Savage FJ, Boulos PB, *et al*. Loss of cell–cell and cell–matrix adhesion molecules in colorectal cancer. *Br J Cancer* 1993;**68**:507–14.

28 Ramkisson Y, Del Buono R, Filipe IM, *et al*. Integrins and their extracellular matrix ligands in gastric cancer. *Int J Oncol* 1996; in press.

29 Hall PA, Coates PJ, Lemoine NR, *et al*. Characterisation of integrin chains in normal and neoplastic human pancreas. *J Pathol* 1991;**165**:33–41.

30 Koukoulis GK, Virtanen I, Moll R, *et al*. Immunolocalisation of integrins in normal and neoplastic colonic epithelium. *Virchows Arch* 1993;**63**:373–83.

31 Gunthert U, Hofmann M, Rudy W, *et al*. A new variant of glycoprotein CD44 confers metastatic potential on rat carcinoma cells. *Cell* 1991;**65**:13–24.

32 Mayer B, Jauch KW, Gunthert U, *et al*. De novo expression of CD44 and survival in gastric cancer. *Lancet* 1993;**342**:1019–22.

33 Hewlich P, Pals S, Ponta H. CD44 in colon cancer. *Eur J Cancer* 1995;**31A**:1110–12.

34 Mulder J-WR, Kruyt PM, Sewnath M, *et al*. Colorectal cancer prognosis and expression of exon v6 containing CD44 proteins. *Lancet* 1994;**344**:1470–2.

35 Schultz RM, Silberman S, Persky B, *et al*. Inhibition by human recombinant tissue inhibitor of metalloproteinases of human amnion invasion and lung colonisation by B16-F10 melanoma cells. *Cancer Res* 1988;**48**:5539–45.

36 Alvarez OA, Carmichael DF, De Clerck YA. Inhibition of collagenolytic activity and metastasis of tumour cells by a recombinant human tissue inhibitor of metalloproteinases. *J Natl Cancer Inst* 1990;**82**:589–95.

37 Tsuchiya Y, Sato H, Endo Y, *et al*. Tissue inhibitor of metalloproteinase 1 is a negative regulator of the metastatic ability of a human gastric cancer cell line KKLS in chick embryo. *Cancer Res* 1991;**53**:1397–402.

38 Hollas W, Blasi F, Boyd D. Role of the urokinase receptor in regulating extracellular matrix invasion by cultured colon cancer. *Cancer Res* 1991;**51**:3690–5.

39 Pyke C, Kristenon P, Ralfkiaer E, *et al*. Urokinase plasminogen activator is expressed in stromal cells and its receptor in cancer cells at invasive foci in human colon adenocarcinomas. *Am J Pathol* 1991;**138**:1059–67.

40 Deluecchio S, Stopelli MP, Carriero MV, *et al*. Human urokinase receptor concentration in malignant and benign breast tumours by *in vitro* quantitative autoradiography. Comparison of urokinase levels. *Cancer Res* 1991;**53**:3198–206.

41 McCulloch P, George WD. Warfarin inhibition of metastasis: the role of anticoagulation. *Br J Surg* 1987;**74**:879–83.

42 Rickles FR, Edwards RL. Activation of blood coagulation in cancer: Trousseau's syndrome revisited. *Blood* 1983;**62**:14–31.

43 Steeg PS, Bevilacqua G, Kopper L, *et al.* Evidence for a novel gene associated with low metastatic potential. *J Natl Cancer Inst* 1988;**80**:200–4.

44 Bevilacqua G, Sobel ME, Liotta LA, *et al.* Association of low nm23 RNA levels in human infiltrating ductal breast carcinomas with lymph node involvement and other histopathological indication of metastatic potential. *Cancer Res* 1989;**49**:5185–90.

45 Nakayama T, Ohtsuru A, Nakao K, *et al.* Expression in a human hepatocellular carcinoma of nucleoside diphosphate kinase activity or homologue of therm 23 gene product. *J Natl Cancer Inst* 1991;**84**:1349–54.

46 Leone A, Flatow U, King CR, *et al.* Reduced tumour incidence, metastatic potential and cytokine responsiveness of nm23 transfected melanoma cells. *Cell* 1991;**65**:1–20.

47 Leone A, Flatow U, Van Houtte K, Steeg PS. Transfection of human nm23-H1 into human MDA-MB-435 breast carcinoma cell line: effects on tumour metastatic potential, colonisation and enzymic activity. *Oncogene* 1993;**8**:2325–33.

48 Leone A, Yasui W, Weston A, *et al.* Somatic allelic deletion of nm23 in human cancer. *Cancer Res* 1991;**51**:2490–3.

49 Wang L, Patel U, Ghosh L, *et al.* Mutation in nm23 gene is associated with metastasis in colorectal cancer. *Cancer Res* 1993;**53**:717–20.

50 Cohn KH, Wang P, Desoto-La Paix F, *et al.* Association of nm23-H1 deletions with distant metastases in colorectal carcinoma. *Lancet* 1991;**338**:722–4.

51 Ridley AJ, Hall A. The small GTP binding protein rho regulates the assembly of focal adhesions and active stress fibres in response to growth factors. *Cell* 1991;**70**:389–99.

52 Habets GCM, Scholtes EHM, Zuydgeest D, *et al.* Identification of an invasion inducing gene, Tiam, that encodes a protein with homology to GDP-GTP exchanges for rho-like proteins. *Cell* 1994;**327**:537–549.

53 Stoker M, Gherardi E, Perryman M, *et al.* Scatter factor a fibroblast derived modulator of cell mobility. *Nature* 1987;**327**:239–42.

54 Stoker M, Gherardi E. Regulation of cell movement: the motogenic cytokines. *Biochem Biophys Acta* 1991;**1072**:81–102.

55 Jiang WG, Hallett MB, Puntis MCA. Motility factors in cancer invasion and metastasis. *Surg Res Commun* 1994;**16**:219–37.

56 Hoff SD, Matsushita Y, Oto DM, *et al.* Increased expression of sialyl-dimeric Le^x antigen in liver metastases of human colorectal carcinoma. *Cancer Res* 1989;**49**:6883–8.

57 Irimura T, Nakamori S, Matsushita Y, *et al.* Colorectal cancer metastasis determined by carbohydrate mediated cell adhesion: role of sialyl-Le^x antigens. *Semin Cancer Biol* 1993;**4**:319–24.

58 Hanski C, Hanski M-L, Zimmer T, *et al.* Characterisation of the major sialyl-Le^x positive mucins present in colon, colon carcinoma and sera of patients with colorectal cancer. *Cancer Res* 1995;**55**:928–35.

59 Fisher B, Wolmark N, Bauer M, *et al.* The accuracy of clinical node staging and of limited axillary dissection as a determinant of histological nodel status in carcinoma of the breast. *Surg Gynecol Obstet* 1981;**152**:765–72.

60 Ochiai T, Sasako M, Mizuno S, *et al.* Hepatic resection for metastatic tumours from gastric cancer: analysis of prognostic factors. *Br J Surg* 1994;**81**:1175–8.

61 Halsted WS. The radical operation for the cure of carcinoma of the breast. *Johns Hopkins Hosp Rep* 1898;**28**:557.

62 MacDonald I. Biological predeterminism in human cancer. *Surg Gynecol Obstet* 1951;**92**:443.

63 Malik ST, East N, Boraschi D, *et al.* Effects of intraperitoneal recombinant interleukin 1 beta in intraperitoneal human ovarian cancer xenograft models: comparison with the effects of tumour necrosis factor. *Br J Cancer* 1992;**65**:661–6.

3: Biology of carcinogenesis: influences and modes of action

J R G NASH

The gastrointestinal tract contains a significant proportion of the epithelial tissue of the whole body. As part of the "external" surface it is thus exposed to a number of extraneous influences and substances, and it is perhaps not surprising that cancer is common at this site. In most Western countries, cancer of the colon and rectum is the second most common malignant cause of mortality, after bronchial and lung cancer, adding together the incidence figures for both sexes (for women only, breast cancer is more common, while for men only, prostate cancer is more common).[1]

There is considerable variation in incidence between different parts of the gastrointestinal tract, with tumours being common in the large intestine, somewhat less common in the stomach and oesophagus, and rare in the small intestine. The reasons for this are not understood: in spite of the fact that the small intestine has the most rapid turnover of its epithelial cells, and therefore a good opportunity for the expression of mutations, its observed low influence of cancer remains a puzzle. Rapid turnover and shedding of the epithelial cells does not seem a sufficient explanation, as there is probably at most a 2–3-fold difference from the colon in this respect. There is speculation that the rapid transit of contents through the small intestine precludes lengthy exposure to noxious chemicals, and reduced time for degradative bacterial action, may partly explain the lower incidence of cancer, but there are likely to be additional protective mechanisms.

On a worldwide scale, primary cancer of the liver (hepatocellular carcinoma) is an extremely common neoplasm, probably until recently *the* most common globally. This high incidence is associated with hepatitis B virus infection,[2] often acquired by vertical transmission or in childhood, at which time it is more likely to progress to a carrier status. Hepatocellular carcinoma remains a relatively rare tumour in the West, where hepatitis B carrier status is uncommon, generally less than 1% in most countries.

This chapter will consider the principal influences active in causing neoplasia in the gastrointestinal tract and liver, outline the evidence and a few speculations on how these influences might cause cancer, and then discuss in more detail the factors operating at particular sites in the gastrointestinal tract.

Principal influences causing neoplastic disease

Epidemiological factors will be only briefly discussed in this chapter, where they are relevant to mechanisms of carcinogenesis. For a detailed review of the epidemiological evidence, please refer to Chapter 1.

Dietary factors

The gastrointestinal tract will naturally come into contact with substances contained in food. Not surprisingly, there has been considerable interest in the role of diet in causing cancer, with possible active dietary substances being investigated; with the exception of obvious carcinogens, the role of dietary deficiencies, especially of micronutrients, has, however, merited more attention. Thus, low or deficient levels of vitamins (particularly the antioxidant vitamins A, C and E) have been implicated as risk factors for cancer.[3] Selenium is also postulated as an important antioxidant and organoselenium compounds can prevent cancer in an animal model.[4] It is postulated that absence of antioxidant effect, or its relative lack, allows oxidative processes, including those due to free radicals, to proceed to an undue extent. Free radical activity may then cause damage to intracellular DNA and thus induce mutations. An absence of antioxidants might also allow oxidation reactions, such as those forming nitrosamines from nitrites and amine residues, to proceed to an undesirable extent. Various measures of oxidative stress are increased in breast, colon, and prostate cancer, tending to support this hypothesis.[5] Patients at increased risk of gastric cancer, by virtue of the presence of superficial gastritis, mild or severe atrophic gastritis, or a previous partial gastrectomy, showed reduced antioxidant effect in the mucosa, not entirely reversed by administration of vitamin E.[6] Nitrosamines are well established as carcinogens; they are probably formed *in vivo* after the ingestion of certain combinations of foodstuffs, such as protein- or amine-containing foods in conjunction with nitrite, often used as a preservative. A study in a high risk area for gastric cancer in southern China showed increased *n*-nitroso compounds in locally made and consumed fish sauce, markedly raised following nitrosation, and resulting in DNA methylation experimentally.[7] A study in Moping County (also in China) showed marked reduction of *in vivo* nitrosation after exposure to fruit juice and green tea; vegetable juice had the opposite effect.[8]

Dietary excesses, particularly of protein and fat in the diet, have been blamed for an increased incidence of large bowel and possibly breast cancer. Postulated mechanisms include increased output of bile salts, which might then become hydrolysed in the large bowel to form methylcholanthrene, and other associated carcinogens. High fat, high protein diets may include a low fibre residue, which may increase bowel transit time and thus the time for action of the hypothesised carcinogens. A prolonged large bowel transit time would therefore presumably potentiate this process. The evidence of many studies has been reviewed[9] and red meat, rather than fat *per se*, appears to be important. A diet with an unnecessarily high energy content emerges as a definite risk factor but the role of refined sugars is less clear cut. Experimental evidence does, however, show enhancement of carcinogenesis by sucrose in mice.[10]

Artificial food additives are thoroughly tested for safety in both microbiological and animal dietary experiments, and some (added antioxidants) are thought to be actively protective against cancer, presumably by mechanisms similar to the natural antioxidants cited above. The role of salt in the diet, a common additive, has, however, been put forward as possibly carcinogenic (in addition to its accepted effects on blood pressure). A study in Puerto Rico found a strong association between salt consumption and gastric cancer.[11] A similar link was found in Japan between salt consumption and large bowel cancer.[12]

Agricultural chemicals such as herbicides and insecticides are a possible hazard, as residues may remain detectable in foodstuffs, as well as entering the water supply. These chemicals will generally be present at very low levels and probably do not play a part in causing the average case of gastrointestinal cancer. The health of farm workers at risk of occupational exposure requires consideration, as exposures could be at considerably higher levels in the event of an accidental exposure or failure of protective measures.

Smoking

The early epidemiological studies on smoking established its strong association with lung and bronchial cancer, amply confirmed by more recent studies, and related work has shown linkage to other types of cancer, including that of the urinary bladder and gastrointestinal tract, particularly oesophagus and (to a lesser extent) stomach. Adenocarcinoma of the lower oesophagus and cardia[13] and elsewhere in the stomach[14] is significantly associated with smoking. In the large bowel, the effect is less clear cut:

Japanese smokers showed a reduced risk of large bowel cancer in the colon but not the rectum.[15] The tar component of smoke has been blamed for the carcinogenic effect, implying that high tar cigarettes, pipes, and cigars are the most likely to be associated with the subsequent formation of tumours. Qat chewing and water-pipe smoking in the Yemen are associated with both mid- and lower-oesophageal and gastric cardia tumours. The effect of smoking appears to be enhanced by alcohol, particularly in the oesophagus. While these two factors may act independently, they also undoubtedly show synergism.[14]

Alcohol

The amount, form, and purity of alcohol ingested appears to be important: spirits appear to carry a higher risk than more dilute forms of alcohol, with large doses being riskier.[16] Congeners and other substances present in alcohol as a result of the manufacturing process may also be implicated. It is not clear what effect wood derived substances may have on carcinogenesis: spirits stored (matured) for lengthy periods of 15–20 years in wooden barrels presumably dissolve substances from the wooden cask. Some of these, notably the flavonoids, may have a protective effect.

Infection

The characterisation of *Helicobacter pylori* in the 1970s (originally known as *Campylobacter pyloridis* or *pylori*) has been followed by considerable interest and research into its mode of action and effects. It is clear that this organism, which grows only on gastric type mucosa and preferentially on antral-type mucosa, has local effects, including the production of urease and thence ammonia, which damages the gastric mucosal barrier. The organism has been implicated in peptic ulcer disease, including both gastric and duodenal ulceration, and also in chronic gastritis, particularly of the antral type.[17] Antibodies cross reacting with gastric mucosa are produced, probably contributing to the chronic gastritis.[18] Chronic infection with the organism, which may often be acquired during childhood, carries particular risks, with increased incidence of intestinal metaplasia, gastric carcinoma eventually following on from this,[19] and primary gastric lymphoma.[20] The mechanism of *epithelial carcinogenesis* is still unclear but local toxins may be implicated. The *lymphomagenesis* may be due to the induction of abnormal gastric lymphoid tissue, not usually present in the stomach (discussed further in the section on inflammatory disease below).

Abnormal overgrowths of bacteria may be relevant in other sites of gastrointestinal tract—for example, causing breakdown of bile salts in the large intestine—and in the blind loop syndrome. In particular situations, such as achlorhydria occurring in pernicious anaemia, bacterial overgrowth may again occur. This may be a factor in the observed increased risk of gastric carcinoma in this condition.[21]

Inflammatory disease

This includes infective disease as well as autoimmune or idiopathic types of inflammation which occur in the gastrointestinal tract. It is probable that inflammatory change acts as a tumour promoter (see below), both because of cytotoxicity and cytolysis caused by the inflammation, resulting in damage, including free radical damage, to DNA, and as a consequence of the resulting regeneration of hyperplasia. The result is likely to be an increased incidence of neoplastic transformation. This is probably a part of the explanation for the high incidence of adenocarcinoma in Barrett's oesophagus, particularly in the type showing intestinal metaplasia (see below).[22]

Lymphoma

This shows separate risk factors from those important in epithelial tumours of the stomach and bowel. Immunosuppression (if present) is important here, as in lymphoma at other sites,[23 24] in allowing the proliferation of Epstein–Barr virus and therefore transformation of lymphoid cells.[25 26] In patients who are immunocompetent, the role of helicobacter in inducing gastric mucosa associated lymphoid tissue (MALT), which may then become lymphomatous, has been documented,[27] this lymphoma showing the unusual feature of being reversible by antibiotic treatment in the early stages. The presence of MALT is regarded as abnormal in the stomach, and is thought to be induced by the chronic inflammation of *H. pylori* infection. The first change is the accumulation of MALT. This is a predominantly B cell population, initially polyclonal, but later becoming monoclonal, presumably by selection of one particular cell by mutation.[28] Further immune stimulation would then eventually result in the formation of a self perpetuating B cell clone. This is reminiscent of the situation in Mediterranean lymphoma, a type of immunoproliferative small intestinal disease that results from longstanding α heavy chain disease,[29] and may also be reversible by treatment with antibiotics in the early stages.[30]

A similar pattern emerges in autoimmune and immune based disease, in which lymphoma may complicate conditions such as Sjögren's disease, Hashimoto's disease, and coeliac disease. The antibody specificities of many plasmacytomas and immunocytomas are directed against self antigens, implying that autoimmune stimulation may be a fairly common origin for B cell neoplasms.[31] Other chronic immune or inflammatory stimuli include the known predilection for developing non-Hodgkin's lymphoma as a long term complication in coeliac disease.[32] The pattern in coeliac disease is different from that of other chronic immune stimulated states: 10% of patients in a large series of individuals with coeliac disease developed lymphoma, usually of large T cell phenotype. No evidence of infection with Epstein–Barr virus could be demonstrated in these cases, whether of T cell or B cell phenotype,[33] in spite of its demonstrable presence in a single case of lymphoma occurring after renal transplant in a middle aged patient with clinically confirmed coeliac disease.[34]

Genetic (inherited) factors

Considerable progress has been made in elucidating inherited factors in cancer. Three main groups are recognised.[35]

1 *Inherited cancer syndromes showing autosomal dominance*: retinoblastoma, adenomatous polyposis and associated carcinoma of the colon, multiple endocrine neoplasia, neurofibromatosis and von Hippel–Lindau syndrome.
2 *Cancers showing a familial clustering tendency*: breast, ovarian, and hereditary non-polyposis colon cancer. (The role of heredity may be unclear in individual cases.)
3 *Autosomal recessive syndromes of defective DNA repair*: xeroderma pigmentosum, ataxia-telangiectasia, Bloom's syndrome, and Fanconi's anaemia.

(*List reproduced with permission of author and publishers from Ponder BAJ*[35].)

While at most anatomical sites studied the incidence of cancers attributable to inherited genetic abnormalities is probably 5% or less, these cases have a tendency to occur at a younger age than sporadic cancers, giving them a disproportionate importance. The first degree relatives may also be affected, requiring screening programmes to detect early disease. Some inherited conditions are well known to predispose to the development of cancer: the strong association of familial adenomatous polyposis with cancer of the colon occurring before the age of 30 years has led to surveillance colonoscopy and frequent prophylactic colectomy. This strong association has been a very productive area for molecular genetic studies (see below). The more recent studies of the BRCA-1 gene and breast cancer in "high risk of cancer" families, showing a high lifetime risk of developing breast cancer, often at an early age,[36] are also relevant to cancer of the stomach and large intestine, as mutations of this gene have been implicated at these sites as well.[37 38] The proportion of total cancers attributed to inherited mutations is small and it is not yet clear what level of preventive action should be taken in these patients. A second form of hereditary large bowel cancer, hereditary non-polyposis colon cancer (HNPCC) has been described, and is associated with a deletion of one allele of a DNA mismatch repair (MMR) gene. Other important inherited somatic mutations, such as deletion of the retinoblastoma gene, and Li–Fraumeni syndrome, associated with p53 mutation,[39] have a more general effect and may sometimes involve the gastrointestinal tract as part of a general propensity to malignancy.

Cellular, chromosomal, gene based and molecular events

A complete understanding of neoplasia will be possible only when the events in different levels of structural organisation can be linked, and effects attributed to causes. It will then be possible to follow changes seamlessly from the tissue all the way to the atoms of which it is ultimately composed. The "coarser grained" end of the spectrum, in which gross appearances of tumours were linked to microscopic (cellular) composition, was studied in the nineteenth and early twentieth centuries, and progress continues. Chromosomal abnormalities followed on, then gene based abnormalities. Many gene alterations can now be correlated with biochemical changes in the nucleic acid, and these in turn can sometimes be traced to particular damaging events. Many gaps in detail remain but the skeleton of the whole picture is there.

Cellular basis of neoplasia

The overall behaviour of a tissue is seen as the product of the individual behaviour of its cells. Thus carcinoma of an organ is seen as a malfunction of the cells of that organ. Current thinking inclines to a single cell (clonal) origin for most malignant tumours, in which a mutated cell acquires a proliferative advantage, forms an established, self perpetuating clone, and outgrows its neighbours. Under this view, all cells in a neoplasm would initially be identical, although with further mutations, subcloning would undoubtedly occur. Cells acquiring a more aggressive phenotype would then gradually come to predominate, leading to corresponding dedifferentiation of the tumour as it became further and further removed from the normal mature phenotype. This does not exclude multiple independent origins of separate tumours and the frequent simultaneous presence of earlier stage, benign proliferations, due to acquired abnormalities affecting a whole epithelium, a process described as "field change".

In order for clonal selection and establishment to occur, non-lethal genetic damage is a prerequisite: if the damage to the DNA structure is too severe, the cell will not replicate any further, and therefore cannot become neoplastic. The principal targets of damage appear to be oncogene units, particularly antioncogenes (oncosuppressor genes), which may become deleted, and proto-oncogenes, which may become activated into cellular oncogenes. Other possible sites are the apoptosis genes, normally acting as a "self destruct" mechanism for damaged or mutated cells, as well as a physiological mechanism for controlling cell numbers and life span. These may be associated with demonstrable chromosomal alterations such as translocation (see below).

Genetic changes—acquired or inherited

The model of Fearon and Vogelstein for the induction of colon cancer has been helpful in organising and structuring the data.[40] This postulates a six-stage process in which the earlier mutations result in minor pathological abnormalities. The model seeks to link the observed genetic changes to the usual progression of events in colorectal carcinogenesis, the "adenoma–carcinoma sequence", reflecting the fact that most sporadic carcinomas appear to arise in a pre-existing adenoma.[41]

The first mutation in this model is in the APC (adenomatous polyposis of colon) gene, a tumour suppressor located on chromosome 5q21. This gene is mutated in familial adenomatous polyposis and also in 60–80% of sporadic colon carcinomas. This stage correlates with the production of proliferative changes in the epithelium but not an adenoma as yet. The second step is hypomethylation of DNA, which has an uncertain role in carcinogenesis but may cause mitotic non-disjunction and chromosomal irregularities.[42] This stage matches the production of an early adenoma with no propensity to invade as yet. The third step, K-ras mutations, is seen in intermediate adenomas. These also occur in about half of sporadic large bowel cancers. This may give a growth advantage over cells with only the APC mutation as point mutations in ras can lead to protein overactivity.[43] The fourth stage is deletion of DCC (deleted in colon cancer), a gene on 18q22 coding for an adhesion molecule.[44] This correlates with the presence of a late adenoma, at the stage leading up to invasion. The gene function may clearly have implications for production of invasion. The DCC gene is mutated in about 70% of colorectal carcinomas.[40] The last stage described by the model is p53 mutation, which is also found to have occurred in up to 70% of colorectal carcinomas. Wild type (non-mutated) p53 protein is important in maintaining the structural integrity of DNA.[45] DNA damage causes arrest in G_1 pending repair of the DNA, or cell destruction by apoptosis if repair is impossible.[46 47]

Figure 3.1 illustrates the mutational events in the development of carcinoma of the large bowel. This model has been very helpful in setting out the cumulative sequence of events resulting in one common type of cancer, and illuminates how the malignant phenotype may emerge as a result of changes at a molecular genetic level. It also incorporates some information on chromosomal changes or damage. The model has been discussed in some detail because it is currently the best worked out sequence of events occurring in carcinogenesis in any organ, and has stimulated research into related processes of carcinogenesis in other tumours showing both a sporadic and a non-sporadic (inherited) pattern. It will form a useful framework into which details of carcinogenic steps at other sites may be fitted. Recent additions to and variations from the model are discussed in the section on the colon below.

Overexpression of the relevant oncogenes will result in abnormal expression of growth factors, disturbed signalling, and loss of control of cellular processes, including cell division, adhesion, and apoptosis. All these potentially contribute to the malignant phenotype. These subjects are not considered in this chapter (see Chapter 4).

Specific roles of oncogenes

Oncogenes may become mutated, resulting in overexpression and over-activity of their protein products. Thus the ras oncogene product causes overexpression of growth factor genes, resulting in secretion of large amounts of growth factors such as transforming growth factor α (TGFα).[48][49] Ki-ras mutations have been implicated—for example, in pancreatic carcinoma,[50] experimental hepatocellular carcinoma induced by aflatoxin,[51] and human colon carcinoma.[52] The H-ras gene, by contrast, has been found mutated in gastric cancer.[53] Mutations of the ras gene family are common in human tumours, and may exceed 50% in carcinomas of the colon.[40] The gene product appears to play an important role in inducing mitosis, and interacts with growth factors such as epidermal growth factor (EGF), platelet derived growth factor (PDGF), and colony stimulating factor. The proto-oncogene C-sis, which encodes the β chain of PDGF, has been found abnormally expressed in gastric carcinomas, accompanying abnormal expression of TGFα mRNA.[54] Messenger RNA for basic fibroblast growth factor (bFGF) and its receptor FGFR1/N-sam has been demonstrated in oesophageal cancer cell lines but not gastric cancer cell lines.[55] While these factors may result in increased cell division, they are not alone sufficient for malignant transformation. A further group of mutations, occurring in growth factor receptors such as erb, which encodes for a mutant EGF receptor, may also interfere with its function. The c-erbB-2 gene (also known as c-neu) is amplified in many types of carcinoma, including that in the stomach.[56] Its abnormally increased protein product can be demonstrated in some gastric and many breast carcinomas by immunohistochemistry using a specific antibody (Figure 3.2).

The myc oncogene, an example of a group of nuclear regulatory protein genes, appears to be commonly involved in neoplasia, and indeed the

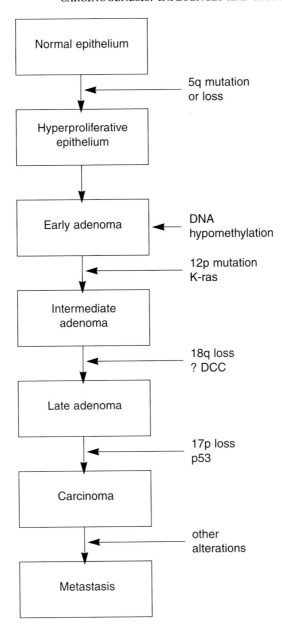

FIGURE 3.1—*Mutational events in the sequence of premalignant and malignant changes in the development of carcinoma of the large bowel. DCC, deleted in colon cancer. (Redrawn; reproduced with permission of the authors and the Cell Press from Fearon and Vogelstein.*[40]*)*

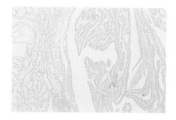 

FIGURE 3.2—*(a) Gastric carcinoma (left) and non-neoplastic epithelium (right), stained for c-erbB-2 protein expression. Both malignant and non-malignant epithelium are negative. (b) Paget's disease of the nipple, stained for c-erbB-2. The adenocarcinoma cells are positive (brown), clearly standing out against the negative squamous epithelium. Magnification factors: 3.2(a) × 24; 3.2(b) × 60.*

normal c-myc proto-oncogene is expressed in almost all cells.[57] This group of proteins shows disturbed function in neoplasia and their normal role is in the control of the cell cycle: the c-myc forms a complex with max, another protein, the complex then binding to specific DNA sequences, resulting in the regulation of transcription of growth control genes.[58] Changes in protein interactions after disregulation of c-myc expression have been observed in certain tumours such as Burkitt's lymphoma, while in small cell lung carcinoma N-myc and L-myc are amplified.[59] Other members of this group include fos, jun, and myb: both c-fos and c-myc have been found amplified in experimental rat hepatocellular carcinoma induced by a chemical (aminoazobenzene) derivative.[60]

Activation of oncogenes

Proto-oncogenes may become activated by a variety of mechanisms, including point mutation, which has been identified particularly in the ras oncogene. It is extremely common in pancreatic and bile duct cancers and also relatively common in colon cancer.[50 52] The abnormally active c-myc oncogene, by contrast, is an example of overactivation caused by chromosomal translocation. This is well documented in certain types of lymphoma, including Burkitt's lymphoma, which invariably contains the translocated gene.[61] The bcl-2 gene, which has an antiapoptosis function, thus preserving cells that would otherwise be lost,[62] may be overexpressed after a chromosomal translocation (to chromosome 14), as in follicular lymphoma.[63] Finally, gene amplification may occur, with production of multiple copies of the DNA sequences of affected genes. These may occur either as new chromosomes composed of amplified genes, known as homogenous staining regions (HSRs), or as multiple small chromosome-like structures called double minutes (DMs). These have been shown to result in amplification of n-myc and c-erbB-2 in neuroblastoma and breast cancer respectively[64 65] and may occur in nearly 50% of these tumours.

Role of oncosuppressor genes

Since discovery of the retinoblastoma (rb) suppressor oncogene, the prototype of this group, several other oncosuppressor genes have been identified and characterised. The findings were explained in the model hypothesis of Knudson.[66] In rb gene deletion, young children inheriting one deletion of the gene were found to be at high risk of developing retinoblastoma, owing to sporadic mutation deletion of their single remaining copy of this antioncogene. Patients with the familial type of retinoblastoma are also at greater risk, later in life, of developing osteosarcomas. Inactivation of the gene is found in tumours in other organs, such as the breast, lung, and bladder.[67] It is clear that the rb gene has wider effects than just in the eye. Oesophageal cancer shows a high rate of partial deletion of rb[68] and associated p53 mutations.[69] Also in the oesophagus, a probable suppressor gene, MTS-1, has been found deleted.[70]

The Knudson type of model can be applied to p53, the most commonly mutated gene in human cancers. Most examples of p53 mutation appear to be acquired, but inherited syndromes are also known, as in the Li–Fraumeni syndrome (see above). The p53 gene product regulates DNA replication, cell proliferation, and cell death, normally acting as a tumour suppressor gene. The exact mechanism of this is not yet elucidated, but it has been postulated that p53 would delay cell division of the genetically damaged cells by accumulating in the nucleus and binding to DNA. This would cause a cell cycle G_1 arrest, allowing time for DNA repair.[71] If this should fail, p53 appears able to trigger apoptosis—the reason for its being called "the guardian of the genome".[45] Normal ("wild" type) p53 has a very short half life and is detectable only with difficulty; however, mutations (usually mis-sense mutations) may result in stabilisation of the protein,[72] which can then be easily demonstrated by immunohistochemistry (Figure 3.3), or deletion leading to total absence. Much of the extensive literature on p53 staining in tumours refers to the positive reaction, in which the stabilised mutant type protein is demonstrated. Total deletion of the protein may, however, result in equally abnormal function. p53 has other roles and may act as an oncogene in certain situations, leading to transformation of cells *in vitro*. Mutant forms of p53 may additionally bind and inactivate normal "wild" type p53.[73] p53 mutations have been reported in human and experimental tumours of the liver,[74 75] in gastric,[76 77] colonic,[52 78] and oesophageal tumours, of both squamous[79 80] and Barrett's types.[81 82] Mutations of the p53 and H-ras genes have been found in nitrosamine induced oesophageal papillomas in the rat.[83]

Other oncosuppressor genes currently under study include the DCC gene located on 18q21. This area shows frequent loss of heterozygosity in colorectal cancers. More recently the DCC gene has been found deleted

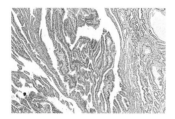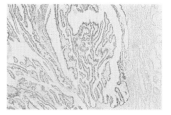

FIGURE 3.3—*(a) Gastric carcinoma of intestinal type (left) and non-neoplastic mucosa (right). (b) The carcinoma, but not the non-malignant area, shows strong nuclear p53 expression (brown). Magnification factors: 3.3(a) × 24; 3.3(b) × 24.*

in some gastric cancers.[84] Mutations of the APC suppressor gene are not confined to colorectal neoplasms, being detectable in gastric carcinoma as well.[85 86]

The molecular level

Radiation carcinogenesis

Radiation, including ultraviolet radiation, is well known to cause mutations, including those in oncogenes and tumour suppressor genes. In the skin, mutant forms of ras and p53 have been found after exposure to ultraviolet B radiation. This is clearly less relevant in the gastrointestinal tract, which will not be exposed to light at this level. Ionising radiation, capable of penetrating the body to the gastrointestinal tract, certainly has the potential and energy to cause DNA damage and therefore mutations, but exposure to radiation, whether therapeutic or accidental, has not been strongly linked with gastrointestinal cancer.

Chemical carcinogenesis: molecular effects

Initiation and promotion It has long been known that chemical carcinogenesis may be conceptually divided into two stages, initiation and promotion. This was originally demonstrated in experimental models of chemical carcinogenesis in the skin of experimental animals, and showed that initiation resulted from primary exposure of cells to an appropriate dose of carcinogenic agent known as the initiator. The cells were found to be altered permanently, making it likely that a tumour would arise at the site later. Initiation on its own was not, however, sufficient to result in tumour formation. It is clear that initiation had caused permanent DNA damage with mutations and was therefore irreversible. The second phase, of promotion, resulted in induction of tumours in initiated cells but not in untreated cells. Although these processes describe experimental data, similar processes appear to be relevant to *in vivo* tumorigenesis.

Initiators are found to be of two types:

1 *Direct acting carcinogens.* The only important examples of a direct acting agents in the human clinical situation are the therapeutic alkylating agents used in the treatment of cancer. The risk of cancer from the use of these agents (including melphalan, chlorambucil, cyclophosphamide, and busulphan) is low but has to be taken into account, particularly when some of these drugs are used for treating non-malignant autoimmune conditions.

2 *Indirect acting procarcinogens.* These chemicals require metabolic activation before they become effective carcinogens. All these substances have highly reactive electrophilic structures which react avidly with electron rich sites in the cell nucleus. These result in the formation of covalent DNA adducts and may produce damage at a lethal level, resulting in the death of the cell, or at a sublethal level, sometimes resulting in a mutation. The DNA adducts may be demonstrable in populations exposed to increased levels of carcinogens. These may indicate an increased risk of developing carcinoma: patients with lung cancer show increased numbers of DNA adducts compared with non-cancer bearing patients with a similar carcinogen exposure.[87] This implies a variation in both adduct formation and cancer susceptibility within the population, possibly due to differences in activation of procarcinogens. The procarcinogens in this group of polycyclic aromatic hydrocarbons are activated by cytochrome *P*-450 dependent mono-oxygenases, whose level may be controlled by inherited or ethnic[88] and environmental factors, such as diet. There is some evidence linking particular mutations, mostly those of the ras oncogene, to particular chemicals. It may eventually be possible to trace the chemical origin of individual tumours.[89] Specific patterns of p53 mutations may reflect exposure to individual carcinogens—for example, specific p53 mutations are seen in lung tumours in smokers, involving many sites in the gene, and characteristic for exposure to polycyclic aromatic hydrocarbons or oxidants. Lung tumours in uranium miners (exposed to radon) show a single and quite different p53 mutation.[90] Characteristic mutations of the p53 gene, which may also be seen after exposure to aflatoxin, are different from those found in tumours induced by exposure to hepatitis B virus.[91]

The remaining known groups of carcinogenic chemicals, including aromatic amines (aniline and benzidine are good examples) and some azo dyes, nitrosamines, and aflatoxin, all require activation, a process generally involving the microsomal cytochrome *P*-450 system (see above). Other known carcinogens, such as asbestos and vinyl chloride monomer, are rare causes of cancer and are particularly relevant to occupational exposure.

Promoters are not by themselves capable of producing a tumour: they are stimulatory substances that may themselves cause DNA breaks owing to the production of free radicals. TPA (12–O–Tetradecanoyl–Phorbol–13–Acetate) for example, a well known phorbol ester,[92] and croton oil are widely used experimental tumour promoters. Examples of promoter substances relevant to human exposure include some drugs, natural or exogenous hormones, and some phenol compounds. Any stimulus of chronic hyperplasia is also likely to have a promoting effect.

A clear and comprehensive review of neoplasia, mutation, and carcinogenesis is contained in a standard pathology textbook (Cotran, Kumar and Robbins[93]). Readers requiring further study in this area may find it helpful to consult this source.

Factors operating at particular sites

Oesophagus

The combination of smoking and alcohol has a well known association with oesophageal cancer,[94 95] and the consumption of hot substances, food or drink, has been implicated.[96 97] Contamination of food, particularly by mould, has been implicated in Chinese studies. Thus fusarin induced tumours in rodent oesophagus;[98] correspondingly high levels of mycotoxins, capable of forming nitrosamines under the right conditions, were identified in foods in a high risk area of China.[99] Nitrates, nitrites, and nitrosamines by themselves in the diet have been implicated in studies of populations in Kashmir and China.[100 101] Dietary deficiencies are deemed important at this (oesophageal) site, with vitamins A, C and E,[102 103] and fruit and vegetables in the diet being protective.[104 105] Maize consumption in Africa and Northern Italy has been linked with a locally increased incidence of oesophageal cancer.[106] A rare genetic cause, inherited as an autosomal dominant condition, is seen in an extended family kindred originally from, and still partly resident in, Liverpool. These affected individuals show the signs of tylosis (hyperkeratosis of the soles of the feet, and to a lesser extent the palms of the hands). There is an associated high risk of developing oesophageal carcinoma in the lower third of the oesophagus, estimated at approaching 95% by late middle age. The autosomal dominant mutation accounting for tylosis has recently been characterised by analysis of restriction fragment length polymorphisms[107] and mapped.[108]

Barrett's oesophagus is important as a predisposing factor for the development of tumours, showing a 40–100-fold increase in adenocarcinoma of this site in affected individuals.[109 110] The development of adenocarcinoma is rare in individuals not showing intestinal metaplasia,[109 111] which in turn appears to be associated with cigarette smoking.[112] Reassuringly, there is no detectable increased risk from commonly used treatments for reflux.[113]

Stomach

The incidence of gastric cancer is decreasing worldwide, especially the intestinal type. The less common diffuse type (signet-ring cell carcinoma) continues at its previous level. This type is not associated with chronic gastritis, unlike the more common intestinal type cancer.[114] Countries showing a high incidence, such as Japan, have demonstrably different local factors, such as smoked fish in the diet. The role of salt may also be important here: one study found the intake of salty food correlated with increased risk of *H. pylori* infection.[115] The incidence of gastric cancer in Japan is decreasing, as elsewhere,[116] and an active screening programme has led to a marked reduction in the death rate from gastric cancer. Other dietary factors implicated include nitrites and therefore nitrosamines, smoked food, and lack of fresh fruit and vegetables, suggesting vitamin deficiency. These factors have been found to be correlated with the presence of intestinal metaplasia and dysplasia, known risk factors for the development of gastric cancer.[117] The strong link between *H. pylori* and gastric cancer is well known, and the organism does seem to have a role in causing gastric cancer, probably in association with other risk factors.[118] The organism is associated with a higher mutation rate in the H-ras oncogene, and a higher expression of ras p21 protein. The DNA content of S phase cells also increases. All these changes favour the development of malignancy.[119] Evidence of infection with the bacterium is found in 75% of patients with gastric cancer, but no difference of bacterial prevalence was observed between intestinal and diffuse types of cancer,[120] in spite of their differing epidemiology. A history of previous gastrectomy, possibly also reflecting the likelihood of *H. pylori* infection, is a risk factor for subsequent development of gastric carcinoma,[121] as is the presence of adenomas of the gastric mucosa. These appear to have a higher rate of conversion to carcinoma than adenomas of the colon.[122] Genetic tendencies are only weakly implicated, showing only epidemiological associations rather than high individual risk, but, interestingly, there is evidence of different genetic susceptibility to *H. pylori* infection.[123] Evidence from experimental induction of gastric carcinoma in a rat model using a nitroso compound shows the importance of genetic polymorphisms in the Buffalo strain of rats used, the evidence suggesting that resistance to the tumours is conferred by a single dominant allele.[124]

Finally, there is some evidence of a link between radiation exposure (both as a result of nuclear attack[125] and from therapeutic sources) and cancer of the stomach.

Small intestine

This is a relatively rare site for cancer, and the causes are correspondingly poorly documented in comparison with the major sites. Less than 1% of the gastrointestinal cancers seen in our institution are at this site. It is not further discussed here.

Large intestine

This site is clinically associated with development of tumours in late middle age, with a peak in the 60–70 year old group. The tumours are more common in males, but this applies only to rectal tumours. While left sided tumours still considerably outnumber those of the right, this ratio is changing, with right sided tumours becoming relatively more common. These, by contrast, show an equal sex incidence. Dietary factors implicated include fat and cooked meat in the diet, with a protective effect shown by higher levels of dietary fibre and dietary calcium, but the source of these components appears to be important.[59] Supplementary calcium reduced tumours in an experimental model.[126] The studies of dietary factors are somewhat conflicting, not all showing a benefit from higher fibre levels in the diet nor from increased dietary diversity.[127 128] An experimental assay using the production of aberrant crypt foci[129] revealed risks from caramelised sugar, thermolysed casein, and single boluses of sucrose and fructose. Micronutrients, particularly selenium,[130] and vitamins have been implicated at this site as elsewhere. The protective role of the antioxidant A, C, and E vitamins has been put forward but is still largely speculative here.[131] Vitamin D_3 has been found to have an anticancer effect in animal models.[132] The role of anti-inflammatory drugs as inhibitors of tumour development has been confirmed experimentally for aspirin,[133] prixocam,[134] and sulindac,[135] while omeprazole, a proton pump inhibitor used in the treatment of excess acid production, also shows the ability to block the production of azoxymethane induced colorectal tumours in the rat. It has been suggested that aspirin prophylaxis might reduce colorectal carcinoma in humans,[136] and it, along with other non-steroidal anti-inflammatory drugs (NSAIDs), reduces the proliferation of colon cancer cells in vitro. The other NSAIDs, but not aspirin, cause apoptosis,[137] possibly leading to shedding of potentially malignant cells.

Known specific risks for colorectal carcinoma include pre-existing chronic idiopathic inflammatory bowel disease, in which there is a small but definite risk of developing carcinoma in longstanding ulcerative colitis. This is often a flat carcinoma not arising in a pre-existing adenoma.[138] Ulcerative colitis associated tumours show different molecular genetic features from those seen in sporadic cancers: they show a lower rate of APC mutation[139] and K-ras mutation.[140] Bcl-2, a gene acting to prevent apoptosis,[141] is less frequently overexpressed in this tumour type, although p53 mutations seem to occur earlier.[142] In the non-colitic bowel, the association with pre-existing adenomas has been known for many years, the villous subtype appearing to pose a particular risk of transformation, often when the polyp has grown to around 3 cm in diameter. Aberrant crypts and microadenomas (dysplastic areas) are found in a carcinogen exposed rodent model, supporting the adenoma–carcinoma hypothesis.[143] There is evidence that not all carcinomas arise in polyps, as adenomatous remnants are found only variably within cancers, and are much less likely to be seen in the ulcerating and infiltrating types than in the polypoid tumours.[144] This raises the possibility that two distinct mechanisms operate in the different morphological types of tumour.

Genetic risks show a weak association, with a previous diagnosis of colorectal carcinomas resulting in a 2–4-fold increased risk in the patient's relatives. The risk of malignant transformation in familial adenomatous polyposis is well documented, and the more recently described syndrome of HNPCC furnishes an additional example of an inherited condition. The original model of Fearon and Vogelstein has been recently reappraised[145] and modified to incorporate the new data on MMR genes mutated in cancer HNPCC (Figure 3.4). This results in replication errors (RER+) seen as "mistakes" in microsatellite sequences, but probably only if both MMR genes are mutated.[146] The condition shows genetic instability, which is likely to worsen as the adenomas of the condition progress towards carcinoma.[147] The mutations are also heterogeneous for the locus involved.[148 149] This (HNPCC) cancer is clinically different from sporadic cancer in generating a higher frequency of poorly differentiated and right sided tumours, which nevertheless do not result in a worse prognosis.[150] Other new factors not included in the original model include loss of heterozygosity, probably modifying the action of suppressor oncogene.[151] Loss of heterozygosity is common in sporadic tumours but much rarer in HNPCC, which is usually near diploid.[145] The 1990 model clearly does not outline the stages of development of every type of colorectal tumour.

Liver (hepatocellular carcinoma)

RNA viruses, of which the best known directly-oncogenic example is HTLV-I, associated with T cell leukaemia/lymphoma, do not so far appear to cause cancer in the gastrointestinal tract, and so will not be considered further. Several *DNA* viruses, including Epstein–Barr virus, human papilloma virus, and hepatitis B virus (HBV) *have*, however, been implicated in human carcinogenesis. The member of this group relevant to the gastrointestinal tract is hepatitis B virus, which is associated with hepatocellular carcinoma in the presence of chronic infection. Such chronically infected individuals may have a greatly increased incidence of

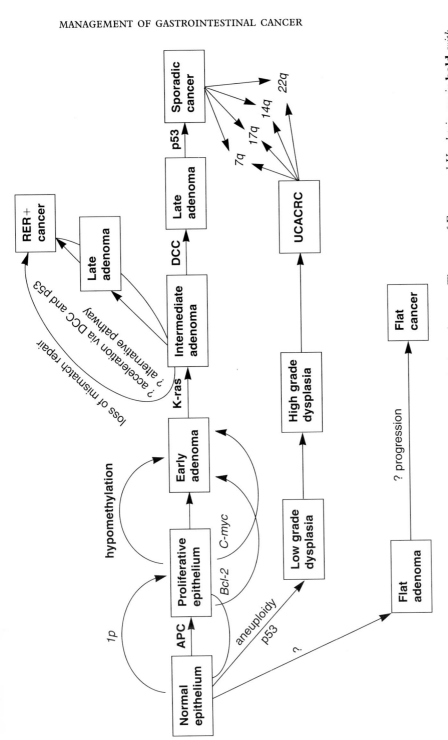

FIGURE 3.4—*An updated scheme of putative models for the development of colorectal cancer. The steps of Fearon and Vogelstein are in* **bold** *with other candidate loci in italics, showing the stage at which they act. Loss of mismatch repair probably occurs after adenomas have developed. It is not known if this simply accelerates development of replication error positive (RER+) tumours along the same pathway as replication error negative (RER−) tumours. Ulcerative colitis associated colorectal carcinomas (UCACRC) show fewer APC and K-ras mutations and may develop along an alternative pathway involving early mutation of p53. The genetic changes involved in the development of flat adenomas and flat carcinomas are not known, although they tend to show fewer K-ras mutations than sporadic cancers. (Reproduced with permission of the authors and Blackwell Science Ltd from Ilyas and Tomlinson.[145])*

hepatocellular cancer, reported as 200-fold greater in Taiwan.[2 152] Epidemiological studies indicate that this tumour is much more common in the Far East than elsewhere, and this, with the known higher carrier rate of HBV, suggests a link to this infection. The link is particularly strong if the chronic active hepatitis form of disease is present, and the age of acquiring the infection appears to be important. Thus neonates infected by vertical transmission seem at much greater risk than those acquiring the infection later in childhood or early adult life. The mechanism is not straightforward, as the HBV genome encodes no oncoproteins, and although the DNA is integrated, there is no consistent pattern of integration, even in tumours in the same patient.[153 154] Several factors have been postulated, including chronic liver cell injury with accompanying regenerative hyperplasia, possibly resulting in spontaneous mutations. The additional presence of aflatoxin in the diet in this situation adds a particular hazard and may cause p53 mutations at the codon 249 mutation hotspot,[155] with inactivation perhaps leading to clonal expansion.[93] There are genetic polymorphisms controlling the enzymatic detoxification of aflatoxin B1 (AFB1), possibly placing individuals with mutant genotypes at increased risk of developing p53 mutations and hepatocullular carcinoma (HCC).[156] A protein known as HBX, encoded by HBV, activates protein kinase C and could therefore act as a tumour promoter,[157] and may prevent p53 mediated apoptosis.[158] The same protein appears to disrupt normal growth control of hepatocytes by transcriptional activation of several host cell proto-oncogenes,[159] including the c-jun proto-oncogene.[160]

The hepatitis C virus (HCV) also appears to be important in HCC: in 63 Japanese patients with HCC, 54% were positive for HCV infection, 27% for HBV, and 9·5% for both viruses.[161] A study in China gave similar results for HBV, HCV, and HDV (the δ agent).[162] In patients with HCC but no expression of HBV surface antigen, HCV was found in 87·5% of 40 patients with HCC, and in 100% of those with a history of blood transfusions in addition to HCC.[163] A case–control study in 51 HCC patients, 34 of whom were cirrhotic, suggested that HCV was related to HCC only indirectly via cirrhosis,[164] casting some doubt on the direct carcinogenicity of HCV.

Other factors that have been implicated include high alcohol intake, reported to account for 13% of HCC in patients studied in Fukuoka, Japan, a somewhat lower rate than the 17% attributed to HBV in the same study.[165] Comparing cirrhotic and non-cirrhotic patients with HCC, the cirrhotic group were more likely to show infection with HBV or HCV, and also more likely to have a heavy alcohol intake.[166] HCC does occur in the non-cirrhotic liver, and is then more likely to spread outside the liver. The presence of aflatoxin in the diet is linked to the incidence of HCC, and the effect appears independent of HBV infection, if this is also present.[167]

The production of DNA adducts of AFB1, a marker of DNA damage, is independent of the presence of HBsAg in these patients.[168] In contrast, a large study in Shanghai suggested interaction between HBV and AFB1 (measured as its urinary metabolites) in patients who developed HCC.[169] Experimental evidence suggests that Ki-ras activation follows AFB1 exposure in the rat,[51] giving a possible mechanism for tumour induction. A p53 mutation at codon 249, found in HCC in both African and Chinese patients, has been attributed to AFB1 exposure, providing an alternative pathway.

A long observed but generally weak association with the use of the oral contraceptive pill, which has occasionally been described in association with hepatic adenomas or hepatocellular carcinoma, is not substantiated by a survey of mortality trends in England and Wales,[170] but increased risk of HCC in patients with an elevated testosterone level[171] point to the possible effects of some steroid hormones. Other unrelated causes include haemochromatosis, in which abnormal amounts of storage iron are present, overspilling the reticuloendothelial system, and so present in hepatocytes as well as Kupffer cells. The iron itself may have a directly carcinogenic effect as a result of its redox effects in the cell, leading to DNA damage.[172] In cirrhotic cases due to iron overload, the risk of HCC is reportedly increased 200-fold.[173] α_1 antitrypsin deficiency, a known precursor of cirrhosis, appears not to have a specific tendency to induce HCC beyond that caused by the accompanying cirrhosis.[174] There may be an association between smoking, raised α_1 antitrypsin levels and HCC.[175] Tyrosinaemia[176] is important if present, but a relatively rare cause of HCC. Dietary deficiencies might be expected to have a similar effect to those seen in other areas of gastrointestinal tract carcinogenesis, but this effect is demonstrable for β carotene and retinol and not for vitamin E.[177] Some effect from tobacco smoking was found in the same study, and homozygosity for the cl/cl genotype for cytochrome P-450, in combination with exposure to tobacco smoke, has been found associated with an increased risk of HCC,[178] a finding reminiscent of that in lung cancer (see above).

Cholangiocarcinoma

Most cases show no known risk factors, but in northeast Thailand, where raw fish is frequently consumed, infestation with the liver fluke *Opisthorchis viverrini* has been found strongly linked to cholangiocarcinoma. Although infestation with the parasite is itself an infrequent cause of death, cholangiocarcinoma is a major cause of death in the region.[179] Elevated nitrate and nitrite levels can be demonstrated in infested humans,[180] an effect mediated by nitric oxide synthetase (at least in a hamster model of infestation[181]). Infestation with the parasite is also found to have a strong promoting effect on hamster liver which has been initiated with dimethylnitrosamine.[182] The parasite's presence could thus be acting as both an initiator and promoter.

Outside this part of Thailand, the aetiology of the average case of cholangiocarcinoma is obscure, although occasional cases have been seen after therapeutic exposure to Thorotrast, a now obsolete thorium-containing radiology contrast medium.[183 184] Occupational exposure to vinyl chloride monomer, even at a low level, is a known risk factor,[185] and vinyl chloride monomer can produce persistent DNA adducts in rat liver.[186]

Gall bladder carcinoma

The old aphorism "fair, fat, female, fecund, and forty", known to medical students for many years as a thumbnail sketch of the risk factors for gall stones, may partly apply to gall bladder cancer too. Parity appears to be a positive risk factor if the first pregnancy was at age less than 25 years,[187] as do calorie intake and cholelithiasis, while vitamins C and E in the diet appeared to lower the risk.[188] Smoking and constipation were found to be risk factors in a Canadian study, while coffee showed an apparent protective effect.[189]

Carcinogenesis in the gall bladder has been associated with demonstrable changes in oncogene protein expression. Thus p53 is elevated in both dysplasia and cancer, suggesting a mutation occurring early in carcinogenesis,[190] while increased levels of c-erbB-2 expression are seen in the cancer stage.[191] There is a rise in ras p21 protein but this is also seen in chronic cholecystitis.[192] More specific are K-ras mutations at codon 12[193] and homozygous deletions of cyclin kinase inhibitor genes, known to be important for cell cycle regulation, and shown in gall bladder cancer cell lines.[194] Loss of heterozygosity at p53, 9p, 8p, and the DCC locus are frequent and early events, at least in at risk population in Chile, in whom similar allele loss was found in non-neoplastic tissue adjacent to tumours.[195]

Pancreas

Neoplasms of the pancreas almost all arise from its ductal epithelial component, and acinar tumours constitute at most a few per cent of the total. The rate of pancreatic carcinoma is rising, and is higher in black individuals and males, at least in the United States.[196] Lifestyle factors implicated as showing increased risk include smoking,[197] dietary factors, particularly a raised protein content in the diet and especially fat,[198] but not the consumption of beverages, including alcohol, tea, and coffee.[199] A study in the USA did however find a link to alcohol intake if it exceeded 10 drinks per month, and to meat in the diet, but no link to the consumption of fruits, vegetables, and grains.[200] Pancreatitis constitutes a risk for pancreatic cancer[201] and the risk increases with the duration of chronic pancreatitis, although not linked to any particular type.[202] Diabetes mellitus has been studied in relation to pancreatic carcinoma and there is a positive link.[203 204] Interestingly, there is some evidence that the cancers occurring in diabetics may show different biological behaviour from the cancers in non-diabetics, and may become apparent near the time of onset of newly diagnosed diabetes.[205] Some of these tumours produce insulin-like growth factor 1, which may itself influence glucose homeostasis.[206]

The molecular genetics of pancreatic cancer have been studied, although not as extensively as those of colorectal cancer. K-ras mutations (of codon 12) are well documented, both in hyperplasia[207] and carcinoma.[50] Intriguingly, such mutations could be detected in material retrieved from stools[208] or pancreatic juice[209] taken from pancreatic cancer patients, suggesting possibilities for screening. p53 mutations at multiple codon sites have also been found in pancreatic carcinoma but not chronic pancreatitis.[210] Genetic instability, evidenced by the presence of replication errors, is highly prevalent in pancreatic carcinoma (six of nine cases), in comparison with tumours at other sites (3–16%).[211] Loss of heterozygosity on chromosome 5q21 has been compared in gastric cancers, where it is frequent, and pancreatic cancers, where it is very infrequent.[212] This region contains the suppressor genes APC and MCC.

Conclusion

Elements of a sequence of mutations, conceptually similar to the Fearon and Vogelstein model, are also determined at other sites in the gastrointestinal tract. Some of the oncogenes or oncosuppressor genes important in the colon evidently operate elsewhere, but it is too early to say whether the model, or a modified version of it, will satisfactorily explain carcinogenesis at non-intestinal sites. The environmental, and to some extent hereditary, risk factors do overlap at the separate sites, so it would be surprising if the mechanism were radically different for each. Progress is rapid and an understanding of carcinogenesis is no longer an impossible dream.

References

1 Boring CC, Squires TS, Tong T, *et al.* Cancer statistics. *CA* 1994;**44**:7–26.
2 Beasley RP. Hepatitis B virus, the major etiology of hepatocellular carcinoma. *Cancer* 1988;**61**:1942–56.
3 Zheng W, Sellers TA, Doyle TJ, *et al.* Retinol, antioxidant vitamins, and cancers of the upper digestive tract in a prospective cohort study of postmenopausal women. *Am J Epidemiol* 1995;**142**:955–60.

4 Reddy BS, Rivenson A, Kulkarni N, *et al.* Chemoprevention of colon carcinogenesis by the synthetic organoselenium compound 1,4-phenylenebis(methylene)-selenocyanate. *Cancer Res* 1992;**52**:5635–40.

5 Hietanen E, Bartsch H, Bereziat JC, *et al.* Diet and oxidative stress in breast, colon and prostate cancer patients: a case–control study. *Eur J Clin Nutr* 1994;**48**:575–86.

6 Beno I, Volkovova K, Staruchova M. Gastric mucosal antioxidant activity in patients at increased risk of gastric cancer. *Neoplasma* 1993;**40**:315–9.

7 Chen CS, Pignatelli B, Malaveille C, *et al.* Levels of direct-acting mutagens, total *N*-nitroso compounds in nitrosated fermented fish products, consumed in a high-risk area for gastric cancer in southern China. *Mutat Res* 1992;**265**:211–21.

8 Xu GP, Song PJ, Reed PI. Effects of fruit juices, processed vegetable juice, orange peel and green tea on endogenous formation of *N*-nitrosoproline in subjects from a high-risk area for gastric cancer in Moping County, China. *Eur J Cancer Prev* 1993;**2**:327–35.

9 Giovannucci E, Willett WC. Dietary factors and risk of colon cancer. *Ann Med* 1994;**26**: 443–52.

10 Stamp D, Zhang XM, Medline A, *et al.* Sucrose enhancement of the early steps of colon carcinogenesis in mice. *Carcinogenesis* 1993;**14**:777–9.

11 Nazario CM, Szklo M, Diamond E, *et al.* Salt and gastric cancer: a case–control study in Puerto Rico. *Int J Epidemiol* 1993;**22**:790–7.

12 Hoshiyama Y, Sekine T, Sasaba T. A case–control study of colorectal cancer and its relation to diet, cigarettes, and alcohol consumption in Saitama Prefecture, Japan. *Tohoku J Exp Med* 1993;**171**:153–65.

13 Kabat GC, Ng SK, Wynder EL. Tobacco, alcohol intake, and diet in relation to adenocarcinoma of the esophagus and gastric cardia. *Cancer Causes Control* 1993;**4**:123–32.

14 Hansson LE, Baron J, Nyren O, *et al.* Tobacco, alcohol and the risk of gastric cancer. A population-based case–control study in Sweden. *Int J Cancer* 1994;**57**:26–31.

15 Guinaid AA, Sumari AA, Shidrawi RG, *et al.* Oesophageal and gastric carcinoma in the Republic of Yemen. *Br J Cancer* 1995;**71**:409–10.

16 Jedrychowski W, Boeing H, Wahrendorf J, *et al.* Vodka consumption, tobacco smoking and risk of gastric cancer in Poland. *Int J Epidemiol* 1993;**22**:606–13.

17 Wyatt JI, Rathbone BJ. Immune response of the gastric mucosa to *Campylobacter pylori*. *Scand J Gastroenterol Suppl* 1988;**142**:44–9.

18 Negrini R, Lisato L, Zanella I, *et al.* Helicobacter pylori infection induces antibodies cross-reacting with human gastric mucosa. *Gastroenterology* 1991;**101**:437–45.

19 Parsonnet J, Friedman GD, Vandersteen DP, *et al.* Helicobacter pylori infection and the risk of gastric carcinoma. *N Engl J Med* 1991;**325**:1127–31.

20 Wotherspoon AC, Ortiz-Hidalgo C, Falzon MR, *et al.* Helicobacter pylori-associated gastritis and primary B-cell gastric lymphoma. *Lancet* 1991;**338**:1175–6.

21 Mosbech J, Videbaek A. Mortality from and risk of gastric carcinoma among patients with pernicious anaemia. *BMJ* 1950;**2**:390–4.

22 Streitz MM Jr. Barrett's esophagus and esophageal cancer. *Chest Surg Clin North Am* 1994; **4**:227–40.

23 Serraino D, Salamina G, Franceschi S, *et al.* The epidemiology of AIDS associated non-Hodgkin's lymphoma in the World Health Organization European Region. *Br J Cancer* 1992;**66**:912–6.

24 Frizzera G, Hanto DW, Gajl-Peczalska KJ, *et al.* Polymorphic diffuse B-cell hyperplasias and lymphomas in renal transplant recipients. *Cancer Res* 1981;**41**:4262–79.

25 Hamilton-Dutoit SJ, Pallesen G, Frantzmann MB, *et al.* AIDS-related lymphoma. Histopathology, immunophenotype, and association with Epstein–Barr virus as demonstrated by in-situ nucleic acid hybridization. *Am J Pathol* 1991;**138**:149–63.

26 MacMahon EME, Glass JD, Hayward SD, *et al.* Epstein–Barr virus in primary AIDS-related central nervous system lymphoma. *Lancet* 1991;**338**:969–70.

27 Wotherspoon AC, Doglioni C, Diss TC, *et al.* Regression of primary low grade gastric B-cell lymphoma of mucosa-associated tissue type after eradication of *Helicobacter pylori*. *Lancet* 1993;**342**:575–7.

28 Isaacson PG. Pathogenesis and early lesions in extranodal lymphoma. *Toxicol Lett* 1993; **67**:237–47.

29 Martin IG, Aldoori MI. Immunoproliferative small intestinal disease: Mediterranean lymphoma and alpha heavy chain disease. *Br J Surg* 1994;**81**:20–4.

30 Ben-Ayed F, Halphen M, Najjar T, *et al.* Treatment of alpha chain disease. Results of a prospective study in 21 patients by the Tunisian–French Intestinal Lymphoma Study Group. *Cancer* 1989;**63**:1251–6.

31 Muller-Hermelink HK, Greiner A. Autoimmune diseases and malignant lymphoma. *Verh Dtsch Ges Pathol* 1992;**76**:96–109.

32 Wright DH. The major complications of coeliac disease. *Baillière's Clin Gastroenterol* 1995; **9**:351–69.

33 Ilyas M, Niedobitek G, Agathanggelou A, *et al.* Non-Hodgkin's lymphoma, coeliac disease and Epstein–Barr virus: a study of 13 cases of enteropathy-associated T- and B-cell lymphoma. *J Pathol* 1995;**177**:115–22.

34 Borisch B, Hennig I, Horber F, *et al.* Enteropathy-associated T-cell lymphoma in a renal transplant patient with evidence of Epstein–Barr virus involvement. *Virchows Arch [A]* 1992;**421**:443–7.

35 Ponder BAJ. Inherited predisposition to cancer. *Trends Genet 1990;*6:213–8.

36 Smith, SA, Ponder, BA. Predisposing genes in breast and ovarian cancer: an overview. *Tumori* 1993;**79**:291–6.

37 Schneider BG, Pulitzer DR, Brown RD, *et al.* Allelic imbalance in gastric cancer: an affected site on chromosome arm 3p. *Genes Chromosomes Cancer* 1995;**13**:263–71.

38 Leggett B, Young J, Buttenshaw R, *et al.* Colorectal carcinomas show frequent allelic loss on the long arm of chromosome 17 with evidence for a specific target region. *Br J Cancer* 1995;**71**:1070–3.

39 Malkin D, Li FP, Strong LC, *et al.* Germ line p53 mutations in a familial syndrome of breast cancer, sarcomas and other neoplasms. *Science* 1990;**250**:1233–8.

40 Fearon ER, Vogelstein B. A genetic model for colorectal tumoregenesis. *Cell* 1990;**61**: 759–67.

41 Muto T, Bussey HJ, Morson BC. The evolution of cancer of the colon and rectum. *Cancer* 1975;**36**:2251–70.

42 Counts J, Goodman J. Alterations in DNA methylation may play a variety of roles in carcinogenesis. *Cell* 1995;**83**:13–5.

43 Bos JL. The ras gene family and human carcinogenesis. *Mutat Res* 1988;**195**:255–71.

44 Hedrick I, Cho KR, Fearon ER, *et al.* The DCC gene product in cellular differentiation and colorectal tumorigenesis. *Genes Dev* 1994;**8**:1174–83.

45 Lane DP. Cancer, p53, guardian of the genome. *Nature* 1992;**358**:15–6.

46 Donehower LA, Bradley A. The tumour suppressor p53. *Biochim Biophys Acta* 1993; **1155**:181–205.

47 El-Deiry WS, Harper JW, O'Connor PN, *et al.* WAF1/CIP1 is induced in p53-mediated G1 arrest and apoptosis. *Cancer Res* 1994;**54**:1169–74.

48 Celano P, Berchtold CM, Mabry M, *et al.* Induction of markers of normal differentiation in human colon carcinoma cells by the v-rasH oncogene. *Cell Growth Differ* 1993;**4**:341–7.

49 Filmus J, Shi W, Spencer T. Role of transforming growth factor alpha (TGF-alpha) in the transformation of ras-transfected rat intestinal epithelial cells. *Oncogene* 1993;**8**: 1017–22.

50 Daus H, Trumper L, Burger B, *et al.* Ki-ras mutation as a molecular tumor marker for carcinoma of the pancreas. *Deutsche Med Wochenschr* 1995;**120**:821–5.

51 Soman NR, Wogan GN. Activation of the c-Ki-ras oncogene in aflatoxin B1-induced hepatocellular carcinoma and adenoma in the rat: detection by denaturing gradient gel electrophoresis. *Proc Natl Acad Sci USA* 1993;**90**:2045–9.

52 Kanamaru R, Ishioka C. Mutations of the p53 gene and other genes involved in human colorectal carcinogenesis. *Tokohu J Exp Med* 1992;**168**:159–66.

53 Koh EH, Chung HC, Lee KB, *et al.* Point mutation at codon 12 of the c-Ha-ras gene in human gastric cancers. *J Korean Med Sci* 1992;**7**:110–5.

54 Chung CK, Antoniades HN. Expression of c-sis/platelet-derived growth factor B, insulin-like growth factor 1, and transforming growth factor alpha messenger RNAs and their respective receptor messenger RNAs in primary human gastric carcinomas: in vivo studies with *in situ* hybridization and immunocytochemistry. *Cancer Res* 1992;**52**:3453–9.

55 Iida S, Katoh O, Tokunaga A, *et al.* Expression of fibroblast growth factor gene family and its receptor gene family in the human upper gastrointestinal tract. *Biochem Biophys Res Commun* 1994;**199**:1113–9.

56 Sasaki K, Tomita Y, Azuma M, *et al.* Amplification and overexpression of the c-erbB-2 protooncogene in human gastric cancer. *Gastroenterol Jpn* 1992;**27**:172–8.

57 Koskinen PJ, Alitalo K. Role of myc amplification and overexpression in cell growth, differentiation and death. *Semin Cancer Biol* 1993;**4**:3–12.

58 Kato GJ, Dang CV. Function of the c-myc oncoprotein. *FASEB J* 1992;**6**:3065–72.

59 Makela TP, Saksela K, Alitalo K. Amplification and rearrangement of L-myc in human small-cell lung cancer. *Mutat Res* 1992;**276**:307–15.

60 Chai KJ, Kim JS, Lee HK. Expressions of c-fos and c-myc genes during 3-methyl-4-dimethylaminoazobenzene (3'-MeDAB)-induced rat hepatocarcinoma. *Yonsei Med J* 1992;**33**:240–8.

61 Magrath I, Jain V, Bhatia K. Epstein–Barr virus and Burkitt's lymphoma. *Semin Cancer Biol* 1992;**3**:285–95.

62 Hockenbery DM, Oltvai ZN, Yin XM, *et al.* Bcl-2 functions in an antioxidant pathway to prevent apoptosis. *Cell* 1993;**75**:241–51.

63 Ladanyi M, Wang S. Detection of rearrangement of the BCL2 major breakpoint region in follicular lymphomas. Correlation of polymerase chain reaction results with Southern blot analysis. *Diagn Mol Pathol* 1992;**1**:31–5.

64 Schwab M. Amplification of N-myc as a prognostic marker for patients with neuroblastoma. *Semin Cancer Biol* 1993;**4**:13–8.

65 Liu E, Thor A, He M, *et al.* The HER2 (c-erbB-2) oncogene is frequently amplified in in situ carcinomas of the breast. *Oncogene* 1992;**7**:1027–32.

66 Knudson AG. Mutation and cancer: a statistical study of retinoblastoma. *Proc Natl Acad Sci USA* 1971;**68**:820–3.

67 Benedict WF, Xu HJ, Hu SX, *et al.* Role of retinoblastoma gene in the initiation and progression of human cancer. *J Clin Invest* 1990;**85**:988–93.

68 Li HC. Mutation and expression of Rb gene in human oesophageal cancer. *Chung Hua Chung Liu Tsa Chih* 1993;**15**:412–4.

69 Huang Y, Meltzer SJ, Yin J, *et al.* Altered messenger RNA and unique mutational profiles of p53 and Rb in human esophageal carcinomas. *Cancer Res* 1993;**53**:1889–94.

70 Zhou X, Tarmin L, Yin J, *et al.* The MTS1 gene is frequently mutated in primary human esophageal tumors. *Oncogene* 1994;**9**:3737–41.

71 Zambetti GP, Levine AJ. A comparison of the biologic activities of wild type and mutant p53. *FASEB J* 1993;**7**:855–65.

72 Kaklamanis L, Gatter KC, Mortensen N, *et al.* p53 expression in colorectal adenomas. *Am J Pathol* 1993;**142**:87–93.

73 Moore M, Teresky AK, Levine AJ, *et al.* p53 mutations are not selected for in simian virus 40 T-antigen-induced tumors from transgenic mice. *J Virol* 1992;**66**:641–9.

74 Ghebranious N, Knoll BJ, Wu H, *et al.* Characterization of a murine p53ser246 mutant equivalent to the human p53ser249 associated with hepatocellular carcinoma and aflatoxin exposure. *Mol Carcinog* 1995;**13**:104–11.

75 Hollstein MC, Wild CP, Bleicher F, *et al.* p53 mutations and aflatoxin B1 exposure in hepatocellular carcinoma patients from Thailand. *Int J Cancer* 1993;**53**:51–5.

76 Hongyo T, Buzard GS, Palli D, *et al.* Mutations of the K-ras and p53 genes in gastric adenocarcinomas from a high-incidence region around Florence, Italy. *Cancer Res* 1995;**55**:2665–72.

77 Poremba C, Yandell DW, Huang Q, *et al.* Frequency and spectrum of p53 mutations in gastric cancer—a molecular genetic and immunohistochemical study. *Virchows Arch* 1995;**426**:447–55.

78 Uchino S, Noguchi M, Ochiai A, *et al.* p53 mutation in gastric cancer: a genetic model for carcinogenesis is common to gastric and colorectal cancer. *Int J Cancer* 1993;**54**:759–64.

79 Liang YY, Esteve A, Martel-Planche G, *et al.* p53 mutations in esophageal tumours from high-incidence areas of China. *Int J Cancer* 1995;**61**:611–4.

80 Chang F, Syrjanen S, Tervahauta A, *et al.* Frequent mutations of p53 gene in oesophageal squamous cell carcinomas with and without human papillomavirus (HPV) involvement suggest the dominant role of environmental carcinogens in oesophageal carcinogenesis. *Br J Cancer* 1994;**70**:346–51.

81 Hamelin R, Flejou JF, Muzeau F, *et al.* TP53 gene mutations and p53 protein immunoreactivity in malignant and premalignant Barrett's esophagus. *Gastroenterology* 1994;**107**:1012–8.

82 Casson AG, Manopolopoulos B, Troster M, *et al.* Clinical implications of p53 gene mutation in the progression of Barrett's epithelium to invasive esophageal cancer. *Am J Surg* 1994;**167**:52–7.

83 Lozano JC, Nakazawa H, Cross MP, *et al.* G→A mutations in p53 and Ha-ras genes in esophageal papillomas induced by *N*-nitrosomethylbenzylamine in two strains of rats. *Mol Carcinog* 1994;**9**:33–9.

84 Uchino S, Tsuda H, Noguchi M, *et al.* Frequent loss of heterozygosity at the DCC locus in gastric cancer. *Cancer Res* 1992;**52**:3099–102.

85 Nakatsuru S, Yanagisawa A, Ichii S, *et al.* Somatic mutation of the APC gene in gastric cancer: frequent mutations in very well differentiated adenocarcinoma and signet-ring cell carcinoma. *Hum Mol Genet* 1992;**1**:559–63.

86 Horii A, Nakatsuru S, Miyoshi Y, *et al.* The APC gene, responsible for familial adenomatous polyposis, is mutated in human gastric cancer. *Cancer Res* 1992;**52**:3231–3.

87 Pereira FP. Uncovering new clues to cancer risk. *Sci Am* 1996;**274**:40–6.

88 Kato S, Shields PG, Caporaso NE, *et al.* Cytochrome P450IIE1 genetic polymorphisms, racial variation and lung cancer risk. *Cancer Res* 1992;**52**:6712–5.

89 Wogan GN. Molecular epidemiology in cancer risk assessment and prevention: recent progress and avenues for future research. *Environ Health Perspect* 1992;**98**:167–78.

90 Harris CC. p53: at the crossroads of molecular carcinogenesis and risk assessment. *Science* 1993;**262**:1980–1.

91 Hsu IC, Metcalf RA, Sun T, *et al.* Mutational hot spot in the p53 gene in human hepatocellular carcinomas. *Nature* 1991;**350**:427–8.

92 Becher R, Lag M, Schwarze PE, *et al.* Chemically induced DNA damage in isolated rabbit lung cells. *Mutat Res* 1993;**285**:303–11.

93 Cotran RS, Kumar V, Robbins SL. *Pathologic basis of disease*, 5th ed. Philadelphia: WB Saunders, 1994:258–90.

94 Vaughan TL, Davis S, Kristal A, *et al.* Obesity, alcohol and tobacco as risk factors for cancers of the esophagus and gastric cardia: adenocarcinoma versus squamous cell carcinoma. *Cancer Epidemiol Biomarkers Prev* 1995;**4**:85–92.

95 Gray JR, Coldman AJ, MacDonald WC. Cigarette and alcohol use in patients with adenocarcinoma of the gastric cardia or lower esophagus. *Cancer* 1992;**69**:2227–31.

96 Gao YT, McLaughlin JK, Gridley G, *et al.* Risk factors for esophageal cancer in Shanghai, China. II. Role of diet and nutrients. *Int J Cancer* 1994;**58**:197–202.

97 Rolon PA, Castellsague X, Benz M, *et al.* Hot and cold mate drinking and esophageal cancer in Paraguay. *Cancer Epidemiol Biomarkers Prev* 1995;**4**:595–605.

98 Li Mx. Fusarin C induced esophageal and forestomach carcinoma in mice and rats. *Chung Hua Chung Liu Tsa Chih* 1992;**14**:27–9.

99 Chu FS, Li GY. Simultaneous occurrence of fumonisin B1 and other mycotoxins in moldy corn collected from the People's Republic of China in regions with high incidences of esophageal cancer. *Appl Environ Microbiol* 1994;**60**:847–52.

100 Siddiqi M, Kumar R, Fazili Z, *et al.* Increased exposure to dietary amines and nitrate in a population at high risk of oesophageal and gastric cancer in Kashmir (India). *Carcinogenesis* 1992;**13**:1331–5.

101 Wu Y, Chen J, Ohshima H, *et al.* Geographic association between urinary excretion of *N*-nitroso compounds and oesophageal cancer mortality in China. *Int J Cancer* 1993;**54**:713–9.

102 Toma S, Losardo PL, Vincent M, *et al.* Effectiveness of beta-carotene in cancer chemoprevention. *Eur J Cancer Prev* 1995;**4**:213–24.

103 Byers T, Guerrero N. Epidemiologic evidence for vitamin C and vitamin E in cancer prevention. *Am J Clin Nutr* 1995;**62**(6 suppl):1385S–92S.

104 Block G, Patterson B, Subar A. Fruit, vegetables and cancer prevention: a review of the epidemiological evidence. *Nutr Cancer* 1992;**18**:1–29.

105 Li, JY, Taylor PR, Li B, *et al.* Nutrition intervention trials in Linxian, China: multiple vitamin/mineral supplementation, cancer incidence, and disease-specific mortality among adults with esophageal dysplasia. *J Natl Cancer Inst* 1993;**85**:1492–8.

106 Franceschi S, Bidoli E, Baron A, *et al.* Maize and the risk of cancers of the oral cavity, pharynx and oesophagus. *J Natl Cancer Inst* 1990;**82**:1407–11.

107 Rogaev EI, Korovaitseva GI, Ginter EK, *et al.* Mapping of the dominant gene of hyperkeratosis palmaris et plantaris in man. *Genetika* 1993;**29**:1180–5.

108 Risk JM, Field EA, Field JK, *et al.* Tylosis oesophageal cancer mapped. *Nat Genet* 1994;**8**:319–21.

109 Hamilton SR, Smith RL. The relationship between columnar epithelial dysplasia and invasive adenocarcinoma arising in Barrett's oesophagus. *Am J Clin Pathol* 1987;**87**:301–12.

110 Haggitt RC, Tryzeluar J, Ellis FH, *et al.* Adenocarcinoma complicating columnar epithelium lined (Barrett's) esophagus. *Am J Clin Pathol* 1978;**70**:1–5.

111 Peuchmaur M, Potet F, Goldfain D. Mucin histochemistry of the columnar epithelium of the oesophagus (Barrett's oesophagus): a prospective biopsy study. *J Clin Pathol* 1984;**37**:607–10.

112 Gray MR, Donnelly RJ, Kingsnorth AN. The role of smoking and alcohol in metaplasia and cancer risk in Barrett's columnar lined oesophagus. *Gut* 1993;**34**:727–31.

113 Chow WH, Finkle WD, McLaughlin JK, *et al.* The relation of gastroesophageal reflux disease and its treatment to adenocarcinomas of the esophagus and gastric cardia. *JAMA* 1995;**274**:474–7.

114 Craanen ME, Blok P, Dekker W, *et al.* Prevalence of subtypes of intestinal metaplasia in gastric antral mucosa. *Dig Dis Sci* 1991;**36**:1529–36.

115 Tsugane S, Tei Y, Takahashi T, *et al.* Salty food intake and risk of *Helicobacter pylori* infection. *Jpn J Cancer Res* 1994;**85**:474–8.

116 Tominaga S. Decreasing trend of stomach cancer in Japan *Jpn J Cancer Res* 1987;**78**:1–10.

117 Zhang L, Blot WJ, You WC, *et al.* Serum micronutrients in relation to precancerous gastric lesions. *Int J Cancer* 1994;**56**:650–4.

118 Dobrilla G, Benvenuti S, Amplatz S, *et al.* Chronic gastritis, intestinal metaplasia, dysplasia and *Helicobacter pylori* in gastric cancer: putting the pieces together. *Ital J Gastroenterol* 1994;**26**:449–58.

119 Yu K, Zhang JK. Study on the association between *Helicobacter pylori* infection and the pathogenesis of gastric cancer by using molecular biological techniques. *J Tongji Med Univ* 1994;**14**:65–70.

120 Sipponen P, Kosunen TU, Valle J, *et al. Helicobacter pylori* infection and chronic gastritis in gastric cancer. *J Clin Pathol* 1992;**45**:319–23.

121 La-Vecchia C, Negri E, D'Avanzo B, *et al.* Partial gastrectomy and subsequent gastric cancer risk. *J Epidemiol Community Health* 1992;**46**:12–4.

122 Dekker W, op den Orth JO. Polyps of the stomach and duodenum: significance and management. *Dig Dis* 1992;**10**:199–207.

123 Graham DY, Malaty HM, Go MF. Are there susceptible hosts to *Helicobacter pylori* infection? *Scand J Gastroenterol Suppl* 1994;**205**:6–10.

124 Sugimura T, Inoue R, Ohgaki H, *et al.* Genetic polymorphisms and susceptibility to cancer development. *Pharmacogenetics* 1995;**5 Spec no**:S161–5.

125 Shumizu Y, Kato H, Schull WJ, *et al.* Lifespan study report 11, Part I: comparison of risk coefficients for site-specific cancer mortality based on the DS86 and T65DR shielded kerma and organ doses. *Radiation Effects Foundation Technical Report 12–87*, Hiroshima, Japan, 1987.

126 Lipkin M, Newmark H. Calcium and the prevention of colon cancer. *J Cell Biochem Suppl* 1995;**22**:65–73.

127 McCann SE, Randall E, Marshall JR, *et al.* Diet diversity and risk of colon cancer in western New York. *Nutr Cancer* 1994;**21**:133–41.

128 Peters PK, Pike MC, Garabrant D, *et al.* Diet and colon cancer in Los Angeles County, California. *Cancer Causes Control* 1992;**3**:457–73.

129 Bruce WR, Archer MC, Corpet DE, *et al.* Diet, aberrant crypt foci and colorectal cancer. *Mutat Res* 1993;**290**:111–8.

130 Nelson RL, Davis FG, Sutter E, *et al.* Serum selenium and colonic neoplastic risk. *Dis Colon Rectum* 1995;**38**:1306–10.

131 Flagg EW, Coates RJ, Greenberg RS. Epidemiologic studies of antioxidants and cancer in humans. *J Am Coll Nutr* 1995;**14**:419–27.

132 Belleli A, Shany S, Levy J, *et al.* A protective role of 1,25-dihydroxyvitamin D_3 in chemically induced rat colon carcinogenesis. *Carcinogenesis* 1992;**13**:2293–8.

133 Reddy BS, Rao CV, Rivenson A, *et al.* Inhibitory effect of aspirin on azoxymethane-induced colon carcinogenesis in F344 rats. *Carcinogenesis* 1993;**14**:1493–7.

134 Singh J, Kelloff G, Reddy BS. Effect of chemopreventive agents on intermediate biomarkers during different stages of azoxymethane-induced colon carcinogenesis. *Cancer Epidemiol Biomarkers Prev* 1992;**1**:405–11.

135 Rao CV, Rivenson A, Simi B, *et al.* Chemoprevention of colon carcinogenesis by sulindac, a nonsteroidal anti-inflammatory agent. *Cancer Res* 1995;**55**:1464–72.

136 Thun MJ, Namboodiri MM, Calle EE, *et al.* Aspirin use and risk of fatal cancer. *Cancer Res* 1993;**53**:1322–7.

137 Shiff SJ, Koutsos MI, Qiao L, *et al.* Nonsteroidal anti-inflammatory drugs inhibit the proliferation of colon adenocarcinoma cells: effects on cell cycle and apoptosis. *Exp Cell Res* 1996;**222**:179–88.

138 Levin B. Ulcerative colitis and colon cancer: biology and surveillance. *J Cell Biochem Suppl* 1992;**16G**:47–50.

139 Tarmin L, Yin J, Harpaz N, *et al.* Adenomatous polyposis coli gene mutations in ulcerative colitis-associated dysplasias and cancers versus sporadic colon neoplasms. *Cancer Res* 1995;**55**:2035–8.

140 Redston M, Papadopoulos N, Caldas C, *et al.* Common occurrence of APC and K-ras mutation in the spectrum of colitis-associated neoplasias. *Gastroenterology* 1995;**108**:383–92.

141 Bissonnette RP, Echeverri F, Mahboubi A, *et al.* Apoptotic cell death induced by c-myc is inhibited by bcl-2. *Nature* 1992;**359**:552–4.

142 Brentall TA, Crispon DA, Rabinovitch PS, *et al.* Mutations in the p53 gene: an early marker of neoplastic progression in ulcerative colitis. *Gastroenterology* 1994;**107**:369–78.

143 Roncucci L. Early events in human colorectal carcinogenesis. Aberrant crypts and microadenoma. *Ital J Gastroenterol* 1992;**24**:498–501.

144 Bedenne L, Faivre J, Boutron MC, *et al.* Adenoma–carcinoma sequence or "de novo" carcinogenesis? A study of adenomatous remnants in a population-based series of large bowel cancers. *Cancer* 1992;**69**:883–8.

145 Ilyas M, Tomlinson IPM. Genetic pathways in colorectal cancer. *Histopathology* 1996;**28**:389–99.

146 Aaltonen LA, Peltomaki P, Mecklion JP, *et al.* Replication errors in benign and malignant tumours from hereditary nonpolyposis colorectal cancer patients. *Cancer Res* 1994;**54**:1645–8.

147 Jacoby RF, Marshall DJ, Kailas S, *et al.* Genetic instability associated with adenoma to carcinoma progression in hereditary nonpolyposis colon cancer. *Gastroenterology* 1995;**109**:73–82.

148 Froggatt NJ, Koch J, Davies R, *et al.* Genetic linkage and analysis in hereditary non-polyposis colon cancer syndrome. *J Med Genet* 1995;**32**:352–7.

149 Lindblom A, Tannergard P, Werelius B, *et al.* Genetic mapping of a second locus predisposing to hereditary non-polyposis colon cancer. *Nat Genet* 1993;**5**:279–82.

150 Jass JR, Smyrk TC, Stewart SM, *et al.* Pathology of hereditary non-polyposis colorectal cancer. *Anticancer Res* 1994;**14**:1631–4.

151 Tanaka K, Yanoshita R, Konishi M, *et al.* Suppression of tumorigenicity in human colon-carcinoma cells by introduction of normal chromosome 1p36 region. *Oncogene* 1993;**8**:2253–8.

152 Beasley RP, Lin C, Hwang LY, *et al.* Hepatocellular carcinoma and hepatitis B virus. A prospective study of 22 707 men in Taiwan. *Lancet* 1981;**ii**:1129–33.

153 Liang XH. Clonal origin of intrahepatic recurrence after resection of hepatocellular carcinoma. *Chung Hua Chung Liu Tsa Chih* 1991;**13**:2–4.

154 Hsu HC, Chiou TJ, Chen JY, *et al.* Clonality and clonal evolution of hepatocellular carcinoma with multiple nodules. *Hepatology* 1991;**13**:923–8.

155 Ozturk M. p53 mutation in hepatocellular carcinoma after aflatoxin exposure. *Lancet* 1991;**338**:1356–9.

156 McGlynn KA, Rosvold EA, Lustbader ED, *et al.* Susceptibility to hepatocellular carcinoma is associated with genetic variation in the enzymatic detoxification of aflatoxin B1. *Proc Natl Acad Sci USA* 1995;**92**:2384–7.

157 Luber B, Lauer U, Weiss L, *et al.* The hepatitis B virus transactivator HBx causes elevation of diacylglycerol and activation of protein kinase C. *Res Virol* 1993;**144**:311–21.

158 Wang XW, Gibson MK, Vermeulen W, *et al.* Abrogation of p53-induced apoptosis by the hepatitis B virus X gene. *Cancer Res* 1995;**55**:6012–6.

159 Kekule AS, Lauer U, Weiss L, *et al.* Hepatitis B transactivator Hbx uses a tumour promoter signalling pathway. *Nature* 1993;**361**:742–5.

160 Twu JS, Lai MY, Chen DS, *et al.* Activation of protoncogene c-jun by the X protein of hepatitis B virus. *Virology* 1993;**192**:346–50.

161 Wild CP, Shrestha SM, Anwar WA, *et al.* Field studies of aflatoxin exposure, metabolism and induction of genetic alterations in relation to HBV infection and hepatocellular carcinoma in The Gambia and Thailand. *Toxicol Lett* 1992;**64–65 Spec no**:455–61.

162 Zeng WZ, Chu RJ, Jiang MD. Clinical evaluation of HBV, HCV and HDV serum markers in patients with liver cirrhosis (LC) and hepatocellular carcinoma (HCC). *Chung Hua Nei Ko Tsa Chih* 1993;**32**:167–9.

163 Enriquez J, Fuchs K, Martinez-Cerezo FJ, *et al.* Demonstration of HCV-RNA and HBV-DNA in the serum of HBsAg negative patients with hepatocellular carcinoma. *Eur J Epidemiol* 1994;**10**:189–94.

164 Goritsas CP, Athanasiadou A, Arvaniti A, *et al.* The leading role of hepatitis B and C viruses as risk factors for the development of hepatocellular carcinoma. A case control study. *J Clin Gastroenterol* 1995;**20**:220–4.

165 Tanaka K, Hirohata T, Takeshita S, *et al.* Hepatitis B virus, cigarette smoking and alcohol consumption in the development of hepatocellular carcinoma: a case–control study in Fukuoka, Japan. *Int J Cancer* 1992;**51**:509–14.

166 Trevisani F, D'Intino PE, Caraceni P, *et al.* Etiologic factors and clinical presentation of hepatocellular carcinoma. Differences between cirrhotic and noncirrhotic Italian patients. *Cancer* 1995;**75**:2220–32.

167 Hatch MC, Chen CJ, Levin B, *et al.* Urinary aflatoxin levels, hepatitis B virus infection and hepatocellular carcinoma in Taiwan. *Int J Cancer* 1993;**54**:931–4.

168 Santella RM, Zhang YJ, Chen CJ, *et al.* Immunohistochemical detection of aflatoxin B1-DNA adducts and hepatitis B virus antigens in hepatocellular and nontumorous liver tissue. *Environ Health Perspect* 1993;**99**:199–202.

169 Ross RK, Yuan JM, Yu MC, *et al.* Urinary aflatoxin biomarkers and risk of hepatocellular carcinoma. *Lancet* 1992;**339**:943–6.

170 Mant JW, Vessey MP. Trends in mortality from primary liver cancer in England and Wales 1975–92: influence of oral contraceptives. *Br J Cancer* 1995;**72**:800–3.

171 Yu MW, Chen CJ. Elevated serum testosterone levels and risk of hepatocellular carcinoma. *Cancer Res* 1993;**53**:790–4.

172 Toyokuni S, Sagripanti JL. Induction of oxidative single- and double-strand breaks in DNA by ferric citrate. *Free Radic Biol Med* 1993;**15**:117–23.

173 Stal P. Iron as a hepatotoxin. *Dig Dis* 1995;**13**:205–22.

174 Propst T, Propst A, Dietze O, *et al.* Prevalence of hepatocellular carcinoma in alpha-1-antitrypsin deficiency. *J Hepatol* 1994;**21**:1006–11.

175 Petridou E, Chapuis-Cellier C, Roukas K, *et al.* Tobacco smoking and other factors in relation to serum alpha-1-antitrypsin. *Hum Biol* 1993;**65**:425–32.

176 Kvittingen EA. Tyrosinaemia—treatment and outcome. *J Inherit Metab Dis* 1995;**18**:375–9.

177 Pan WH, Wang CY, Huang SM, *et al.* Vitamin A, vitamin E or beta-carotene status and hepatitis B-related hepatocellular carcinoma. *Ann Epidemiol* 1993;**3**:217–24.

178 Yu MW, Gladek-Yarborough A, Chiamprasert S, *et al.* Cytochrome P450 2E1 and glutathione *S*-transferase M1 polymorphisms and susceptiblity to hepatocellular carcinoma. *Gastroenterology* 1995;**109**:1266–73.

179 Sithithaworn P, Haswell-Elkins MR, Mairiang P, *et al.* Parasite-associated morbidity: liver fluke infection and bile duct cancer in Northeast Thailand. *Int J Parasitol* 1994;**24**: 833–43.

180 Haswell-Elkins MR, Satarug S, Tsuda M, *et al.* Liver fluke infection and cholangiocarcinoma: model of endogenous nitric oxide and extragastric nitrosation in human carcinogenesis. *Mutat Res* 1994;**305**:241–52.

181 Ohshima H, Bandaletova TY, Brouet I, *et al.* Increased nitrosamine and nitrate biosynthesis mediated by nitric oxide synthase induced in hamsters infected with liver fluke (*Opisthorchis viverrini*). *Carcinogenesis* 1994;**15**:271–5.

182 Thamavit W, Pairojkul C, Tiwawech D, *et al.* Strong promoting effect of *Opisthorchis viverrini* infection on dimethylnitrosamine-initiated hamster liver. *Cancer Lett* 1994;**78**: 121–5.

183 Masbou J, Valmary J, Bili H, *et al.* Simultaneous hepatic cholangiocarcinoma and bone fibrosarcoma 45 years after ingestion of Thorotrast. *Gastroenterol Clin Biol* 1995;**19**: 120–2.

184 Hayasaka K, Amoh K, Kakisaka A, *et al.* MRI appearance of Thorotrast-induced cholangiocarcinoma in a case of thorotrastosis. *Radiat Med* 1993;**11**:60–2.

185 Laplanche A, Clavel-Chapelon F, Contassot JC, *et al.* Exposure to vinyl chloride monomer: results of a cohort study after a seven year follow-up. The French VCM Group. *Br J Ind Med* 1992;**49**:134–7.

186 Swenberg JA, Fedtke N, Ciroussel F, *et al.* Etheno adducts found in DNA of vinyl chloride-exposed rats are highly persistent in liver. *Carcinogenesis* 1992;**13**:727–9.

187 Lambe M, Trichopoulos D, Hsieh CC, *et al.* Parity and cancers of the gallbladder and the extrahepatic bile ducts. *Int J Cancer* 1993;**54**:941–4.

188 Zatonski WA, La-Vecchia C, Przewozniak K, *et al.* Risk factors for gallbladder cancer: a Polish case–control study. *Int J Cancer* 1992;**51**:707–11.

189 Ghadirian P, Simard A, Baillargeon J. A population-based case–control study of cancer of the bile duct and gallbladder in Quebec, Canada. *Rev Epidemiol Santé Publique* 1992; **41**:107–12.

190 Kamel D, Paakko P, Nurova K, *et al.* p53 and c-erbB-2 protein expression in adenocarcinomas and epithelial dysplasia of the gall bladder. *J Pathol* 1993;**170**:67–72.

191 Suzuki T, Takano Y, Kakita A, *et al.* An immunohistochemical and molecular biological study of c-erbB-2 amplification and prognostic relevance in gallbladder cancer. *Pathol Res Pract* 1993;**189**:283–92.

192 Yukawa M, Fuijimori T, Hirayama D, *et al.* Expression of oncogene products and growth factors in early gallbladder cancer, advanced gallbladder cancer, and chronic cholecystitis. *Hum Pathol* 1993;**24**:37–40.

193 Watanabe M, Asaka M, Tanaka J, *et al.* Point mutation of K-ras gene codon 12 in biliary tract tumours. *Gastroenterology* 1994;**107**:1147–53.

194 Yoshida S, Todoroki T, Ichikawa Y, *et al.* Mutations of p16Ink4/CDKN2 and p15Ink4B/ MTS2 genes in biliary tract cancers. *Cancer Res* 1995;**55**:2756–60.

195 Wistuba II, Sugio K, Hung J, *et al.* Allele-specific mutations involved in the pathogenesis of endemic gallbladder carcinoma in Chile. *Cancer Res* 1995;**55**:2511–5.

196 Gold EB. Epidemiology of and risk factors for pancreatic cancer. *Surg Clin North Am* 1995;**75**:819–43.

197 Ji BT, Chow WH, Dai Q, *et al.* Cigarette smoking and alcohol consumption and the risk of pancreatic cancer: a case–control study in Shanghai, China. *Cancer Causes Control* 1995;**6**:369–76.

198 Meryn S. Pancreatic carcinoma—epidemiology and risk factors. *Wien Klin Wochenschr* 1994;**106**:694–7.

199 Bueno-de-Mesquita HB, Maisonneuve P, Moerman CJ, *et al.* Lifetime consumption of alcoholic beverages, tea and coffee and exocrine carcinoma of the pancreas: a population-based study in The Netherlands. *Int J Cancer* 1992;**50**:514–22.

200 Zheng W, McLaughlin JK, Gridley G, *et al.* A cohort study of smoking, alcohol consumption, and dietary factors for pancreatic cancer (United States). *Cancer Causes Control* 1993;**4**:477–82.

201 Bansal P, Sonnenberg A. Pancreatitis is a risk factor for pancreatic cancer. *Gastroenterology* 1995;**109**:247–51.

202 Lowenfels AB, Maisonneuve P, Cavallini G, *et al.* Pancreatitis and the risk of pancreatic cancer. International Pancreatitis Study Group. *N Engl J Med* 1993;**328**:1433–7.

203 Kalapothaki V, Tzonou A, Hsieh CC, *et al.* Tobacco, ethanol, pancreatitis, diabetes mellitus, and cholelithiasis as risk factors for pancreatic carcinoma. *Cancer Causes Control* 1993;**4**:375–82.

204 Everhart J, Wright D. Diabetes mellitus as a risk factor for pancreatic cancer. A meta-analysis. *JAMA* 1995;**273**:1605–9.

205 Girelli CM, Reguzzoni G, Limido E, *et al.* Pancreatic carcinoma: differences between patients with or without diabetes mellitus. *Recenti Prog Med* 1995;**86**:143–6.

206 Basso D, Plebani M, Fogar P, *et al.* Insulin-like growth factor-I, interleukin-1 alpha and beta in pancreatic cancer: role in tumor invasiveness and associated diabetes. *Int K Clin Lab Res* 1995;**25**:40–3.

207 Tada M, Ohashi M, Shiratori Y, *et al.* Analysis of K-ras gene mutation in hyperplastic duct cells of the pancreas without pancreatic disease. *Gastroenterology* 1996;**110**:227–31.

208 Caldas C, Hahn SA, Hruban RH, *et al.* Detection of K-ras mutations in the stool of patients with pancreatic adenocarcinoma and pancreatic ductal hyperplasia. *Cancer Res* 1994;**54**:3568–73.

209 Kondo H, Sugano K, Fukayama N, *et al.* Detection of point mutations in the K-ras oncogene at codon 12 in pure pancreatic juice for diagnosis of pancreatic carcinoma. *Cancer* 1994;**73**:1589–94.

210 Casey G, Yamanaka Y, Friess H, *et al.* p53 mutations are common in pancreatic cancer and are absent in chronic pancreatitis. *Cancer Lett* 1993;**69**:151–60.

211 Han HJ, Yanagisawa A, Kato Y, *et al.* Genetic instability in pancreatic cancer and poorly differentiated type of gastric cancer. *Cancer Res* 1993;**53**:5087–9.

212 McKie AB, Filipe MI, Lemoine NR. Abnormalities affecting the APC and MCC tumour suppressor gene loci on chromosome 5q occur frequently in gastric cancer but not in pancreatic cancer. *Int J Cancer* 1993;**55**:598–603.

4: Molecular biology

NICHOLAS R LEMOINE and ARTHUR B McKIE

Understanding of the genetic basis of malignant disease has advanced spectacularly since the mid-1980s, largely through investigation of the model of colorectal neoplasia, and as a result we are now at the dawn of a new era of clinical practice in which molecular genetics will be translated into benefits for diagnosis, screening, and treatment of this disease. As our knowledge increases, we can anticipate similar developments for tumours at other sites in the gastrointestinal tract, particularly cancers of the stomach and pancreas, and here we review the current state of knowledge and the potential for clinical application.

Cancer results from the clonal proliferation of cells which accumulate genetic defects that activate dominant oncogenes and inactivate tumour suppressor genes. In general, oncogenes encode growth factors, receptors, or other components of signal transduction pathways that can be activated either by overexpression or by mutations that alter the activity of the protein. Tumour suppressor genes encode a wide variety of proteins that are required for the control of cell division and behaviour, including cell cycle control factors, DNA repair proteins, and cell adhesion molecules. There are both similarities and differences in the pattern of genes involved in various tumour types, which reflect not only the type of genotoxic agent involved in carcinogenesis but also the normal control mechanisms at work in each organ.

Colorectal cancer

Inherited susceptibility to colorectal cancer

Familial adenomatous polyposis (FAP) and the APC gene

Approximately 1 in 8000 individuals is born with the familial polyposis mutation, which is inherited in an autosomal dominant fashion, leading to a characteristic clinical syndrome. That Gardner's syndrome is associated with abnormalities of the long arm of chromosome 5 was first reported in 1986; in 1991 the APC (for adenomatous polyposis coli) gene was cloned and sequenced. Although its cellular role remains uncertain, the observation that the protein product associates with catenin molecules involved in the control of E-cadherin function suggests that it may be involved in cell adhesion. It was found that most germline mutations affect the first half of the gene and result in truncation of the protein product; this observation has led to the development of a mutation detection system that can detect the shortened protein in over 80% of cases. The exact site of the mutation appears to correlate to some extent with the disease phenotype, such as the presence of congenital hypertrophy of the retinal pigment epithelium, the density of polyp formation in the colon, and the attenuated adenomatous polyposis coli and hereditary flat adenoma syndromes. Knowledge of the mutation in index cases can therefore be very helpful in management and counselling of the families.

Since FAP is a single gene disorder affecting a limited number of organs, it is a potential candidate for gene therapy to restore expression of a functional APC gene. This might be particularly appropriate for the rectal mucosa after ileorectal anastomosis, and for the prevention of upper gastrointestinal polyposis and desmoid disease. Clearly there will be difficulties in achieving gene transfer to the entire population of stem cells in the organs at risk and in ensuring appropriate transcriptional control using current technologies, but we can anticipate developments in this area that could make gene therapy for FAP a realistic therapeutic option.

Hereditary non-polyposis colorectal cancer and DNA mismatch repair enzyme genes (hMSH2, hMLH1, hPMS1, and hPMS2)

Hereditary non-polyposis colorectal cancer (HNPCC) is an autosomal dominant disorder with high penetrance that accounts for perhaps 5–15% of cases of colorectal cancer. In 1993 a concerted multinational effort identified a locus on chromosome 2p as responsible for HNPCC in two large kindreds, and shortly afterwards the gene, known as hMSH2, was cloned. This gene is the human homologue of genes in yeast and bacteria that had recently been shown to encode enzymes critical to the repair of DNA mismatches, and all of the mutations that occur in the hMSH2 gene lead to an aberrant or truncated product with loss of function. Subsequent investigation showed that three other related genes, hMLH1, hPMS1, and hPMS2, which all encode other DNA mismatch repair enzymes, are mutated in cases of HNPCC not linked to hMSH2, and so it appears that this disease phenotype is the result of a global defect in DNA replication fidelity. Recently it has been found that somatic deletions in microsatellite markers (the hallmark of the replication error phenotype) are present in 12% of sporadic colorectal tumours including adenomas, particularly those in the right side of the colon, and that there is an inverse correlation between these abnormalities and other genetic defects such as K-ras and p53 mutations. Thus, as well as being important for management of families known to have HNPCC, these discoveries may have implications for screening of the population for colorectal neoplasia. Therapeutic intervention for individuals at risk of cancer due to abnormalities in one of the DNA mismatch repair genes might in the future involve the development of drugs that could reduce replication errors, as well as gene therapy to restore normal gene expression.

Other types of familial colorectal cancer

There are other inherited genes that predispose to colorectal and other cancers. Inherited mutations in the p53 tumour suppressor gene are responsible for the Li–Fraumeni cancer predisposition syndrome; this gene is considered in more detail below. Another class of gene that may be important in predisposition to colorectal cancer is the family of genes encoding enzymes involved in drug detoxification; for instance, individuals with "fast" acetylator status have a twofold increased risk of colorectal cancer relative to those with the "slow" status (the acetylator locus is involved in detoxification of arylamines in cooked protein). Similarly, some alleles of the glutathione-*S*-transferase and the cytochrome *P*-450 family genes appear to be associated with excess risk. Although these genes may have a less powerful effect than the autosomal dominant genes responsible for FAP and HNPCC, their higher prevalence may mean that they contribute to a higher proportion of cases of colorectal cancer.

Kirsten ras (K-ras) oncogene

The K-ras gene is one of a family of three human ras genes (K-ras, H-ras, and N-ras) that encode small GTP-binding proteins that are localised to the inner leaflet of the cell membrane and are involved in transducing signals from receptor tyrosine kinases such as the epidermal growth factor (EGF) receptor. The receptors are coupled to ras proteins through an intermediate complex of GRB and SOS2 proteins, while downstream elements of the signal transduction pathway include the cytoplasmic RAF serine-threonine kinase and the mitogen-activated proteins (MAP)-kinase cascade. The ras proteins are activated on binding GTP and returned to the resting state by stimulation of their intrinsic GTPase activity by two GTPase activating (GAP) proteins. One of these is known as ras-GAP p120, while the other is neurofibromin, product of the NF1 tumour suppressor gene. The ras oncogenes are activated by point mutations that prevent the stimulation of GTPase function and so leave the ras proteins locked in the active GTP-bound conformation.

Mutations occur in more than 50% of colorectal cancers, with an increasing frequency in larger and more advanced lesions. Adenomas less than 1 cm in diameter have a K-ras mutation in less than 9% of cases, and the frequency of mutation increases with the size. Mutations occur at comparable frequency in lesions from patients with FAP, as in the sporadic disease, but as mentioned above the frequency appears to be lower in lesions from patients with HNPCC.

K-ras mutations are also found in aberrant crypt foci at high frequency, raising the possibility that such lesions, which have conventionally been considered hyperplastic, might in fact represent (pre)neoplastic events.

It is now possible to detect mutant K-ras oncogenes in DNA extracted (using highly sensitive DNA amplification techniques) from faecal samples containing cells exfoliated from neoplastic lesions of the gastrointestinal tract. Hence it may be possible to screen for the presence of early or even pre-neoplastic lesions using such molecular genetic techniques.

Mutant K-ras may represent a target for specific therapy using drugs that interfere with HMG-CoA reductase or other enzymes involved in cholesterol metabolism. Lovastatin is an example of this class of agent, and it has been shown to inhibit the growth and tumorigenicity of K-ras transformed cancer cells. Another approach is to apply antisense technology specifically to inhibit the expression of K-ras, using either synthetic oligonucleotides or recombinant genes introduced using gene transfer vectors such as viruses or liposome-complexed DNA.

Growth factors and growth factor receptors

Epidermal growth factor receptor and erb-B family

A large proportion of colorectal carcinomas and cell lines overexpress the epidermal growth factor receptor (EGFR) as well as several of its ligands, including transforming growth factor α (TGFα), amphiregulin, betacellulin and heparin-binding epidermal growth factor (HB-EGF), so forming potential autocrine loops.

Overexpression of EGFR seems to occur frequently (50–70%) in invasive colorectal adenocarcinomas, compared with the adjacent non-neoplastic mucosa, and is associated with malignant progression. Coexpression of EGFR and EGF has been seen at higher frequencies in colorectal tumours that show vascular and lymphatic invasion. Immunoreactive TGFα has also been detected in more than 80% of invasive colorectal adenocarcinomas, compared with only 24% of colorectal adenomas, but no correlation with clinical outcome has been demonstrated.

Recent studies have shown that amphiregulin is more frequently expressed in normal colorectal epithelial cells (100%) than in adenomatous polyps (60%) or invasive colorectal adenocarcinomas (50%). Amphiregulin immunoreactivity has been correlated with the degree of morphological differentiation (for example, tumour grade) of colorectal carcinomas but not with Dukes's stage and survival.

Cripto is a factor structurally related to the EGF family whose receptor has not yet been identified. Overexpression of cripto has been detected in more than 80% of invasive colorectal adenocarcinomas and in 60% of adenomatous polyps. Tumours with flat and excavated morphology show cripto immunoreactivity more frequently than the polypoid tumours. Interestingly, overexpression of cripto at the tumour-mucosal junction seems to be associated with lymph node involvement, bowel wall penetration, and poor survival.

erb-B3 is expressed in about 70% of colorectal carcinoma cell lines and tumour tissues but the significance of these findings is uncertain since normal colorectal epithelial cells express erb-B3 at similar levels.

Tumour suppressor genes

p53

Abnormalities of p53 are probably the most frequent genetic events associated with human cancer. It is now known that p53 plays a key role in protecting cells against DNA damage by producing cell cycle arrest followed by repair or (if the level of damage is too extreme) programmed cell death. Hence loss of function of p53 by mutation or deletion allows cells to accumulate mutations throughout the genome and short-circuits the protective mechanism of apoptosis.

Interest in p53 in colorectal cancer was stimulated by the finding that there was a high frequency (65%) of allele loss on chromosome 17p, which included the area carrying this gene. In cases in which one copy of p53 is deleted the remaining copy is frequently mutated to produce loss of function, but mutations also occur in tumours that retain a normal allele. Overall, about 75% of colorectal cancers have p53 abnormalities, but the frequency appears to be lower in mucinous carcinomas and right sided cancers than in other types. Mutations are rare and deletions are uncommon in adenomas of all sizes, unlike the situation for K-ras where lesions over 1 cm have a mutation frequency equivalent to cancers. This suggests that p53 may play a role in tumour progression, but clearly it is not an absolute requirement for malignancy because a significant proportion of cases have no detectable abnormality.

APC

Somatic mutation of the APC tumour suppressor gene is thought to be an important and relatively early event in sporadic as well as inherited colorectal cancer. Most of the heterozygosity and inactivating mutations are found in approximately 60% of both colorectal adenomas and carcinomas, and such changes can be found in adenomas as small as 5 mm in diameter; however, abnormalities of APC are not found in aberrant crypt foci, except in patients with FAP, suggesting that APC mutation could be a factor in their infrequent progression to a true adenoma.

DCC

The deleted in colon cancer (DCC) gene was discovered through positional cloning of the region on chromosome 18q which showed a very high rate (70%) of allele loss in colorectal cancer. The predicted structure of its protein product is homologous to neural cell adhesion molecules and there is accumulating evidence that it plays a role in controlling cell adhesion. It is lost as a relatively late event in colorectal cancer progression and hence may be involved in the processes of invasion and metastasis.

Pancreatic cancer

K-ras oncogene

Mutation at codon 12 of the K-ras oncogene is found in at least 75% of ductal adenocarcinomas of advanced stage, and pancreatic cancer is notable not only for the very high frequency of activation but also for the tight restriction of mutations to codon 12 alone (mutations in other tumour types may affect K-ras, H-ras, or N-ras and involve codons 13 and 61 in addition to codon 12). The most common base change at K-ras codon 12 in pancreatic cancers is a guanine to adenine (G to A) transition, similar to the situation for K-ras mutations in colorectal cancer but in marked contrast to the pattern observed in lung tumours, in which guanine to thymine (G to T) transversion is the most common lesion. The high prevalence of G to T transversions in lung cancer can be ascribed to the action of the carcinogen benzpyrene, which forms adducts with guanine residues and causes misrepair. The prevalence of G to A transitions in pancreatic cancer could be due to the action of a different class of carcinogen found in cigarette smoke, such as the aromatic amines and N-nitrosamines, and indeed there is evidence to suggest that the prevalence of K-ras point mutation is higher in patients who have smoked cigarettes than in those who have never smoked. Molecular epidemiology may reveal geographical or ethnic differences in the pathogenesis of this disease because the pattern of K-ras mutations has been reported to be markedly different in Japanese compared with European patients, and to show regional variations even within Europe.

It appears that K-ras point mutation is an early event in pancreatic tumorigenesis, associated with initiation or establishment of preinvasive carcinoma and in situ neoplastic lesions, and several reports suggest that mutations may be found in clonal lesions involving severe dysplasia of the ductal epithelium. Amplification of DNA by the polymerase chain reaction allows detection of mutation in cytological preparations or lesions comprising a few cells microdissected from histological slides. Recently there have been reports of K-ras mutations even in mucous cell hyperplasia without dysplasia, particularly in patients with a family history of pancreatic cancer, which is interesting in view of reports of increased risk of pancreatic cancer in those with chronic pancreatitis. The high frequency and specificity of K-ras mutations in early pancreatic cancer makes their detection an attractive approach to early diagnosis, and possibly even to screening in populations at risk (elderly smokers and those with chronic pancreatitis, for instance). Several groups have shown that polymerase chain reaction based techniques can successfully detect K-ras mutation in exfoliated tumour cells present in the pancreatic juice collected at endoscopic retrograde cholepancreatography of patients suspected of having pancreatic cancer. It is possible that this could also be applied to detect pancreatic cancer cells shed into the intestinal tract and it may be extended to pick up tumour cells in the peripheral blood.

Growth factors and growth factor receptors

Epidermal growth factor receptor and erb-B family

High levels of both EGFR and several of its ligands are seen in almost all ductal adenocarcinomas of the pancreas with the formation of potential autocrine loops. Coexpression of the EGF receptor with EGF and/or TGFα in individual tumour cells has been reported to be associated with shorter postoperative survival in a small series of patients. It has been proposed that upregulation of this ligand–receptor system may involve paracrine stimulation of the p75 and p55 TNFα receptors on tumour cells by cytokine produced by stromal cells. A recent study has shown that TGFα is abundant within the nerves in the pancreas, suggesting that the EGFR system may also be involved in the perineural invasion classically seen in pancreatic cancer.

Amphiregulin protein is present only in the nuclei of normal duct cells but it appears in the cytoplasm of malignant cells, sometimes exclusively and sometimes combined with nuclear immunoreactivity, and cases with amphiregulin immunoreactivity only in the cytoplasm have a poorer prognosis than those in which there is also nuclear immunoreactivity. Heparin-binding EGF mRNA has been detected in pancreatic cancer cells in vitro and the level of HB-EGF expression is usually higher in pancreatic cancer tissue than in the normal organ. Upregulation of cripto expression is seen in most pancreatic tumours, including invasive ductal adenocarcinomas, intraductal papillary mucinous tumours, and cystic tumours.

Increased expression of erb-B2 due to transcriptional upregulation is seen in 20–50% of pancreatic cancers and it remains uncertain whether there are associations with grade or stage. Overexpression of erb-B2 is very frequent in intraductal papillary mucinous tumours and appears to correlate with the grade of epithelial dysplasia. The tumour specific nature of high level erb-B2 overexpression has been exploited for the development of a novel form of gene therapy for cancer, namely genetically directed enzyme prodrug therapy. Constructs are made in which a gene encoding a non-mammalian enzyme capable of activating a prodrug to a cytotoxic agent (such as cytosine deaminase, which converts 5-fluorocytosine to 5-fluorouracil) is connected to the human erb-B2 promoter so that expression is driven specifically in tumour cells and only these cells are rendered susceptible to the toxic effects of the prodrug. If suitable gene delivery vehicles can be developed, this strategy could ultimately be used for the systemic treatment of metastatic pancreatic cancer.

The third member of the type 1 growth factor receptor family, the erb-B3 gene, is overexpressed in both pancreatitis and in pancreatic cancer, with the levels being higher in malignant disease. Upregulated expression may correlate with poor patient survival in invasive pancreatic cancer.

Hepatocyte growth factor and the MET receptor

Hepatocyte growth factor is found in the stromal elements of the normal pancreas by immunohistochemistry, and mRNA levels are reported to be elevated as much as 10-fold in pancreatic cancers, probably derived from cells in the stroma or possibly the islets of Langerhans as no expression can be detected in pancreatic cancer cells. Hepatocyte growth factor produces phosphorylation of the MET receptor in human pancreatic cancer cells in vitro and stimulates them to both scatter and proliferate; in cell lines that overexpress the MET receptor there is constitutive autophosphorylation, even in the absence of exogenous ligand. Upregulated expression of the MET receptor is frequently observed in pancreatic cancers, both in vitro and in vivo, and there is thus the possibility of paracrine stimulation of growth and abnormal motility, which may enhance invasion and metastasis.

Transforming growth factor β

Upregulated expression of transforming growth factor β (TGFβ) isoforms has been correlated with poor postoperative survival in a small series of patients with pancreatic cancer, and the expression of the TGFβ2 isoform has been associated with advanced tumour stage. Immunohistochemistry and RNA analysis shows that about 65% of cases express one or more of the three TGFβ isoforms at levels greater than or equal to those found in normal pancreatic tissues, with TGFβ1 being upregulated most dramatically; however, degenerating non-neoplastic cells involved by invasive tumour also show upregulated TGFβ expression, so this should not be regarded as a tumour specific phenomenon. The role played by TGFβ in epithelial–stromal interaction is likely to be complex because this cytokine is able to increase the production of extracellular matrix components, alter expression of adhesion molecules, and stimulate angiogenesis and fibrosis.

Fibroblast (heparin binding) growth factors and their receptors

The involvement of the large family of fibroblast growth factors (FGF1–9) and their high affinity receptors (FGFR1–4) in pancreatic pathology is complex. Low levels of FGF1 have been reported to be produced by exocrine pancreatic epithelial cells in chronic pancreatitis. An association of high level FGF1 expression and advanced stage ductal adenocarcinoma has been reported. In the normal pancreas the extracellular matrix shows immunoreactivity for FGF2 derived from acinar cells, and to a much lesser extent ductal cells, and expression is enhanced in chronic pancreatitis. Upregulated expression of FGF2 is found in the tumour cells of about 50% of cases of pancreatic cancer and there may be some association with advanced stage. Expression of FGFR1, 3, and 4 is found in the acinar cells and some vascular endothelium of the normal adult pancreas, and expression of one or more of these receptors is seen in the tumour cells of about 60% of pancreatic cancers, with a number of different splice variants observed.

Tumour suppressor genes

p53

Overall more than 50% of pancreatic tumours have some alteration of this gene. The p53 locus at chromosome 17p13 shows allelic loss (deletion of one copy of the gene) in up to 80% of cases of pancreatic cancer, while mutations are seen in over 50%. In contrast to the type of mutation affecting K-ras (mis-sense mutations restricted to a single codon), a wide variety is seen in p53. The vast majority (about 80%) are point mutations in the coding sequence of the gene, particularly the evolutionarily conserved exons 5–9 and other conserved residues, while the rest are intragenic deletions or (less commonly) microinsertions or splice site mutations that result in truncated proteins. The deletions and insertions appear to be a special feature of pancreatic cancer compared with other tumour types and typically are concentrated in homocopolymer tracts. Transitions are the most frequent type of point mutation (about 55% overall) and occur particularly at CpG sites, which probably reflects spontaneous deamination at methylated cytosine residues.

p16

The p16 gene that lies at chromosome 9p21 is variously referred to as p16^{ink4}, CDKN4I, CDKN2, and MTS1. Mutations of this gene are commonly observed in established cancer cell lines but appear to be relatively rare in most primary tumour types, except pancreatic cancer in which 80% of cases show inactivation. In about half of these cases there is a loss of function mutation in one allele accompanied by deletion of the other, while the rest have homozygous deletion of both alleles. The deleted fragment commonly includes the adjacent candidate tumour suppressor gene p15, another cell cycle inhibitor closely related in sequence to p16, and it is possible that this gene is also important in the pathogenesis of the condition. The possibility that inactivation of the p16 gene occurs almost exclusively in pancreatic cancer and not in other gastrointestinal tumours could make it possible to design multiplex genetic assays which localise the origin of shed neoplastic cells.

DPC4

Inactination of this putative tumour suppressor gene on the long arm of chromosome 18 occurs in at least 30% of cases of pancreatic cancer. Its protein product is predicted to be involved in control of TGFβ signalling.

DCC

Allelic imbalance is observed fairly frequently on the long arm of chromosome 18 (18q), but while expression levels of DCC may vary substantially in pancreatic cancers, complete extinction is rare and deletion of the DCC locus is uncommon.

RB1

This gene appears to be only rarely affected even in advanced pancreatic cancer. Although one study reported aberrations in Rb expression in some pancreatic cell lines, subsequent work suggests that genuine loss of Rb function is very uncommon in either cell lines or clinical material. Recently it has been suggested that the high prevalence of allelic imbalance around the RB1 locus at chromosome 13q14 reflects the involvement of the breast cancer susceptibility gene 2 (BRCA2) at 13q12.

APC

There have been conflicting reports of the involvement of this gene in human pancreatic cancer, and it may be that Japanese cases show an especially high frequency compared with American or European patients. It is interesting that APC gene mutations are apparently frequent in ampullary cancers, and it is possible that the origin of some cases of pancreatic cancer is misclassified.

DNA mismatch repair genes (hMSH2, hMLH1, hPMS1, and hPMS2)

As with abnormalities of the APC and DCC genes, there may be distinct differences between the Japanese and other populations in the involvement of this class of tumour suppressor gene: while a Japanese group reported a few cases of microsatellite instability indicative of defects in DNA mismatch repair, American and European studies have found this to be a relatively rare phenomenon.

Gastric cancer

K-ras and other ras oncogenes

Mutations of ras oncogenes are relatively uncommon in gastric cancer, only around 20% of gastric cancers having activating mutations, and these have been described at codons 12, 13, or 61 of K-ras, N-ras, or H-ras. This is in sharp contrast to the situation for colorectal and pancreatic cancer where the majority of cases possess activating mutations restricted to K-ras at codon 12. The gastric tumours that possess mutations are usually intestinal in type, including a proportion of gastric adenomas. In countries where the incidence of gastric cancer is very high (such as South Africa), ras mutations are rarely found and hence it is possible that different genotoxic carcinogens are involved.

Growth factors and growth factor receptors

Epidermal growth factor receptor and erb-B family

Overexpression of the EGF receptor is relatively common in gastric adenocarcinomas, being reported at frequencies of 30–50% in most series, and appears to be more frequent in intestinal type than diffuse type tumours. The mechanism of overexpression appears to involve transcriptional upregulation, as amplification of the EGFR gene is rare in gastric cancer. Occasionally there may be moderate EGFR upregulation in simple intestinal metaplasia and immunoreactivity for this receptor cannot therefore be considered to be a marker of neoplasia in the stomach.

Of the ligands for the EGFR, at least TFGα, amphiregulin and (to a lesser extent) EGF are reported to be frequently expressed at an elevated level in gastric cancer. TGFα is found in 50–75% of cancers and about 20% of cases of intestinal metaplasia, particularly in the mucosal field surrounding a cancer. Coexpression of this ligand with the EGFR in cancers is associated with increased proliferative activity, invasive tumour phenotype, and poor patient survival. Transgenic mice engineered to overexpress TGFα in the stomach develop severe adenomatous hyperplasia, similar to Ménétrier's disease in the human, supporting a role for this autocrine circuit in gastric tumorigenesis. Amphiregulin is expressed in about 30% of intestinal metaplasia and 50% of gastric cancers, often in association with EGFR expression. Cripto is commonly coexpressed with TGFα and amphiregulin in both intestinal metaplasia (50% of cases) and in gastric cancer (50% of cases overall), with higher frequencies observed in advanced compared with early cancers, and in intestinal compared with diffuse type cancers in Japanese series.

The erb-B2 gene is amplified in about 10% of gastric cancers and overexpression (due to transcriptional upregulation as well as gene amplification) is found in about 20% of cases overall, more commonly in intestinal type (50% of cases) than in diffuse type cancers (5% of cases). Although it remains a controversial issue, it appears that erb-B2 overexpression may be associated with poor prognosis in patients with intestinal type cancers. Overexpression of erb-B2 is also found in about 10% of intestinal type adenocarcinomas arising in Barrett's mucosa of the oesophagus. Upregulated expression of erb-B2 appears to be restricted to malignant lesions of the stomach, and is found neither in gastric adenomas nor in intestinal metaplasia.

erb-B3 is expressed only in the parietal cells of the normal gastric glands, and is found at elevated levels in around 70% of gastric cancers overall, with higher frequency in intestinal than diffuse type tumours. There is also slightly elevated expression in intestinal metaplasia, although the immunoreactivity in such cases tends to be cytoplasmic rather than membrane-bound so its functional significance is presently uncertain.

Hepatocyte growth factor and the MET receptor

The MET oncogene is frequently amplified in advanced gastric cancer, and overexpression of the MET receptor due to gene amplification is correlated with advanced tumour stage (including the presence of lymph node metastases) and poor prognosis. Abnormalities of MET are particularly frequent in diffuse and scirrhous cancer, all of the scirrhous carcinoma cell lines in one study showing gene amplification.

Fibroblast (heparin binding) growth factors and their receptors

A variant of the FGFR2 gene, known as K-sam, is frequently amplified in diffuse gastric cancers, and it is likely that there is some connection between the expression of this receptor and the phenotype of this tumour type. It has been shown that this FGF receptor variant may be expressed in at least four forms, two of which are membrane-bound and two of which are potentially secreted to interact with ligands at other sites.

A locus on chromosome 11q13 contains a cluster of genes that are amplified together in a proportion of gastric cancers as well as in the majority of oesophageal cancers. Two of the genes in the amplicon (HST1 and INT2) encode members of the FGF family (FGF3 and FGF4 respectively) but it appears that neither is overexpressed, despite them being present in up to 30 times the normal copy number. Instead, it is the cell cycle control gene cyclin D1 lying close by that is actually overexpressed, resulting in inappropriate cell division.

Transforming growth factor β

More than 80% of gastric cancers show a reduction in expression of the type 1 TGFβ receptor, as well as inappropriately low levels of the TGFβ inhibitory element binding protein. There appears to be a correlation between this expression pattern and the depth of invasion through the stomach wall, leading to the suggestion that invasion is favoured by escape from the growth inhibition normally exerted by TGFβ.

Tumour suppressor genes

p53

Allele loss and mutations of the p53 tumour suppressor gene occur in more than 60% of gastric cancers and (although there is some controversy on this issue) appear to be more common in the intestinal than in the diffuse type. The mutations are mostly mis-sense mutations producing a change in the p53 protein sequence, but a significant proportion are nonsense mutations producing premature truncation. Frameshift mutations resulting from microdeletions and insertions are relatively uncommon, in contrast to pancreatic cancer. Mutations at CpG dinucleotides are particularly frequent, and this has been taken as evidence in support of the involvement of ingested nitrosamines and the chronic production of nitric oxide in response to *Helicobacter pylori* infestation because these factors favour deamination of cytosine residues. Mutations have been observed in approximately 10% of cases of gastric dysplasia and up to 30% of gastric adenomas, implying that p53 abnormalities could be relatively early events in gastric tumorigenesis.

APC

Abnormalities of the APC tumour suppressor gene are very frequent in intestinal type cancers, allele loss and gene mutation being found in around 45% of such cases. In contrast, it does not appear to occur at all in diffuse type cancers and is relatively rare in signet ring cell cancers. The type of mutation of this gene in gastric cancer is interesting because almost all of them are mis-sense mutations, in contrast to the nonsense (truncation producing) mutations seen in both inherited and sporadic colorectal cancers. Further evidence of the potential importance of the cell adhesion system involving APC in gastric cancer is the observation that reduction or loss of expression of α catenin (the molecule with which APC interacts to control E-cadherin function) occurs in at least 60% of cases. While E-cadherin expression appears to be normal in intestinal type cancers, there is almost always loss of expression in diffuse cancers, sometimes accompanied by structural mutations of the E-cadherin gene.

DNA mismatch repair genes (hMSH2, hMLH1, hPMS1, and hPMS2)

Microsatellite instability, the hallmark of the replication error phenotype, is found in 64% of diffuse type gastric cancers and in 17% of those of intestinal type. Interestingly, the frequency of such abnormalities is even higher in cases with multiple gastric cancers, implying that failure of DNA repair is particularly important in predisposition to the development of independent clonal lesions in the gastric mucosa. Microsatellite instability has also been found in some cases of gastric adenoma, again pointing to early involvement in tumorigenesis by allowing the accumulation of abnormalities at multiple genetic loci. Screening for microsatellite instability may be useful for selecting patients who are at high risk of developing multiple cancers, both within the stomach and elsewhere.

Future prospects

Analysis of the genes involved in the different types of gastrointestinal cancer gives us clues about the pathogenesis of the disease as well as offering opportunities for application in clinical settings. Not only do we now have the appropriate tools for the development of molecular genetic tests for early diagnosis and screening for malignant disease but we also have the prospect of identifying those at high risk of developing particular types of gastrointestinal cancer at a point when clinical intervention, perhaps by life style alteration or even gene therapy, could prevent the disease altogether. The 1990s have seen dramatic developments in the cancer research laboratories of the world; we look forward to the future when these should be translated into the clinic.

Further reading

Bishop DT, Hall NR. The genetics of colorectal cancer. *Eur J Cancer* 1994;**13**:1946–56.

Lemoine NR. Molecular pathology of pancreatic duct neoplasms. In: Sirica AE, Longnecker DS, eds. *Biliary and pancreatic ductal epithelia: pathobiology and pathophysiology.* New York: Marcel Dekker, 1996.

Lemoine NR, Neoptolemos JP, Cooke T, eds. *Cancer: a molecular approach.* Oxford: Blackwell Scientific, 1994.

Neoptolemos JP, Lemoine NR, eds. *Pancreatic cancer: molecular and clinical advances.* Oxford: Blackwell Scientific, 1996.

Stemmermann G, Heffleflinger SC, Noffsinger A, *et al.* The molecular biology of esophageal and gastric cancer and their precursors: oncogenes, tumor suppressor genes and growth factors. *Hum Pathol* 1995;**25**:968–81.

5: Oesophagus

Epidemiology, investigation, and surgical management

JOHN BANCEWICZ and HARUSHI OSUGI

Oesophageal cancer is a challenging disease with a poor outlook. There is thus some justification for the widespread pessimism that affects clinicians who manage these patients. Not every patient, however, has a bad prognosis: there are many whose disease can be cured, and for those who are incurable methods of palliation continue to improve.

At present surgical resection remains the major curative treatment. Radiotherapy is also potentially curative, particularly for squamous carcinomas above the lower third of the oesophagus. Although never tested by formal randomised study, the reported results of radiotherapy are generally felt to be inferior to those of surgical resection (see Peake and Cottier below).

Care in patient selection and meticulous attention to technical detail are essential if the best results are to be achieved. To this end many European surgeons have looked with interest to the results of Japanese surgeons because these seem better than is often achieved in Europe and the USA. Japanese colleagues have a well developed tradition of accurate preoperative staging and emphasise radical surgical resection with meticulous surgical display, accurate anatomical dissection, and avoidance of blood loss.

This chapter is presented from both Japanese and British surgical viewpoints. The two contributors have built up a close personal and professional relationship since the early 1980s and think that the different surgical attitudes in the two countries harbour a debate that is of crucial importance for the effective management of oesophageal cancer.

Epidemiology

Squamous cell cancer and adenocarcinoma are different diseases with a different aetiology. Worldwide, squamous cancer is the more common condition, but adenocarcinoma due to malignant change in Barrett's oesophagus has become increasingly common in many Westernised countries. In some, adenocarcinoma is now more common than squamous cancer and its incidence is rising steadily. The reason for this change is unknown. The incidence of cancer of the gastric cardia is also increasing, suggesting that this is probably the same disease.

The guidelines for clinical and pathological studies of carcinoma of the oesophagus of the Japanese Society for Esophageal Diseases define oesophageal cancer as one that originates in the oesophagus or whose centre is in the oesophagus or at the oesophagogastric junction when the lesion involves the cardia.[1] This simple and convenient definition is used in this chapter. Contrary to popular opinion oesophageal cancer is more common in the United Kingdom than in Japan, the incidence being 7·4 per 100 000 and 5·7 per 100 000 respectively. In 1992 it accounted for over 2·5% of all cancers registered in males and almost 2% of registrations in females in the United Kingdom (Office of Population Censuses and Surveys). Provisional statistics for 1993 show that cancer of the oesophagus caused 6480 deaths (3880 males and 2600 females), accounting for approximately 4·0% of all cancer deaths. Squamous cancer accounts for 94% of Japanese cases, most of which are located in the middle third, but adenocarcinoma now accounts for more than 60% of British cases, which are mostly in the lower third. Smoking and alcohol consumption are relevant aetiological factors in both countries.

In 11% of Japanese cases more than one cancer is found in the oesophagus. Metachronous lesions also occur. Accurate figures are not available for the United Kingdom.

Investigation: clinical presentation and diagnosis

Most oesophageal cancer presents with dysphagia. Non-specific dyspepsia or reflux-like symptoms may occur in early cases. Advanced disease may cause anaemia, respiratory infection due to overflow or fistulation, and chest pain. There is growing emphasis on early endoscopy for those with non-specific upper gastrointestinal symptoms and for systematic screening of high risk cases. In Western countries it is now common to screen patients with Barrett's oesophagus by annual endoscopy and mucosal biopsy. In Japan the emphasis is on screening for gastric cancer, because that is a common disease, but more attention is being paid to careful inspection of the oesophagus. In 1982 in Japan only 2% of patients with oesophageal cancer were detected at the presymptomatic stage. An unpublished analysis by Endo has shown that 71% of 500 cases of early mucosal cancer of the oesophagus resected between 1984 and 1989 were detected during either screening endoscopy or the investigation of unrelated symptoms. No Japanese national figures are available for the proportion of cases that are currently detected in the presymptomatic stage, but it is expected that this is now significantly greater than 2%.

In the West, screening of patients with Barrett's oesophagus is also yielding a proportion of cases at an early stage, but it has been a little disappointing. Adenocarcinoma of the oesophagus seems a more aggressive disease than squamous cell cancer. Considerable effort is being invested in improving current results.

Diagnosis of most symptomatic oesophageal cancer is not difficult. Modern video endoscopy gives excellent views of the whole of the oesophagus and even small lesions can be seen; however, very early lesions give trouble in both countries and may be extremely difficult to find.

In the United Kingdom the major problem is the diagnosis of malignant transformation in Barrett's oesophagus. Early malignancy may occur with no gross change and multiple routine biopsies are essential. The minimum recommendation at present is quadrantic biopsies at 2 cm intervals.

In Japan the early diagnosis of oesophageal cancer is emphasised as much as the early diagnosis of gastric cancer. A nationwide study of resected oesophageal cancer from 1983 to 1989 showed that 18% of patients had Tis (in situ) or T1 tumours. Detection of such small lesions is difficult and the use of iodine staining at endoscopy is recommended. The endoscopist looks for minute changes in the mucosa, such as slight coarseness, reddening, or depression or elevation of the mucosa. Unstained areas greater than 10 mm in diameter should be biopsied. For assessment of Barrett's oesophagus vital staining with iodine or other stains has not increased the detection of early cancer because there is a greater preponderance of non-specific change that alters patterns of staining.

Early cancer of the oesophagus behaves in a more aggressive manner than early cancer of the stomach, presumably because of the different stuctures of the two organs. Lymph node metastasis and lymphatic and vascular permeation is particularly high in cancer that extends to the submucosal layer of the oesophagus. Carcinoma limited to the epithelium or mucosal layer has the same incidence of lymphatic invasion as carcinoma of the stomach that extends into the submucosal layer.[2] Thus the challenge of early diagnosis is greater for the oesophagus than for the stomach.

Patient assessment and tumour staging

Once the diagnosis of oesophageal cancer has been made, all patients should be assessed as candidates for curative treatment. The twin aims of this are:

- to offer potentially curative treatment to those in whom there is a reasonable expectation of cure
- to avoid inappropriately aggressive treatment in those who are not likely to be cured.

In some cases it will be quite obvious on superficial examination that cure is impossible, because of extreme age, poor general health, or advanced disease. Detailed investigation should not be performed in such circumstances. In most newly diagnosed cases systematic investigation will, however, be required.

Assessment of the tumour (staging)

The most important aspect of staging is a painstaking search for metastatic disease that would preclude cure. Such a search should include:

- clinical examination with careful examination of the neck for lymphadenopathy, including ultrasonography in doubtful cases
- chest x ray
- ultrasonography of the liver and upper abdomen
- computed tomography (CT) of the neck, thorax, and abdomen
- bronchoscopy to detect tracheobronchial invasion that may occur in lesions of the middle or upper thirds
- laparoscopy for adenocarcinomas of the lower oesophagus or cardia.

If evidence of metastasis is found at an early stage of investigation it will usually be inappropriate to complete the above list of investigations.

In the United Kingdom the discovery of distant metastases is usually taken as an indication for palliative treatment, such as laser or intubation. In Japan palliative resection is much more widely used but the surgical approach may be altered—for example, transhiatal resection.

Endoscopy

In patients undergoing assessment for radical treatment it is useful for the surgeon to repeat the endoscopy. It is essential to have accurate localisation of the tumour in order to plan surgical resection appropriately. Accurate knowledge of the site and extent of the tumour is especially important for tumours of the lower oesophagus and cardia because of the variety of surgical approaches to these tumours. Synchronous lesions of the aerodigestive tract may be present and should always be sought.

In Japan endoscopic staging is emphasised much more strongly than in the United Kingdom. This is largely because more effort is invested in detecting and treating early lesions. The superficial flat type lesion that is confined to the epithelium appears as a mucosal reddening with an unclear border or a whitish mucosal thickening with disappearance of the normal arborescent appearance of the small mucosal vessels. Superficial protuberant lesions less than 1 mm in height and superficial depressed lesions less than 0·5 mm deep are usually limited to the epithelium or to the mucosa if they do not spread more than 5 cm. Lesions with a nodular or irregular surface tend to invade deeper than those with a granular or fine surface. Thus lesions that are easily detectable by conventional endoscopic observation have already invaded into the submucosal layer or deeper. It is for this reason that oesophageal irrigation and iodine staining is widely used in

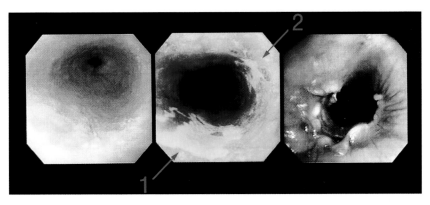

FIGURE 5.1—*Left—an endoscopic picture showing a slightly depressed lesion with granular surface (mucosal). Middle—iodine staining shows the lesion detected by conventional observation (1) and revealed another unstained area (2) which was a superficial flat cancer (epithelial). Right—lesion 1 was resected by endoscopic mucosal resection; lesion 2 was resected later.*

Japan (Figure 5.1). All cancerous lesions at any depth of invasion remain unstained with iodine; however, not all unstained lesions are cancer, and iodine staining has proved less helpful in the West.

Since 11% of patients with oesophageal cancer have more than one lesion, Japanese surgeons recommend iodine staining even in patients with an advanced lesion.

Barium radiology

Barium radiology has a less dominant role than formerly. Nevertheless, it provides a useful "road map" of malignant lesions. It is particularly useful if it has been impossible to pass an endoscope through the tumour. In advanced lesions a barium swallow gives the best documentation of oesophagobronchial fistulation or of deep ulceration. The finding of axis deviation of the oesophagus, in which the normal anatomical line of the oesophagus changes abruptly at the tumour, indicates a high chance of invasion of neighbouring structures.

Ultrasonography

Ultrasonography is useful for the detection of liver metastasis, which most surgeons would regard as precluding surgical resection. Ultrasonography and CT are complementary techniques for the diagnosis of liver metastases and ideally both should be performed.

Computed tomography

CT is at its best for the detection of metastatic disease to the liver or lungs and is mandatory before embarking on a resection.

CT of the thorax to examine the primary tumour is not sufficiently accurate to indicate incurability or irresectability.[3] It is at its least accurate for the assessment of lymph node invasion. A study performed in Osaka City University Hospital involved detailed pathology on 3661 nodes removed from 72 patients having extended lymphadenectomy. Receiver operator curve (ROC) analysis suggested that 8 mm diameter gave the best discrimination between invaded and non-invaded nodes, with a sensitivity of 65% and a specificity of 76%. CT and magnetic resonance imaging (MRI) can detect nodes of 1 cm diameter so many invaded nodes are missed. Enlarged nodes detected by CT have an 86% chance of being invaded; however, nodes below the tracheal bifurcation may be larger, yet still not invaded.

CT is more accurate for the detection of tracheobronchial invasion or aortic invasion, but the criteria for making this assessment are critical and require careful audit in individual institutions. In the United Kingdom it is now unusual to see aortic invasion, and tracheal invasion is much less common than formerly. Individual CT reports should therefore be regarded with suspicion and reviewed in a specialist centre.

Magnetic resonance imaging

MRI has not yet been shown to improve the accuracy of preoperative staging,[4] but this is a continuously evolving technology and some improvement may be expected. MRI may be better than CT for detecting tracheobronchial invasion if the criteria for a positive examination include disappearance of the high intensity signal between the oesophageal wall and the trachea or bronchus. This strong signal is thought to be generated by the normal tracheobronchial membrane.

Endoscopic ultrasonography

Endoscopic ultrasonography (EUS) is the best method of staging the primary lesion and evaluating lymph node spread.[45] It is a mature technology in Japan and is widely available in most European countries and the USA, but in only a few centres in the United Kingdom.

The normal oesophageal wall is seen as a five layer structure (sometimes seven layers with high frequency probes) of alternating hyperechoic and

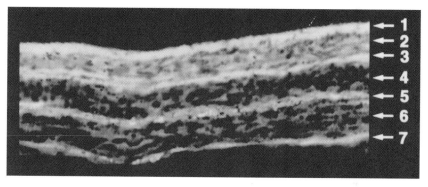

FIGURE 5.2—*Ultrasonographic structure of the oesophageal wall delineated with a 20 MHz sonoprobe. Layers 1 and 2 correspond to mucosa, layer 3 to submucosa, layers 4, 5, and 6 to the muscularis propria, and layer 7 to the adventitia.*

hypoechoic bands (Figure 5.2). The depth of tumour invasion can be assessed with 85% accuracy by EUS (Figures 5.3 and 5.4). Lymph node invasion can be detected with 87% accuracy because smaller nodes can be seen and the internal architecture can be assessed.

Lymph nodes are detected as oval hypoechoic areas. Nodes as small as 3 mm can be detected. The diagnosis of metastasis is based on the diameter of the nodes and the ratio of the smaller:larger diameter (≥ 0.5 indicates invasion). The characteristics of the border and the internal echo of the node are also helpful (Figures 5.5–5.7). Nodes with a clear border and uneven, coarse, or scattered internal echo can be diagnosed as metastatic with an accuracy of 87%.[6]

EUS seems particularly useful for assessing very early cancers that may be amenable to mucosal resection or ablation. It should also have a place for the selection of groups of patients who might be entered into prospective randomised studies of preoperative treatment with drugs or radiation.

103

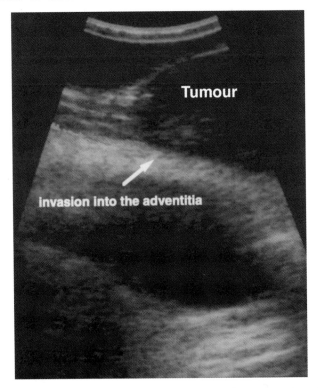

FIGURE 5.3—*Endoscopic ultrasonogram (7·5 MHz) showing tumour invasion into the adventitia.*

The main limitation of EUS at present is that the instrument has a 4 cm rigid tip, 13 mm in diameter, and it may not be possible to pass it through the tumour. Newer probes that can be passed down the biopsy channel of a standard endoscope have, however, been developed. Ironically, these have a limited depth of view and are better for assessing superficial lesions than the deeply invading lesion that is likely to produce marked stenosis.

Laparoscopy

Laparoscopy is used by a minority of clinicians at present but it is a simple technique that gives useful information in those patients with adenocarcinomas of the lower oesophagus and cardia, particularly the latter.[78] Its main strength is in the assessment of transperitoneal spread; hence its value in lesions that may extend below the phreno-oesophageal ligament. It still has a place for the diagnosis of metastatic disease of the liver, which is occasionally missed by non-invasive imaging.

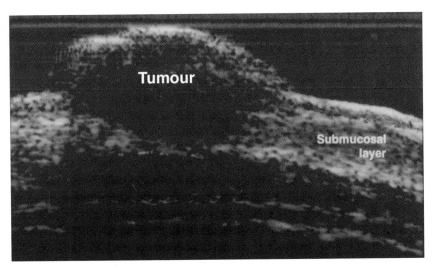

FIGURE 5.4—*Tumour invading deep into the submucosa revealed by 20 MHz sonoprobe.*

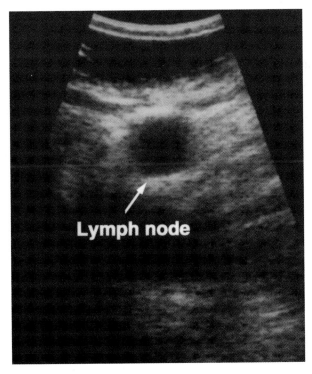

FIGURE 5.5—*Endoscopic ultrasonogram showing a lymph node without metastasis.*

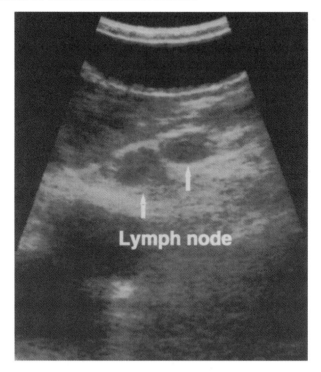

FIGURE 5.6—*Lymph node with metastasis showing clear border and coarse internal echo.*

Importance of histology

The presence of metastatic disease detected by any method of imaging should be confirmed by biopsy if at all possible. None of the imaging methods is 100% reliable[9] and it is a tragedy to refuse potentially curative treatment to a patient because of overinterpretation of computed tomograms or ultrasonograms.

Assessment of the patient

Radical treatment for oesophageal cancer is hazardous and it is therefore particularly important to assess the fitness of patients for any treatment that is proposed. Mortality after oesophageal resection is related to age, tumour size, and lung function (forced expiratory volume in one second, FEV_1).[10] Simple lung function tests, routine cardiovascular tests, and overall assessment by an experienced clinician give a reasonably accurate assessment of the risk of resection. In the United Kingdom respiratory function is usually the major limiting factor. It is impossible to give hard and fast rules because estimating respiratory reserve is somewhat imprecise

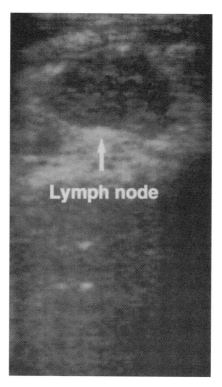

FIGURE 5.7—*Lymph node with metastasis showing clear border and scattered internal echo.*

and biological age may differ from chronological age; however, a useful rule of thumb runs as given in Table 5.1.

TABLE 5.1—*Respiratory function in patient assessment*

Age (years)	FEV$_1$ (litres)	Action
<70	>1·5	Resect
70–75	1·3–1·5	Think
75–80	1·0–1·3	Think carefully
>80	<1·0	Do not resect

Clearly such rules are for general guidance only and their applicability will vary with the prevalence of cardiopulmonary disease in individual areas. The British author works in an area with a particularly high prevalence of severe cardiac and respiratory disease and many patients with oesophageal cancer are obese. The Japanese author sees a greater proportion of relatively

107

fit patients, of whom most are lean. Both authors were surprised to learn that there is an enormous difference in the incidence of perioperative venous thrombotic disease between Britain and Japan. In Osaka, as elsewhere in Japan, no prophylaxis for deep vein thrombosis is used because the incidence is so low! It is to be hoped that more accurate methods of operative risk assessment will evolve. As well as being useful for decision making in the individual patient, they would aid objective international comparison of results. The POSSUM scoring system may well meet this need.[11]

Nutritional status and nutritional support

Severe malnutrition usually indicates advanced cancer. If it occurs there is no point in attempting restoration to normal nutritional status before resection as this takes too long to be practical. Partial nutritional restoration has not been shown to reduce the risks of oesophageal resection, but this remains a controversial topic.[12 13]

Despite these comments, good nutritional advice and the sensible use of dietary supplements and substitutes, particularly liquid diets, is an important aspect of treatment.

General support

Oesophageal cancer and the process of assessment and treatment are extremely stressful to patients and their relatives, even when cure is achieved. Considerable effort therefore needs to be directed to general care, to counselling, and to psychological support. Clinicians, hospital nurses, district nurses, specialised cancer care nurses, such as the MacMillan nurses in the United Kingdom, and patient support groups all have a part to play. This aspect of treatment tends to be neglected and needs to be improved.

Surgical management

Surgical excision of the oesophagus for the treatment of cancer has improved considerably in recent years because of developments in anaesthetic management, surgical techniques, and perioperative care, including pain relief. This has produced lower operative mortality rates, and several series report increased long term survival, but there is still intense debate as to whether this is due to better treatment, case selection, or simply chance variation in disease severity. There is a very wide variation in reported operative mortality rates and five year survival rates. Assessment of the relevant literature must also be qualified by the fact that most published reports are from enthusiastic experts who think that their results are good. There are very few examples of population based survival statistics that allow accurate assessment of the value of various treatments.

Despite these reservations, the bias of both authors is that reasonable results can be achieved with surgical resection provided that careful attention is paid to case selection and to the details of operative technique.

Because of the disappointing results of surgical resection it has become fashionable to refer to surgical palliation rather than to surgical cure; however, good palliation of dysphagia can now be produced without resection and it is therefore pertinent to ask why one should embark on a major operation if short term palliation is the only aim. In Japan there is still a strong feeling that surgical resection produces the best palliation. The British author feels that resection should not be performed if there is no chance of cure, or only a minimal chance. Whichever policy is adopted, both authors feel that the concept of curative surgery is an important one and that the primary aim of surgical resection should be cure whenever possible.

Radical excision

Radical excision involves removal of the primary tumour and other tissues that might be invaded. Tumours in the oesophagus have a propensity for extensive proximal spread in the submucosal lymphatics. Surgical clearance should therefore take account of this and generous proximal clearance is commonly recommended. McKeown popularised the concept of subtotal oesophagectomy in the United Kingdom. In this operation only a small proximal stump is left behind and proximal tumour clearance is invariably complete for lesions as high as the middle third. This was popularised by McKeown in the 1970s and was associated with five year survival of approximately 30% at a time when the average was 10–15%.[14] Not all surgeons subscribe to this principle, but the evidence is persuasive and an additional benefit is that gastrointestinal function is better with an oesophagogastric anastomosis above the level of the aortic arch.

In Japan there is a longer tradition of safe oesophagectomy than in the United Kingdom. Nakayama was the first to report low operative mortality rates, but the cost of this to the patient was a staged resection and reconstruction, which took several months to complete and involved a temporary oesophagostomy. This never gained favour outside Japan, but Nakayama's results provided a benchmark against which to measure the results of single stage resection and reconstruction.

Lesions of the cardia may be dealt with by subtotal oesophageal resection provided that the tumour in the proximal stomach can be cleared adequately and still leave enough stomach for a satisfactory reconstruction. Total gastrectomy and distal oesophagectomy is an alternative approach favoured by the British contributor. DeMeester has suggested subtotal oesophagectomy and total gastrectomy with reconstruction by colonic interposition in fit patients with potentially curable disease.[15] This is a very major undertaking and only suitable for very carefully selected cases.

With careful case selection and an experienced team, reasonable survival figures can be obtained. Salama and Leong in Nottingham report an overall five year survival of 36% for squamous cancers, but only 3% for adenocarcinomas.[16] The latter figure is unusually low and may reflect local referral patterns. The operative mortality was 10·6%. Menke-Pluymers *et al* report 24% five year survival after resection for adenocarcinoma in Barrett's oesophagus, with 6% operative mortality.[17] These figures confirm that cancer of the oesophagus is a bad disease, but they show that it is not untreatable. Survival, as with all cancers, is stage related and overall survival figures reflect the stage mix within individual series.

Survival figures and operative mortality rates vary markedly in the surgical literature. While some of the variation must be due to stage mix and general risk factors, there is a growing body of evidence that suggests that the best results come from centres that treat the disease regularly.[18]

"Standard" resection: the Lewis–Tanner procedure

There are many methods of oesophagectomy and reconstruction but the Lewis–Tanner procedure is probably the most widely practised. The stomach is first mobilised at laparotomy and intra-abdominal lymph node dissection is done at the discretion of the surgeon. The patient is then turned into the lateral position and the right chest is opened. This allows easy mobilisation of the whole of the intrathoracic oesophagus. The only major anatomical structure between the surgeon and the oesophagus is the azygos vein, which is easily divided.

Although a variety of other approaches may be used, this is arguably the most straightforward and versatile method of access. A popular alternative is to use a left thoracotomy or thoracoabdominal approach. This allows access to the oesophagus below the aortic arch and is often used for lesions of the distal oesophagus or cardia. The attraction of this is that it is a single incision operation that allows limited resection with a low mortality rate. The disadvantage is that postoperative reflux symptoms may be very troublesome and cure may be compromised. Reported series with a high proportion of left thoracic resections have a high local recurrence rate and disappointing five year survival rates.[19]

Once access has been gained, the subsequent procedure varies widely between individual surgeons. Some resect only a limited portion of the oesophagus and stomach, others perform subtotal oesophagectomy. The bias of the authors is in favour of subtotal oesophagectomy because this gives optimum clearance of the submucosal lymphatics and produces an excellent functional result with a low incidence of troublesome reflux. The

British contributor performs an anastomosis in the chest at the thoracic inlet. The Japanese contributor performs an anastomosis in the neck, often including a lymph node dissection in the lower part of the neck as part of a three field operation.

The principle of subtotal oesophagectomy seems an important one for function and clearance. It adds little to the operation because most of the operative trauma is related to access rather than the removal of a few extra centimetres of oesophagus. It also seems sensible to excise the upper part of the lesser curve of the stomach to include the left gastric group of lymph nodes in the specimen. Protagonists of very limited resection do not always do this, but again this adds nothing to the trauma of the operation.

Transhiatal oesophagectomy

Transhiatal oesophagectomy without thoracotomy has enjoyed considerable popularity, but its routine use has not been effective in reducing postoperative morbidity or mortality. A randomised trial in France showed no difference between the results of resection by thoracotomy or by transhiatal dissection.[20] It is our impression that enthusiasm for transhiatal dissection has declined, and a recent European study has suggested that transhiatal dissection produces inferior survival in patients with early lesions.[21]

The argument against transhiatal resection is that it is more difficult to perform a truly radical resection. Certainly a complete lymphadenectomy is impossible by transhiatal surgery. It is likely that the place of this operation will be a matter of debate for many years.

The authors' practice is to reserve transhiatal dissection for those who are unfit or for whom palliation is all that can be achieved.

Minimal access surgery (minimally invasive surgery)

The advent of minimal access surgery has created enormous interest. Completely endoscopic resection of the oesophagus, including gastric mobilisation and anastomosis, has been performed but it is an extraordinarily prolonged procedure and is at present impractical for routine use. Several groups have resected the oesophagus by thoracoscopy, while mobilising the stomach by conventional laparotomy. The anastomosis has most commonly been performed in the neck, but intrathoracic stapled anastomosis has also been performed. Avoiding formal thoracotomy seems rational, but as yet surgical morbidity has not been reduced by endoscopic surgery and the procedure remains experimental.

For the moment, techniques are still evolving and surgeons are improving their skills. If a useful method is developed it is vital that minimal access oesophagectomy is submitted to formal prospective randomised study at the earliest opportunity.

Three field lymph node dissection

There is controversy about the role of radical resection with methodical clearance of regional lymph nodes and adjacent tissues. The ultimate lymph node clearance involves radical dissection in the abdomen, chest, and neck (three field dissection). This is widely practised in Japan, with a low postoperative mortality rate, and Japanese surgeons are the strongest protagonists of this procedure.

The rationale for the procedure was the relatively unsatisfactory outcome of conventional oesophagectomy with lymph node dissection in the middle and inferior mediastinum.[22] Japanese national statistics indicated a five year survival rate of 23·8%; recurrence commonly occurred in the upper mediastinum and neck. In three field lymph node dissection the nodes are dissected in the following territories: internal jugular chain, supraclavicular, recurrent laryngeal nerve, paratracheal, tracheal bifurcation and pulmonary hilum, paraoesophageal, para-aortic, pulmonary ligament, superior and inferior diaphragmatic, perigastric (pericardiac), lesser curve of stomach, left gastric, common hepatic and coeliac axis.

The upper mediastinal nodes are dissected via a right thoracotomy and the recurrent laryngeal nerves are taped. The dissection is carried up through the thoracic inlet as far as possible. A collar incision is then made in the neck and the dissection is continued to the level of the omohyoid muscle superiorly and the external jugular vein laterally. This denudes the trachea and bronchi, apart from one third of the circumference in the left anterior section. The right bronchial artery is preserved as far as possible to maintain tracheobronchial circulation.

In Osaka City University Hospital 138 patients underwent this procedure between 1986 and 1993, with a hospital mortality of 5%. The five year survival is currently 42%, survival being stage related and ranging from 100% for Tis lesions to 34% for T4 lesions (Figures 5.8 and 5.9). Survival seemed more dependent on lymph node invasion than on adventitial invasion (Figure 5.10). Lymph node invasion could not be predicted by the depth of invasion of the primary lesion.

The most important lymph node groups seem to be the paraoesophageal, perigastric and recurrent laryngeal nerve groups. The first two groups are easy to dissect, but the others in the cervicothoracic region are technically difficult.

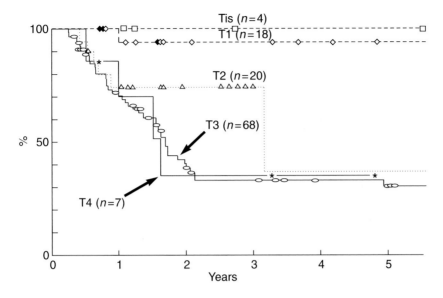

FIGURE 5.8—*Cumulative survival curves in relation to the T factor of the TNM classification.*

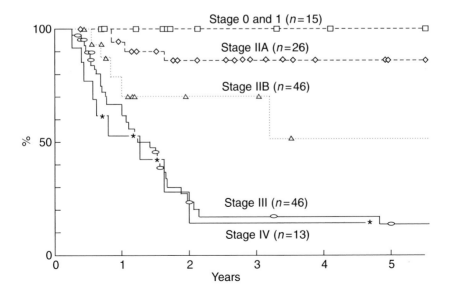

FIGURE 5.9—*Cumulative survival curves in relation to TNM tumour stages.*

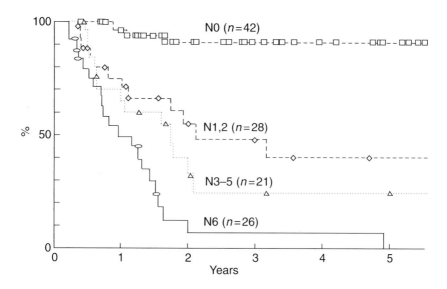

FIGURE 5.10—*Cumulative survival curves in relation to the total number of metastasised nodes. N0=no metastasis; N1, etc=number of invaded nodes.*

The classification of the lymph node groups according to the Japanese *Guidelines for the Clinical and Pathologic Studies of Carcinoma of the Esophagus* is shown in Figure 5.11. The relationship between the site of lymph node involvement and the site of the primary lesion is shown in Table 5.2. The pattern of lymph node metastasis in patients who had only one or two lymph nodes involved was quite unpredictable. In cases of lymph node involvement that did not extend to the cervical or coeliac axis groups, survival was better if the paraoesophageal nodes close to the lesion (juxtanodes, Figure 5.12) were not involved.

Of the 49 patients who have died of recurrence so far, the initial site of recurrence was the liver in 21, lung in 10, lymph nodes in eight, bone in five, brain in one, and pleuroperitoneal dissemination in four.

After three field lymph node dissection pulmonary complications occurred in 16% of cases, which is similar to the local rate in two field dissection. Three field dissection denervates the mediastinal trachea and the mainstem bronchi. Because of the impairment of the cough reflex it is the practice in Osaka to perform fibreoptic bronchoscopy once or twice a day for the first five postoperative days. Thirty per cent of patients developed recurrent laryngeal nerve dysfunction postoperatively. This probably contributed to a significant incidence of regurgitation and pneumonia late in the recovery process.

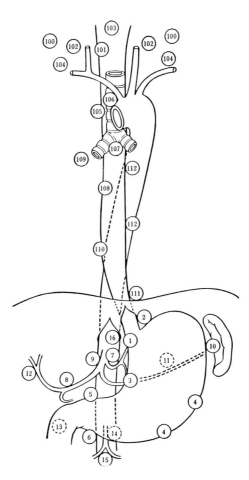

FIGURE 5.11—*Location and numbering of lymph nodes for surgical dissection according to the Japanese* Guidelines for the Clinical and Pathologic Studies of Carcinoma of the Esophagus.

Enthusiasm for three field lymph node dissection is minimal in the United Kingdom. Certainly there are significant differences in the incidence of postoperative respiratory infection between Salford and Osaka. In Salford 37% develop a chest infection following conventional oesophagectomy and most have pre-existing respiratory disease. More extensive use of radical surgery would therefore need to be restricted to carefully selected cases.

In Belgium Lerut has adopted the Japanese methods and has reported results comparable with those obtained in Japan.[23] In order to obtain proof of the validity of three field lymph node dissection, formal prospective randomised study would be required. Such a study would be very difficult

115

TABLE 5.2—*Frequency of metastasis to each lymph node group by location of the primary lesion*

Nodes		Rate of metastasis by location of primary lesion			
Numbering	Location	All (%)	Upper (%)	Middle (%)	Lower (%)
100	Superficial cervical	1	0	0	2
101	Cervical paraoesophageal	3	8	4	0
102	Deep cervical	3	8	4	0
104	Supraclavicular	2	0	4	0
105	Upper thoracic paraoesophageal	12	42	11	8
106	Thoracic paratracheal	4	0	5	2
107	Tracheal bifurcation	13	8	17	8
108	Middle thoracic paraoesophageal	20	25	22	14
109	Pulmonary hilar	8	8	7	8
110	Lower thoracic paraoesophageal	20	8	14	30
111	Diaphragmatic	1	0	0	4
112	Posterior mediastinal	5	8	1	10
1	Right cardiac	26	8	17	44
2	Left cardiac	22	16	13	36
3	Lesser curvature	13	0	13	14
7	Left gastric artery	13	0	13	16
9 8	Coeliac artery Common hepatic artery	2	8	1	2
	Right recurrent laryngeal nerve	18	33	16	18
	Left recurrent laryngeal nerve	12	25	11	10
	Infra-aortic arch	4	0	1	8

to mount because the number of patients who are candidates for the operation is relatively small and there are still institutional differences in the procedure. The British and Dutch trials of R2 gastric resection were both very important, but showed how difficult it is to control complex surgical techniques in large studies.

In Osaka current practice is to reserve transhiatal resection for very high risk patients or for palliation. If cure seems possible, but there are significant operative risk factors, three field lymph node dissection is performed in two stages: oesophagectomy and mediastinal dissection is first, followed by cervicoabdominal dissection and reconstruction three weeks later.

Endoscopic mucosal resection

One side effect of the Japanese enthusiasm for lymph node dissection has been the accumulation of high quality staging information and identification of groups that do not require lymph node dissection at all,

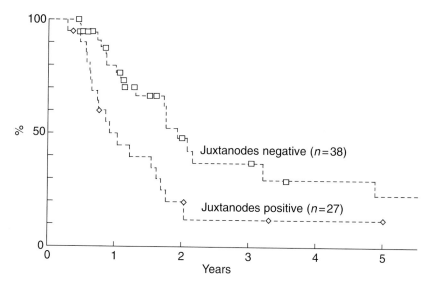

FIGURE 5.12—*Cumulative survival curves of patients with and without involvement of the paraoesophageal lymph nodes close to the primary lesion (juxtanodes).*

or even formal oesophagectomy. If the lesion invades the submucosa the incidence of lymph node metastasis is 40–60%, and of lymphatic permeation 70–80%. If the lesion is confined to the mucosa the incidence is 4–7% and 7–10% respectively, and if the lesion is epithelial no metastasis occurs. In recent years enthusiasm has grown for the technique of endoscopic mucosal resection in very early cases—that is, epithelial or mucosal—especially in elderly or unfit patients.

Endoscopic mucosal resection (EMR) involves raising the lesion by submucosal injection of saline and diathermy excision of the affected portion. Various methods have been employed; the procedure is simplified by the use of an overtube to suck the mucosa into the range of the diathermy snare. At present EMR is recommended if there are five or fewer lesions, the lesion is smaller than 6 cm, or it does not occupy the whole circumference of the oesophagus.

Observations on the differences between Japan and the United Kingdom

It is our feeling that the differences between these countries require careful attention. The different patient populations probably account for some of the differences in results. As has been previously mentioned, patients with oesophageal cancer in the United Kingdom tend to be older and have a higher incidence of cardiorespiratory disease. Major surgery will therefore have greater risks than in Japan, but simply dismissing the Japanese experience as unattainable is too simplistic.

There are distinct differences in surgical practice, surgical training and surgical techniques between Japan and the United Kingdom. There is less pressure on operating theatre time in Japan, allowing time to be taken to do the job thoroughly and well. There is also much less emphasis on the economical use of resources and patients stay in hospital for much longer (mean duration, including chemotherapy, 11 weeks postoperatively). Junior surgeons spend longer in one department and major surgery is therefore usually carried out with well trained assistants, which is often not the case in the United Kingdom. Japanese surgical teams stay together for longer and there is better continuity in the day to day routine of both preoperative and postoperative care. Surgeons tend to be more specialised in Japan, although British practice is changing rapidly. The most impressive features for overseas visitors to Japan are the obsessional emphasis on good surgical technique, avoidance of blood loss, and care in anatomical display, and the meticulous collection of data on clinical care that can be used to monitor the quality of treatment. These have been an inspiration to the British contributor for many years.

Organisation for treating oesophageal cancer

In achieving good results in oesophageal cancer it is important to be realistic about what can be achieved in the community. There is a growing amount of information that suggests that oesophageal resection should only be performed by surgeons who are doing it regularly. The results of those who perform less than six oesophageal resections per year show a considerably higher operative mortality than the results of those who perform six or more.[18] This may be due as much to the quality of perioperative care and anaesthetic management as to the quality of surgery itself. Oesophageal resection is a complex exercise: once a month seems a reasonable minimum to maintain surgical expertise; the optimum may well be more frequently, but there are no data demonstrating this as yet.

Oesophageal resection should only be performed in hospitals with adequate facilities for the assessment and care of patients having such major surgery, including the care of any postoperative complications. These must include a fully staffed intensive care unit and access to sophisticated imaging and good interventional radiology. Occasional oesophageal resection in community hospitals should be discouraged.

Other methods of treatment

Later in this chapter Peake and Cottier discuss the roles of chemotherapy and radiotherapy in detail. The following remarks are chiefly aimed at giving a surgical perspective on the current place of these and other modalities in relation to that of surgery.

Radiotherapy

Radiotherapy and surgical resection are the only means of achieving cure at the present time. For squamous cell cancers of the thoracic oesophagus there is persistent controversy about the relative merits of radiotherapy and surgery, particularly in the United Kingdom. Survey of the literature suggests better cure rates by resection than by irradiation, provided that operative mortality is low, but the comparability of the treatment groups is questionable (see Peake and Cottier below). We believe that radiotherapy is currently the treatment of choice for cancers of the cervical oesophagus, because results appear to be at least equivalent and laryngectomy is avoided. Resection in such cases is reserved for local recurrence.

In theory, combinations of surgery and radiotherapy should improve cure rates because each has different limitations in treating the primary lesion. Preoperative radiotherapy has been examined in eight randomised studies with conflicting results, but an overview suggests a possible small benefit from combined treatment. The Medical Research Council Oesophageal Cancer Working Party is currently performing a meta-analysis of all of the known trials.

Postoperative radiotherapy has not been shown to have any benefit, but trials are few and lack statistical power. Non-randomised studies have suggested a possible deleterious effect.

Chemotherapy

Chemotherapy has improved considerably in recent years but is still not curative on its own. Several studies of preoperative chemotherapy are in progress in the United Kingdom, USA, and continental Europe. Entry of patients into such trials should be encouraged.

Chemotherapy now gives response rates that are clinically useful and morbidity has been greatly reduced. It has a definite place in the management of symptomatic metastatic or recurrent disease. There is considerable scope for development in the future.

Palliation

A substantial proportion of patients with oesophageal cancer is beyond the scope of curative treatment at the time of presentation. This may be because of advanced disease, age, or general medical condition. Undoubtedly the best quality palliation is seen in those who have recovered from an oesophageal resection. Resection is, however, traumatic, and has a significant morbidity and mortality rate. The two contributors are in agreement that when expected survival is reasonably long, say two years, surgical resection should be attempted. For shorter expected survival there are, however, significant differences in practice. In Japan there is much more emphasis on aggressive treatment in the expectation of occasional long term survival and of satisfying patients and relatives that everything possible has been done. Tubes and local palliative measures are therefore procedures of last resort.

In the United Kingdom the prevailing feeling is that if radical treatment is unlikely to achieve a cure it is better to have swallowing restored in the least traumatic manner so that, if survival is short, the remaining time is not spent recovering from a big operation. The decision to pursue a palliative course of action is therefore taken in a greater proportion of cases and the technology of palliation is a subject of much greater interest.

Several methods are now available for relief of dysphagia and the choice is still increasing. All have their advantages and disadvantages and it is impossible to make categorical statements. Laser therapy has been shown to have a small advantage over endoluminal prosthetic tubes. Bipolar diathermy has similar results to laser treatment for circumferential lesions. Endoluminal radiotherapy (brachytherapy) and endoscopic tumour necrosis with ethanol injection are also effective. Expanding metal stents are a recent innovation with promising potential.

Dilatation

Endoscopic dilatation is simple and relatively safe, but gives only temporary relief. It can be very useful for tiding a patient over a period of assessment but has become much less popular for palliation now that there are reasonably satisfactory endoprostheses and other methods of intraluminal treatment.

Intubation

Endoluminal tubes have been used for generations but it is only in the last 20 years or so that tube design and methods of insertion have improved sufficiently to make this technique reasonably effective and safe.

In the United Kingdom the Atkinson tube is probably the most widely used. This is a relatively soft, funnel shaped tube that is inserted endoscopically. It gives reasonable palliation but most patients are restricted to semisolid food and there is a significant perforation rate of the order of 5–10%.

120

Laser

Laser recanalisation is now widely practised and many would regard it as the current method of choice. Good quality palliation can be achieved with little morbidity, and comparative trials have shown it to have small but significant advantages over intubation; however, the procedure usually has to be repeated regularly, the equipment is expensive and requires regular maintenance, and a considerable investment of time is required.

Bipolar diathermy

Bipolar diathermy with the BICAP tumour probe has been shown to produce similar results to laser with circumferential tumours. The equipment is much less expensive than laser but it is not applicable for polypoid tumours that do not encircle the oesophagus. A probe with a 180° contact plate is available for polypoid lesions, but it is difficult to use in practice.

Alcohol injection

Endoscopic tumour necrosis with 100% ethanol is simple and cheap and may have results similar to laser and diathermy, although there have been no comparative trials. A simple endoscopic injection needle is used to inject small aliquots of alcohol into the tumour throughout its length. Relief of dysphagia may take a few days but good quality palliation can be produced.

Endoluminal radiotherapy

Endoluminal radiotherapy with a source that produces little tissue penetration (brachytherapy) is a simple and effective method of palliation with a low complication rate (see Peake and Cottier below). In common with laser, the equipment is expensive, but relief of dysphagia can be prolonged.

Expanding stents

Expanding metal stents are the latest addition to the armamentarium. They are expensive but have the advantage of producing excellent relief of dysphagia with a single procedure. Our own experience in Salford has been that cumulative hospital costs are lower, because repeat treatments are not usually required, and there have been no serious complications during the insertion of approximately 100 stents in the last two years. Prospective comparative trials are in progress and further work is required to determine which of the many available designs is best.

External beam radiotherapy

The role of external beam radiotherapy in palliation is uncertain. "Curative" doses are inappropriate for patients with incurable disease, particularly if the likely life expectancy is less than one year. Lower "palliative" doses have an uncertain effect on the tumour. They may have some role in combination with, say, laser treatment, but the dose that is given seems critical. Clinical trials of various intraluminal modalities combined with external beam therapy are in progress.

Surgical palliation

Palliative resection gives excellent relief of dysphagia, but is a major procedure with significant disadvantages when expected survival is short. Surgical bypass is also a major undertaking and has a very limited role.

The British contributor feels that surgical resection should be discouraged when preoperative investigation indicates that cure is not possible. The only exception to this rule is when the tumour is found to be incurable once surgical exploration is well under way and most of the trauma of an operation has already been inflicted.

Oesophagorespiratory fistula

Tracheo-oesophageal fistulas are best managed by intraluminal tubes incorporating a balloon that seals the fistula. The expandable metal stents may be an even better option, but this remains to be determined in comparative trials.

Summary and conclusions

Treating carcinoma of the oesophagus remains a challenge. The prevailing attitude is one of despair, and it has to be admitted that the results fall short of what one would like to achieve. Considerable progress has, however, been made since the 1970s. Diagnosis is made at an earlier stage, complications such as oesophagobronchial fistulation are less common, mortality following surgical resection has been significantly reduced, methods of palliation have improved, and chemotherapy has a much more predictable response rate. This is not a disease that is untreatable. A great deal can be done.

Achieving the best results requires an experienced multidisciplinary team. It is also important to be aware of the potential for further improvement that is offered by developments in oncology and by evolving surgical techniques, such as the Japanese approach to radical resection.

References

1 Japanese Society for Esophageal Diseases. *Guidelines for the clinical and pathologic studies of carcinoma of the esophagus.* 8th ed. Tokyo: Kanehara, 1992.

2 Goseki N, Koike M, Yoshida M. Histopathologic characteristics of early stage esophageal cancer. A comparative study with gastric carcinoma. *Cancer* 1992;**69**:1088–93.

3 De Manzoni G, Laterza E, Urso SU. Endosonography and computerized tomography in the evaluation of tumor invasion in esophageal cancer after preoperative chemo- and radiotherapy. In: Nabeya K, Hanaoka T, Nogami H, eds. *Recent advances in diseases of the oesophagus.* Heidelberg: Springer, 1993:532–9.

4 Takashima S, Takeuchi N, Shiozaki H, *et al.* Carcinoma of the esophagus: CT vs MR imaging in determining resectability. *Am J Roentgenol* 1991;**156**:297–302.

5 Botet JF, Lightdale CJ, Zauber AG, *et al.* Preoperative staging of esophageal cancer: comparison of endoscopic US and dynamic CT. *Radiology* 1991;**181**:419–25.

6 Osugi H, Sakai K, Higashino M, *et al.* Preoperative staging of esophageal cancer by endoscopic ultrasonography. In: Siewert JR, Hölscher AH, eds. *Diseases of the esophagus.* Heidelberg: Springer, 1987:169–73.

7 Dagnini G, Caldironi MW, Marin G, *et al.* Laparoscopy in abdominal staging of esophageal carcinoma. Report of 369 cases. *Gastrointest Endosc* 1986;**32**:400–2.

8 Shandall A, Johnson C. Laparoscopy or scanning in oesophageal and gastric carcinoma? *Br J Surg* 1985;**72**:449–51.

9 van Overhagen H, Berger MY, Meijers H, *et al.* Influence of radiologically and cytologically assessed distant metastases on the survival of patients with esophageal and gastroesophageal junction carcinoma. *Cancer* 1993;**72**:25–31.

10 Chan K-H, Wong J. Mortality after esophagectomy for carcinoma of esophagus: an analysis of risk factors. *Dis Esophagus* 1990;**3**:49–53.

11 Copeland GP, Jones D, Walters M. POSSUM: a scoring system for surgical audit. *Br J Surg* 1991;**78**:356–60.

12 Heys SD, Park KGM, Garlick PJ, *et al.* Nutrition and malignant disease: implications for surgical practice. *Br J Surg* 1992;**79**:614–23.

13 Campos ACL, Meguid M. A critical appraisal of the usefulness of perioperative nutritional support. *Am J Clin Nutr* 1994;**55**:117–30.

14 McKeown KC. Carcinoma of the oesophagus. *J R Coll Surg Edinb* 1979;**24**:253–74.

15 DeMeester TR, Zaninotto G, Johansson KE. Selective therapeutic approach to cancer of the lower esophagus and cardia. *J Thorac Cardiovasc Surg* 1988;**95**:42–54.

16 Salama FD, Leong YP. Resection for carcinoma of the oesophagus. *J R Coll Surg Edinb* 1989;**34**:97–100.

17 Menke-Pluymers MBE, Schoute NW, Mulder AH, *et al.* Outcome of surgical treatment of adenocarcinoma in Barrett's oesophagus. *Gut* 1992;**33**:1454–8.

18 Matthews HR, Powell DJ, McConkey CC. Effect of surgical experience on the results of resection for oesophageal carcinoma. *Br J Surg* 1986;**73**:621–3.

Chemotherapy, radiotherapy, palliative care, and new approaches

DAVID R PEAKE and BRIAN COTTIER

Historically, patients with oesophageal carcinoma (in common with many other cancers) have been treated by either a surgeon *or* an oncologist. More recently, with the advent of endoscopic methods of palliation, some patients are also now treated by physicians. Despite advances in both surgery and oncology the prognosis for patients with oesophageal carcinoma remains dismal, with an overall five year survival of approximately 5%. Many centres, particularly in North America, are now employing multimodality treatment regimens in order to try to improve the outlook for those with this disease. This modern approach will almost certainly require closer cooperation between the specialties.

The text that follows presents current opinion on the use of radiotherapy and chemotherapy (individually, combined, and in conjunction with surgery); that which should be regarded as standard treatment, and that which remains experimental.

Radical treatment

This section considers the role of radical radiotherapy either as a primary treatment for oesophageal carcinoma or as an adjuvant therapy to surgery. The potential of chemotherapy to improve the therapeutic ratio will also be discussed. The term "radical" indicates treatment given with an intention to cure, in those patients in whom this is considered a realistic possibility. Palliative treatments will be considered separately.

It is generally considered that surgery offers a greater chance of cure than radiotherapy, but at a greater cost in morbidity and mortality. There

124

are, however, no randomised trials comparing the two modalities. The Medical Research Council trial was abandoned because of poor accrual, and it is unlikely that the attempt will be repeated.

The evidence that radiotherapy is inferior to surgery comes from comparisons of published series and must, therefore, be viewed with some caution. The major bias is that of patient selection. In general, it is the patients considered unfit for surgery, either because they are old and frail, or because of concurrent medical problems, who are referred for radiotherapy. This group has a poorer prognosis whatever the treatment. The second problem is that of staging. Non-invasive investigations may underestimate the extent of disease. Patients undergoing surgery will be more accurately staged and some will be considered unsuitable for a radical procedure. It is not possible to make this distinction in patients receiving radiotherapy, who will, therefore, be a more heterogeneous group. Some surgical series exclude patients who have not undergone radical surgery, again biasing the results in favour of surgery.

Radiotherapy

Radiotherapy alone

Patient selection The ideal candidate for radical radiotherapy would also be the ideal patient for surgery—that is, generally fit and healthy, well nourished, with a small primary tumour. There are, however, certain staging considerations that differ between the approach to radical surgery and that to radical radiotherapy. Tumours of the upper and mid-thoracic oesophagus are best suited to irradiation. Carcinoma of the lower oesophagus is better treated by resection because the upper part of the stomach (which is included in the target volume) tolerates radiation relatively poorly, limiting the dose, and early metastatic spread to the coeliac nodes occurs, which cannot easily be encompassed within the treatment volume. Management of carcinoma of the cervical oesophagus is controversial: surgery is complicated and often requires laryngectomy, but irradiation is also technically more difficult than when treating the thorax.

Any patient being considered for radical treatment, whether radiation or surgery, must be staged as accurately as possible. The box lists those investigations the authors regard as mandatory and those considered optional.

Distant metastatic disease or the presence of significant mediastinal lymphadenopathy are absolute contraindications to radical radiotherapy. Mediastinal lymphadenopathy of equivocal significance does not exclude radical therapy. Other generally accepted contraindications to radiotherapy are the presence of a tracheo-oesophageal or broncho-oesophageal fistula,

---

Investigations before radical therapy for oesophageal carcinoma

Mandatory
- Full blood count
- Liver function tests
- Chest *x* ray
- Barium swallow
- CT—mediastinum and liver
- Oesophagoscopy and biopsy

Optional
- CT—lungs
- Liver ultrasonography
- MRI—mediastinum
- Endo-oesophageal ultrasonography
- Bronchoscopy
- Isotope bone scan

---

established mediastinitis, or haemorrhage. Whether involvement of the trachea or bronchus without fistula formation is a contraindication remains controversial, but this implies locally extensive disease and these patients have a poor prognosis and are probably better served by palliative treatment; as the tumour regresses a fistula may be produced.

Relative contraindications to radical therapy are excessive weight loss and serious concurrent pathology, particularly cardiorespiratory disease. Chest or back pain suggest mediastinal infiltration but in themselves are not contraindications to radical therapy. The size of the primary tumour is a significant independent prognostic factor, tumours less than 5 cm long having a better prognosis. It is difficult to irradiate larger tumours to a radical dose (see below). Sex is a further independent prognostic variable, females having a better prognosis.

The principles of radical radiotherapy are the same when treating any region. The aim is to irradiate both the apparent tumour and the sites at high risk of microscopic involvement (the target volume) homogeneously to a dose sufficient to eradicate the tumour, while limiting the dose to the surrounding normal tissues. The thoracic oesophagus lies in close proximity to the lungs and spinal cord, both of which must be considered as dose limiting normal tissues.

Toxicity is related not only to the total dose but also to the volume of tissue receiving that dose. It is vital to limit the *total dose* to the spinal cord to prevent myelopathy, but it is more important to limit the *volume* of lung treated as it is possible to irradiate a small volume to a high dose without causing significant symptoms. When treating the thoracic oesophagus these aims are best achieved by a three field arrangement, treating with an anterior field and two posterior oblique fields (Figure 5.13). A different technique is necessary when treating the cervical oesophagus.

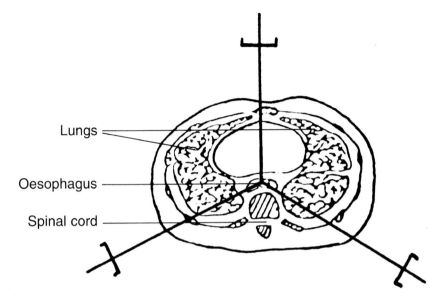

Lungs

Oesophagus

Spinal cord

FIGURE 5.13—*Field arrangement for radiotherapy to the thoracic oesophagus.*

Thoracic oesophagus: technique The patient is planned in the simulator, lying supine with hands clasped and placed on top of the head. An isocentric technique is employed. CT planning is not routine practice in the authors' department, but it may offer an advantage in selected patients. The tumour is localised by asking the patient to swallow a mouthful of barium paste before screening. Anteroposterior and left lateral localisation films are taken. Further planning information is obtained from the diagnostic barium swallow, CT, and endoscopic findings.

The target volume must include a 5 cm margin of apparently normal oesophagus, both superiorly and inferiorly, because of the propensity of this tumour to spread early through the submucosal lymphatics. This means that there is a limit to the size of primary tumour that can be safely considered for radical therapy, otherwise the treatment volume and the associated risk of toxicity become too great. An apparent tumour length of 6–7 cm should be regarded as a maximum for radical treatment. The width of the fields should be sufficient to cover the mediastinal nodes. A typical target volume will measure 15–17 cm in length and 6–7 cm in width and depth (Figure 5.14).

A central axis plan is produced using a planning computer, showing the position of the lungs and spinal cord in relation to the target volume and the isodose distribution (Figure 5.15). A correction factor must be included in the calculation of the dose contribution from the posterior oblique fields

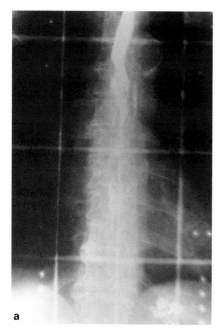

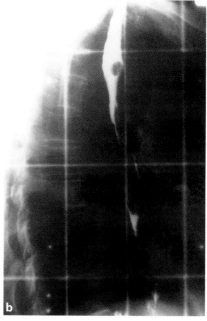

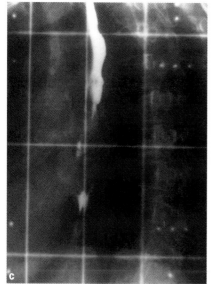

FIGURE 5.14—*(a) Anterior and (b) lateral localisation simulator films; (c) simulator film exposed from posterior oblique position.*

to compensate for reduced attenuation through the lungs. A daily fraction size of no greater than 2 Gy is commonly recommended (because bigger daily fractions are considered to increase the risk of late tissue toxicity), treating to a total dose of 60–64 Gy in 30–32 fractions over 6–6·5 weeks.

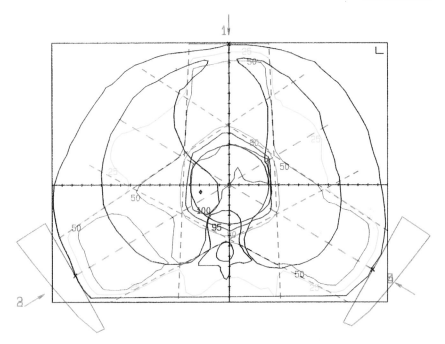

FIGURE 5.15—*Isodose plan for treatment to the thoracic oesophagus using a 3 field technique.*

More condensed schedules are still employed in some centres, including the authors' department, where a total dose of 52·5 Gy in 20 fractions over four weeks is routinely prescribed. The most recent recommendation from the international commission on radiation units is that the dose is prescribed at the isocentre, and with modern computer planning it should be possible to achieve a homogeneous dose with less than 5% variation throughout the target volume.

The patient is treated daily five days a week on a linear accelerator, treating all fields each day. Some units treat oesophageal cancer in two phases: the mediastinum is first treated with parallel opposed anterior and posterior fields to a dose of 40 Gy in 20 fractions, before conversion to a standard three field plan to take the total dose to 60–64 Gy. The apparent disadvantages of this technique are the extra time consumed in planning the patient twice and the higher dose delivered to the spinal cord.

The above description oversimplifies the problem of irradiating the oesophagus. The oesophagus and spinal cord are not straight, parallel structures lying at a constant depth in relation to the isocentre. A thoracic kyphosis means that a length of spinal cord is often included in the high dose volume. It may be possible to remedy this by applying tube head rotation to the posterior oblique fields, but it must be remembered that the localisation films are taken with the gantry angle at 90° and a geometric calculation is necessary to determine the correct tube head rotation as the machine is brought round into the posterior oblique position. A second problem caused by tube head rotation is the phenomenon of the shifting isocentre—that is, the longitudinal central axis is not at a constant distance from the treatment couch. The methods by which these problems may be overcome are described elsewhere.[19] In practice, a maximum of 5° tube head rotation is acceptable on the lateral localisation view without making any corrections as this does not significantly affect dose distribution.

Toxicity Irradiating the oesophagus to a radical dose has a significant morbidity and occasional mortality. The major acute toxicity is radiation oesophagitis. Patients usually develop symptoms at the end of the second week or during the third week of treatment, the timing of symptoms depending more on the cellular kinetics of the mucosa than the dose fractionation schedule employed. The patient complains of discomfort, pain or difficulty on swallowing, indigestion, or heartburn. The severity of the symptoms is usually maximal at 4–5 weeks after the start of treatment. During a six week course of treatment, symptoms may actually start to improve during the final week as the mucosa begins to heal as a result of accelerated repopulation. Within two weeks of completion of treatment there has normally been a significant improvement.

Simple dietary advice is important and patients often benefit from a consultation with a dietician. A bland, soft diet is recommended. It may be necessary to liquidise the food, or provide supplements such as Fortisip. The patient is weighed weekly and, if more than 10% of ideal body weight is lost, enteral feeding via a fine bore nasogastric tube is recommended. This may also be necessary if dysphagia is severe. Very occasionally it is not possible to pass a nasogastric tube, or it cannot be tolerated, and a gastrostomy or parenteral nutrition must be considered.

The situation should be reappraised before starting parenteral nutrition, as this may be considered inappropriate for some patients.

Symptomatic relief is obtained by the use of antacid mixtures. Mucaine suspension (an aluminium and magnesium based antacid containing oxethazaine, a topical anaesthetic) is recommended. Simple analgesics, such as paracetamol or compound preparations containing paracetamol and a weak opiate (preferably soluble), may be necessary.

Sucralfate suspension can be effective for radiation mucositis, not only in the oesophagus but also for the oral cavity. This drug, usually prescribed for gastric or duodenal ulceration, is not absorbed significantly but binds to ulcerated mucosa, producing a protective barrier.

Paradoxically, indomethacin, well known for its gastrointestinal toxicity, has been shown to have a protective effect on radiation induced oesophageal damage in animal studies, probably by blocking the prostaglandin mediated inflammatory response. There is, however, no evidence at present that non-steroidal anti-inflammatory agents are of any clinical value in managing radiation oesophagitis. Cigarette smoking during treatment should be strongly discouraged as this exacerbates oesophagitis. Alcohol (other than spirits), in moderation, is probably allowable. As with radical treatment at any site, patients often complain of general lethargy and lassitude. Nausea and vomiting are not usually significant problems unless the lower oesophagus is being treated; they are usually controlled by simple oral antiemetics, such as metoclopramide or domperidone. If the symptoms of oesophagitis do not improve as expected, it may indicate a superimposed candida infection. Ideally this should be confirmed by endoscopy but may be treated on clinical grounds. Treatment is with an antifungal agent, such as fluconazole, in suspension.

A complication of irradiating part of the lungs is radiation pneumonitis. This often goes unnoticed but the patient may complain of a non-productive cough 1–3 months after completion of treatment. Symptoms are usually minimal unless an unusually large volume of lung has received a significant dose, when the cough may be productive of clear sputum and associated with dyspnoea, pleuritic chest pain, and fever. Auscultation at this stage sometimes elicits inspiratory crepitations but is often unremarkable. The condition is self limiting but steroids may occasionally be necessary. Prednisolone EC should be started at a dose of 30 mg daily and reduced as rapidly as symptoms allow. Steroids probably do not influence the progression to fibrosis but symptomatic late pulmonary toxicity is rare.

One of the more serious complications of irradiating the oesophagus is perforation or a fistula with the tracheobronchial tree, leading to mediastinitis or aspiration pneumonia. Fistula formation occurs more frequently when there is invasion of the trachea or bronchus. This is not strictly a side effect of treatment but a result of tumour regression. Management should include oesophageal intubation, intravenous fluids, and antibiotics, but despite these measures most patients succumb. Similarly, regression may expose a major blood vessel, causing massive, often fatal, haemorrhage.

The most common long term complication is oesophageal stricture. O'Rourke et al have reported on the incidence and significance of stricture in a series of 80 patients treated with radiotherapy, including those treated to both radical and palliative doses.[20] Only 57 patients were followed for long enough to be assessed. Of these, 17 (30%) developed a benign stricture and 16 (28%) a malignant stricture. There was a suggestion that the incidence of benign stricture is higher in the group receiving radical treatment but the difference was not statistically significant. The median

131

time interval between the start of treatment and the development of a benign stricture was six months, and five months for a malignant stricture. The development of a benign stricture did not have an adverse effect on prognosis. The authors comment on the fact that the reported incidence of oesophageal stricture in patients receiving radiotherapy to the mediastinum for other malignancies is much lower. Strictures are probably more common in this group as a result of fibrosis and scarring as the tumour regresses.

Strictures that cause significant dysphagia require dilatation, often repeatedly, and some patients are better served by oesophageal intubation.

Cervical oesophagus: technique   Radiotherapy to the cervical oesophagus is technically more complicated than treatment to the thoracic oesophagus. Not only are the oesophagus and spinal cord in closer proximity at this level, the irregular contour of the neck and shoulders produces a difference in beam attenuation, and hence potential dose inhomogeneity along the length of the target volume. Several techniques have been devised to overcome these problems. A four field box technique has been developed at the University of Florida.[21] A wax compensator is made to fill the gap above the shoulders and the lateral fields are shaped using metal blocks to define the volume more precisely. Treatment is in two phases. The initial four field phase treats the primary and nodes to a dose of 45 Gy in 25 fractions over five weeks. In the second phase the spinal cord is shielded on the lateral fields and the anterior and posterior fields are discontinued. The total dose is taken to 70–75 Gy at the same dose per fraction.

The main advantages of this technique are that spinal cord dose can be calculated more accurately and the portal verification films are much easier to interpret than those for oblique fields. The disadvantages are that skin sparing is lost because of bolus, the shoulders and lung apices are included in the lateral portals, and high energy photons are preferable because of the separation at the shoulders. A more standard technique, and the one with which the authors are familiar, is an anterior oblique wedged pair field arrangement (Figure 5.16). The patient is positioned supine, in a cast, with the spinal cord as straight as possible. As with the Florida technique, the first phase of treatment includes the lymph nodes, but only anterior and posterior fields are employed. These fields are fully compensated to ensure a homogeneous dose distribution. The dose is taken to 44 Gy in 22 fractions over 4·5 weeks. The second phase is CT planned and treats the primary tumour using fully compensated wedged anterior oblique fields (Figure 5.17).

The total dose prescribed is 66–70 Gy at 2 Gy/fraction.

The disadvantages of this method are that it is time consuming to make the compensators and calculate the tube head rotation and couch rotation,

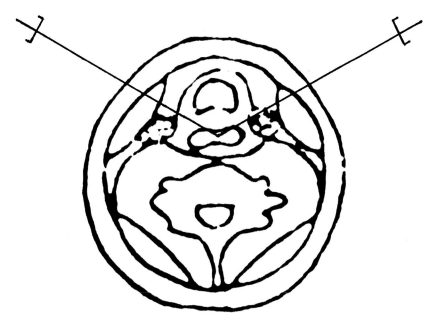

FIGURE 5.16—*Field arrangement for radiotherapy to the cervical oesophagus.*

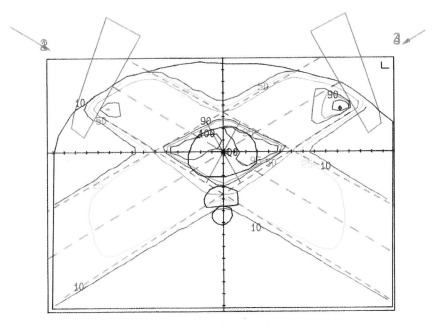

FIGURE 5.17—*Isodose plan for treatment to the cervical oesophagus using wedged anterior oblique fields.*

133

which are usually necessary to avoid the spinal cord. It is also more difficult to interpret oblique portal films, and hence assess the position of the spinal cord. Despite these limitations this technique has been found to be effective and relatively straightforward to implement. Toxicity is similar to that described for the thoracic oesophagus. The patient is more likely to complain specifically of a sore throat.

Symptomatic relief is obtained from soluble aspirin gargles, benzydamine hydrochloride (Difflam) mouthwash or spray, and Mucaine suspension.

Hypothyroidism may occur as a late toxic effect and thyroid function should be monitored after treatment. Of greatest concern when treating either cervical or thoracic oesophagus is spinal cord toxicity. Fortunately, with the above techniques radiation myelopathy is extremely rare.

Lhermitte's syndrome, a result of subacute spinal cord toxicity, is due to temporary demyelination of the cord, and is well recognised following radiation to the cervical oesophagus. Typically the patient complains of shooting pains down the arms or tingling in the hands and fingers, especially on movement of the neck. The symptoms start several weeks or months after completion of treatment. The condition is self limiting and there is no specific therapy; it does not predict myelopathy.

Outcome Locoregional treatment, whether surgery or radiotherapy, can potentially cure only the minority of patients with truly localised disease. There is no conclusive evidence that either modality is superior in this group.

Commonly quoted survival figures are those of two overviews of the treatment of oesophageal cancer, published in 1980, by Earlam and Cunha-Melo.[22 23] The first paper considered data on 83 783 patients (122 papers) treated surgically, and the second on 8489 patients (49 papers) treated by radiotherapy. The authors attempted to standardise the results by quoting survival figures for each modality as a percentage of the total population of patients diagnosed as having oesophageal carcinoma, not of those actually treated.

The overall mean survival at one year, two years, and five years was 18, 8, and 6% respectively for radiotherapy. It was estimated that approximately 50% of these patients would have been treated radically. At first sight the equivalent survival figures for surgery appear remarkably similar, at 18, 8, and 4%; however, if only those patients *undergoing* surgery are considered, the survival is 31% at one year, 14% at two years, and 9% at five years. Furthermore, at the time of surgery, a proportion of these patients will be found to have tumours that are inoperable. If this group is also excluded, the survival of those patients having a radical oesophageal resection is 45% at one year, 20% at two years, and 12% at five years. It is these figures with which radical radiotherapy must be compared.

As discussed previously, this is a highly selected group and it is not possible to identify an equivalent patient population that has received radiotherapy. The authors suggest, however, that three papers on radiotherapy included only patients regarded as comparable with those in surgical series, and that for this group of highly selected cases survival was equivalent to surgical resection, with approximately 44% alive at one year, 8–27% at two years, and 6–20% at five years.

Oliver et al recently reported on 268 patients treated in Nottingham between 1982 and 1985.[24] Radical radiotherapy was attempted in 13%, with a median survival of 190 days, and a one, two, and three year survival of 14, 6, and 6% respectively. These results were based on the initial treatment intention, and hence may include patients who did not complete treatment. An audit on the treatment of oesophageal cancer in Leeds has been reported by Sagar et al.[25] The survival of patients having a resection was equivalent to that quoted by Earlam and Cunha-Melo. Of 29 patients completing radical radiotherapy, the median survival was 175 days and the longest survivor lived only 15 months.

The authors comment that the two groups are not comparable, and that in general it was patients considered unfit for surgery who received radiotherapy.

It has been reported that survival rates after radiotherapy in cancer of the cervical oesophagus are superior to those for thoracic oesophageal carcinoma. Newaishy et al reported the results of a retrospective study of 444 patients with squamous carcinoma of the oesophagus treated with radical radiotherapy in Glasgow between January 1956 and December 1974.[26] The five year crude survival rate, according to site, was almost 19% for tumours of the cervical oesophagus, compared with approximately 10% for thoracic oesophageal tumours. The authors comment that this supported previously reported experience, but that the numbers were small and the results should be viewed with caution. Direct comparison between disease at the two sites is difficult.

Table 5.3 summarises these statistics. It may be concluded that, in the small minority of patients with early, localised disease, cure may be achieved by either radiotherapy or surgery; however, if the prognosis for the majority of patients is to be improved, combined modality treatment, including chemotherapy, must be considered.

Intraluminal brachytherapy As a treatment for oesophageal cancer, intraluminal brachytherapy is not new: radium bougies were used as long ago as the 1920s. In the 1950s radium needles were placed under direct vision and fixed proximally to a tooth and distally through a gastrostomy. A variety of other methods were attempted, but because of the technical difficulties and the associated morbidity, brachytherapy was never widely accepted for treatment of oesophageal cancer. With the advent of fibreoptic endoscopy and remote afterloading machines the procedure is now simpler and less hazardous for both the patient and staff; sources with higher specific activity are now available, shortening treatment times. Because of these advances there is now renewed interest in brachytherapy for oesophageal cancer.

The rationale for the use of brachytherapy is that as the dose rate falls rapidly with increasing distance from the source it is possible to deliver a high dose to the oesophageal wall with minimal risk of toxicity to the surrounding normal tissues, in particular the spinal cord. Clearly, intraluminal therapy alone is inadequate as a radical treatment because disease is rarely limited to the oesophageal wall. In order to treat the mediastinal lymph nodes, brachytherapy must be used in conjunction with external beam therapy. The usual scheduling is to treat initially with external beam therapy and to use intraluminal therapy as a boost to residual disease.

Using this combined approach it is possible to deliver a higher dose of radiation to the oesophageal wall than by using external beam therapy alone; however, unless all residual disease after external beam therapy is included in the high dose volume, it is unlikely that the addition of brachytherapy will be advantageous. The literature suggests that this is often the case. In a significant proportion of patients undergoing oesophageal resection after external radiotherapy, residual disease is confined to the oesophageal wall, which, having a thickness of 4 mm, will be adequately treated by brachytherapy.

Despite these theoretical advantages and the relative simplicity and safety of modern techniques, the role of brachytherapy as a radical treatment remains undefined.

Several phase II studies have been reported, of which three have evaluated over 100 patients. Each of these included patients with limited and extensive disease. Table 5.4 summarises their results.

TABLE 5.3—*Survival after radiotherapy for oesophageal carcinoma*

Authors	Median survival	Survival (%)			
		1 year	2 years	3 years	5 years
Earlam and Cinha-Melo[26][27]					
Overall		18	8		6
Selected		44–46	8–27		6–20
Oliver et al[28]	190 days	14	6	6	0
Sagar et al[29]	175 days		0		
Newaishy et al[30]					
Thoracic					10
Cervical					19

TABLE 5.4—*Results of selected series of patients treated by external beam therapy and intraluminal brachytherapy*

	Flores *et al*[31]	Hishikawa *et al*[32]	Hareyama *et al*[33]
Dose (Gy)			
External	40	60	55–60
Brachytherapy	15	6×2	$4–10 \times 1–3$
Survival (%)			
1 year	33		
2 years	26	37—limited disease (actuarial) 7—extensive disease	
3 years	19		
5 years		18—limited disease	43—stage I (actuarial) 21—stage II (actuarial)
Complication rate (%)			
Fistula	4·7	14	
Ulceration		28	3 { ulceration or
Stricture		10	stricture

Flores *et al* published the results in 211 patients treated (of whom 171 were evaluated) between 1985 and 1988.[27] Their only exclusion criteria were direct invasion of the bronchi or trachea. Patients received initial intraluminal therapy with remotely afterloaded caesium-137 pellets. A cylinder 10 cm long and 2 cm in diameter was treated to a dose of 15 Gy (dose rate 10 Gy/h). Subsequent external beam irradiation was delivered employing a three field technique to a dose of 40 Gy in 15 fractions over three weeks. The treatment was well tolerated, without any mortality directly related to the procedure. Oesophagitis was mild or moderate in the majority of patients, but severe in 25 (14%). All patients with severe oesophagitis had progressive uncontrolled disease. Eight patients developed a fistula but in each case this was thought to be a consequence of disease progression; 56% of patients had restoration of normal swallowing.

Hishikawa *et al* reported 148 patients treated initially by external beam therapy (60 Gy in 30 fractions), followed by two fractions of intraluminal therapy a week apart (6 Gy/fraction prescribed 1 cm from the source, 0·5 cm deep to the mucosal surface).[28] The source was cobalt-60 and the dose rate fell from 6·6 to 2·6 Gy/min (approximately) during the course of the study. Hishikawa observed a fistula rate of 14% (21 patients), but in only six patients (4%) was this not associated with progressive disease. A third series of 161 patients was reported by Hareyama *et al.*[29] There was some variation in the dose delivered by external beam therapy but the most frequent doses employed were 55 Gy in 22 fractions, treating four days a

137

week, or 60 Gy in 30 fractions, treating five days a week. This was followed by brachytherapy, delivering 4–10 Gy to a point 0·5 cm deep to the oesophageal mucosa (the source was radium and the calculated dose rate was 2 Gy/h at the surface of the mucosa). If necessary the insertion was repeated up to three times, but the indications for this are not documented. A complete response was observed in 86 (53·4%) of the 161 patients one month after completion of treatment.

Each of these studies suggested a survival advantage attributable to intraluminal therapy; however, this is based on a comparison with historical controls and hence should be interpreted with caution. Flores observed a survival rate of 33, 26, and 19% at one, two, and three years respectively. Hishikawa recorded a median survival of 13 months, and a two and five year actuarial survival of 37 and 18% respectively, in patients with limited disease (International Union against Cancer (UICC) stage I or II). In patients with stage I disease Hareyama reports an actuarial five year survival of 43%, compared with 21% in stage II disease. Only one randomised study comparing external beam therapy alone with external beam therapy plus intraluminal therapy has been published (as an abstract).[30] One hundred and twenty eight patients were randomised (64 in each arm) to receive 70 Gy in 35 fractions over seven weeks external beam therapy, or 50 Gy in 25 fractions over five weeks with three or four weekly insertions using caesium-137, delivering 6·54 Gy/fraction concurrently with the external therapy. Although there were more survivors at five years in the group treated with intraluminal therapy, this did not reach statistical significance. Brachytherapy is therefore safe, well tolerated, and provides good palliation of dysphagia. Before it can be recommended as a routine addition to external beam therapy as a radical treatment, however, further trials are necessary. Important issues are the scheduling of treatment and the relative merits of low dose rate and high dose rate therapy.

Combined radiotherapy and surgery

Although the majority of patients will develop metastatic disease, there remains a significant proportion who develop locoregional relapse as the only site of disease evident at postmortem examination. This group may benefit from a combined approach to treatment. There are two alternatives: radiotherapy may be given before (neoadjuvant) or after (adjuvant) surgery.

The aim of neoadjuvant therapy is to downstage the tumour and hence increase the chance of a complete resection. A pathologically complete response is found in as many as 15% of patients having a resection after radiotherapy.

Microscopic disease outside the surgical field may also be sterilised, and any clonogenic cells implanted at surgery are less likely to be viable.

Adjuvant radiotherapy is, by definition, given after an apparently complete resection to eradicate any possible residual microscopic disease. The advantages of this approach are that definitive treatment is not delayed, the disease is fully staged, and the surgeon is able to mark the areas most at risk of recurrence with radio-opaque clips. It may also be possible to define a group of patients in whom adjuvant treatment is not necessary. On the negative side, if the disease is found to be more extensive than thought preoperatively the chance to downstage has been missed.

Surgical intervention interferes with the usual routes of metastatic spread via the lymphatics and the target volume becomes more difficult to define. If the stomach has been pulled up into the chest the dose of radiation is limited because of the relative intolerance of the gastric mucosa. Probably because of these disadvantages postoperative radiotherapy has not been evaluated as frequently as preoperative therapy. Most authors conclude that it cannot be recommended routinely and that it should be reserved for those patients who have undergone a complete macroscopic resection but are found to have histologically positive resection margins, or where the surgeon considers a well defined localised area to be at high risk of residual microscopic disease. Doses of up to 60 Gy have been tolerated in this situation but many authors consider 50 Gy at 2 Gy/fraction as the safe limit.

Postoperative radiotherapy for bulk residual tumour should be regarded as palliative and the indications for treatment considered accordingly.

The results of preoperative radiotherapy are more controversial. Some authors report a survival benefit in small non-randomised studies, but this has not been supported by the data from four randomised trials comparing preoperative radiotherapy with surgery alone. The dose fractionation schedules and the relative timing of surgery and radiotherapy in these trials can, however, be criticised. Launois et al reported an increased postoperative mortality rate (although not statistically significant) in the group receiving radiation.[31] This study employed an unconventional regimen of 39–45 Gy over 8–12 days and surgery was performed after an interval of only eight days. No survival benefit was shown, although surgery was performed too soon for maximal regression from the radiotherapy to have been obtained. A European Organisation for the Research and Treatment of Cancer (EORTC) study employed the same timing of surgery but a lower radiation dose of 33 Gy in 10 fractions over 12 days.[32] Results in 201 patients showed equivalent resectability, operative mortality, and survival in both groups. Arnott et al randomised 176 potentially operable patients to surgery alone or preoperative radiotherapy.[33] The dose of radiation prescribed was only 20 Gy in 10 fractions over two weeks. This low dose was chosen on previous evidence that it would not adversely affect the operative morbidity. The only positive finding in favour of radiotherapy was decreased size of the

139

resected lymph nodes, but there was no difference in the proportion of histologically positive nodes. No difference between the two groups was observed in terms of operability or survival. A trial by Wang and Huang found no survival advantage for preoperative radiotherapy compared with surgery alone.[34] On present evidence routine preoperative radiotherapy cannot be recommended. More recent studies have evaluated the role of neoadjuvant chemoradiation.

Chemotherapy

There are several theoretical reasons why the addition of chemotherapy to the treatment of oesophageal cancer may be advantageous. Locoregional relapse and distant metastatic disease are both frequent findings at postmortem examination in patients treated radically for apparently localised disease: oesophageal cancer is therefore likely to be a systemic disease at diagnosis in the majority of cases. Chemotherapy can potentially eradicate microscopic disease but not clinically apparent metastases. An analogous situation is the treatment of breast cancer, in which the advantages of adjuvant cytotoxic chemotherapy are now well established. Neoadjuvant chemotherapy may improve local control for the same reasons as preoperative radiotherapy. There are additional theoretical advantages to concurrent administration of cytotoxic chemotherapy and radiation therapy. The clonogenic cell population within an individual tumour is not homogeneous and there is therefore a natural variation in the sensitivity to chemotherapy and radiotherapy within the tumour. There may therefore be an additive effect from combining the two modalities. Certain cytotoxic agents are thought to potentiate the effects of radiation (radiosensitisers) and, when given concurrently, a synergistic effect may be obtained. This assumes that the toxicity profiles of the two modalities are sufficiently dissimilar to avoid an unacceptable level of normal tissue toxicity.

Clinical experience with concurrent chemoradiation is that toxicity is significantly increased but can be acceptable.

The arguments for the use of chemotherapy are meaningless without effective cytotoxic drugs, but historically oesophageal carcinoma has been considered to be chemoresistant. A number of drugs have nevertheless been reported to be active against this tumour. Kelson reviewed the role of chemotherapy in oesophageal cancer in 1984[35] and updated this 10 years later.[36] In the early studies the criteria for defining response were not always objective measures of tumour regression—as determined for example, by endoscopy or radiology. A subjective improvement in swallowing was sometimes accepted as a response to treatment, although this correlates poorly with tumour regression.

As judged by WHO criteria, 10 agents have been shown to achieve at least a partial response (>50% but <100% regression, measured in at least two dimensions) in more than 15% of subjects (see box). Much of this data comes from small phase II studies, and the 95% confidence limits are wide.

Cytotoxic drugs with demonstrated activity against oesophageal carcinoma

- Bleomycin
- Cisplatin
- Doxorubicin
- 5-Fluorouracil
- Lomustine

- Methotrexate
- Mitoguazone
- Mitomycin
- Paclitaxel
- Vindesine

Combination chemotherapy is now being investigated. Because the number of patients treated by chemotherapy remains small, there is no consensus on the most active single agent or the best combination. Cisplatin is the most widely investigated drug and is included in the majority of modern regimens, often combined with 5-fluorouracil (5FU). The added advantage of these drugs when combined with radiotherapy is that they are considered to be radiosensitisers and hence to potentiate the effect of radiation; however, mucositis may be expected to be more severe when 5FU is given concurrently with radiation as this is a major toxic effect of both treatments.

Mitomycin is the preferred drug of some authors, either replacing or in conjunction with cisplatin, because of the positive results of combining mitomycin and radiation as primary treatment for anal carcinoma. Mitomycin is also more toxic to hypoxic cells, which are relatively radioresistant.

Bleomycin was one of the earliest drugs to be found to be effective against oesophageal carcinoma, but it can no longer be recommended because of the risk of pulmonary fibrosis. There is evidence that previous or combined radiotherapy to the chest increases the risk of fibrosis, as does subsequent surgery, possibly as a result of relative hyperoxia during anaesthesia.

Combined chemotherapy and radiotherapy

Chemotherapy may be delivered before, with, or after radiotherapy. There are no studies that have employed post-radiation chemotherapy alone, but some investigators giving concurrent treatment have continued chemotherapy for several cycles after completion of radiation.

141

Neoadjuvant chemotherapy The use of neoadjuvant chemotherapy before radiotherapy has not been widely investigated. The advantage of this scheduling is that it is less toxic than concurrent chemoradiation. There are, however, theoretical disadvantages. The response rate to present chemotherapy regimens remains disappointingly low, and patients with unresponsive disease gain no benefit from chemotherapy; by delaying definitive treatment the prognosis of this group may be compromised. In those patients with chemosensitive disease, accelerated repopulation may be induced by chemotherapy, reducing the probability of control with radiation. A phase II study reported by Valerdi *et al* employed a regimen of two cycles of cisplatin, bleomycin, and vindesine before radiotherapy.[37] The median survival was 11 months, which is no better than might be expected with radiation alone. More significantly, the local failure rate was 67%, which is higher than in series of patients treated by concurrent chemoradiation.

There are insufficient data to reach any conclusions, but a comparison can be made with the experience of this approach in the treatment of squamous carcinoma of the head and neck. Despite a high response rate (up to 70%) to cisplatin and 5FU, a survival benefit has not been demonstrated.

Concurrent chemoradiation The results of several phase II studies and randomised trials comparing concurrent chemoradiation with radiation alone have now been published (Table 5.5). A non-randomised study was published by Stewart *et al* in 1989.[38] Patients considered fit for surgery were referred for oesophagectomy after receiving chemoradiation. A regimen of 5FU, cisplatin, and mitomycin was given concurrently with radiation to a dose 45 Gy over 4·5 weeks. Of 25 patients with squamous carcinoma, 12 (48%) achieved a complete clinical response and a further nine (36%) a partial response. Thirteen patients had an oesophagectomy and, of these, five had a pathologically complete response. In a further two the only residual disease was outside the radiotherapy treatment volume. The authors concluded that the overall tumour sterilisation rate was 7 of 13 (54%) in those patients undergoing surgery. Patients with metastatic disease were included and this was reflected in the poor survival figures. The median survival was 10 months for the group undergoing surgery and five months for the no surgery group. Because of this it is not really possible to draw any conclusions regarding survival benefit, but this study did show that concurrent chemoradiation is tolerable and that it will eradicate the tumour in a significant proportion of patients.

The Wayne State University group published the results of a non-randomised study in 1994.[39] Previously this group had operated on all suitable patients after chemoradiation, but they abandoned routine surgery

TABLE 5.5—*Selected trials of concurrent chemoradiation*

Authors	Radiotherapy	Chemotherapy	Survival
Non-randomised			
Stewart et al[12]	45 Gy in 4·5 weeks	Cisplatin 5FU Mitomycin	10 months (median)
Poplin et al[13]	50 Gy in 25 fractions	Cisplatin 5FU	24 months (median, actuarial) 1 year 65% 2 years 50% (estimated)
Coia et al[14]	60 Gy in 30 fractions	5FU Mitomycin	18 months* (median) 3 years 29% (actuarial) 5 years 18% (actuarial)
Randomised—compared with radiation alone			
Sischy et al[15†]	60–64 Gy in 30–32 fractions	5FU Mitomycin	Advantage in combined therapy
Herskovic et al[16‡]	50 Gy in 25 fractions	Cisplatin 5FU	Advantage in combined therapy
Arauja et al[47§]	50 Gy in 25 fractions	5FU Mitomycin Bleomycin	Difference not statistically significant

* Stage I and II only (disease specific median survival was 20 months).
† Control arm—same radiation dose.
‡ Control arm—radiation dose 64 Gy in 32 fractions.
§ Control arm—same radiation dose.

because of an unacceptable operative mortality. In this study, therefore, surgery was reserved for those patients not achieving a complete response to chemoradiation. The chemotherapy regimen chosen was 5FU and cisplatin because earlier work by the same group had suggested that this combination was superior to 5FU and mitomycin. Radiation was given to a total dose of 50 Gy in 25 fractions. Concurrent chemoradiation was followed by further chemotherapy, and after four cycles the patient was reassessed. If a complete response had been achieved then chemotherapy was continued for a further three months. If there was neither a complete response nor evidence of metastatic disease, an oesophagectomy was performed. Of the 26 patients entered into the study, 17 (65%) achieved a complete response, as judged by endoscopic inspection. Eight of these had negative biopsies, but biopsy was not performed on all patients. The median actuarial survival was 24 months. The survival rate at one year was 65% and the estimated two year survival 50%. The toxicity of this regimen was considerable: 15 patients required a dose reduction or a delay in chemotherapy; 19 patients required hospitalisation because of toxicity, although there were no treatment related deaths.

A further non-randomised study of concurrent chemoradiation was reported by Coia et al.[40] Again, patients with advanced disease were included. Of the 90 patients treated, 57 had stage I or II disease (1978 American joint committee staging criteria), and were considered potentially curable.

Two cycles of chemotherapy were given during the first and fifth weeks of radiation, consisting of 5FU, 1000 mg/m^2/24 h given as a 96 hour infusion commencing on days 2 and 29 and mitomycin, 10 mg/m^2, given on day 2 only. The radiation dose for those patients with stage I or II disease was 60 Gy at 2 Gy/fraction over 6–7 weeks. Those with stage III or IV disease received the same chemotherapy but the radiation dose was modified (median dose was 50 Gy).

The median disease specific survival for the patients with stage I and II disease was 20 months. The actuarial disease specific survival was 74% at one year, 44% at two years, 41% at three years, and 30% at five years. The actuarial local relapse free survival was 70% at three years and remained constant at five years. The authors concluded that chemoradiation, although toxic, is relatively well tolerated and does have an impact on survival.

A randomised trial by the Eastern Cooperative Oncology Group (ECOG) has been published in abstract by Sischy et al.[41] A regimen comprising 5FU and mitomycin plus radiotherapy was compared with radiation alone. The radiation dose was 60–64 Gy at 2 Gy/fraction. The results demonstrated a survival advantage in the group receiving the combined treatment, the median survival being 15 months compared with nine months. An option to refer the patient for surgery at the discretion of the attending physician could potentially have caused some bias due to case selection, and the results should therefore be regarded with some caution.

A more significant result in favour of chemoradiation was reported by Herskovic et al.[42] Patients were randomised to receive 5FU and cisplatin concurrently with radiation to a dose of 50 Gy in 25 fractions, or radiation alone to a dose of 64 Gy in 32 fractions. In both arms radiation was given in two phases. The initial phase included the supraclavicular fossae within the fields. Patients with metastatic disease (other than supraclavicular lymphadenopathy) were excluded. Chemotherapy was given during weeks 1, 5, 8, and 11, and each cycle consisted of cisplatinum, 75 mg/m^2, on day 1, and 5FU, 1000 mg/m^2/day, on days 1–4.

The trial was terminated early, after 129 patients had been entered, because interim analysis of the first 121 patients found a statistically significant survival advantage in the group receiving the combined treatment. The median survival for the group receiving chemoradiation was 12·5 months, compared with 8·9 months for the group treated by irradiation alone (p<0·001). The estimated survival at one and two years was 33% and 10% respectively in the radiotherapy group, compared with 50% and 38% respectively for those receiving combined therapy. As in other studies, the authors comment on the toxicity of treatment. One patient receiving chemoradiation died of bone marrow and renal failure. Side effects were considered severe in 44% and life threatening in 20% of the combined modality group, compared with 25% and 3% respectively in the radiation alone group.

The authors concluded that, although a survival advantage is seen with chemoradiation, this must be considered in relation to the significant morbidity of treatment. One further randomised trial reporting a survival benefit for chemoradiation has been reported by Arauja et al.[43] The five year survival for the group treated with a regimen of mitomycin, 5FU, and bleomycin given concurrently with radiation was 16%, compared with a five year survival of 6% in the group treated with radiation alone. This difference did not reach statistical significance and the trial can be criticised because the radiation dose was 50 Gy in 25 fractions in both arms and this is undoubtedly suboptimal if not combined with chemotherapy.

There are several ongoing trials addressing chemoradiation.

Interim analysis of two large multicentre trials has suggested that these may show a survival advantage in favour of chemoradiation.

Combined chemotherapy and surgery

The rationale for the use of adjuvant or neoadjuvant chemotherapy in conjunction with surgery is to improve locoregional control by downstaging before surgery, and to reduce distant relapse by eradication of micrometastases. The arguments, discussed above, against the use of neoadjuvant chemotherapy before radiotherapy can be applied to neoadjuvant chemotherapy before surgery, in particular the risk of delaying definitive treatment and thereby compromising the prognosis of those with chemoresistant disease. Because of this, most investigators limit preoperative chemotherapy to two cycles.

Most of the available data are from small, non-randomised studies; only two randomised trials have been published. Roth et al compared a regimen of two cycles of cisplatin, vindesine, and bleomycin preoperatively and six months of cisplatinum and vindesine postoperatively with surgery alone.[44] Schlag gave three cycles of cisplatin and 5FU to those randomised to neoadjuvant therapy.[45] Neither study reported an advantage in terms of resectability or survival for those receiving chemotherapy. Although Schlag reported a higher rate of postoperative complications in the group treated with chemotherapy, this was not confirmed either in Roth's study or in other series. Both of these trials included small numbers of patients (<50). There are at present at least three large ongoing multicentre trials investigating the role of neoadjuvant chemotherapy. Two American trials exclude patients with adenocarcinoma. A British, Medical Research Council trial (OEO2) includes patients with squamous carcinoma, adenocarcinoma, and undifferentiated carcinoma of the upper, middle, or lower oesophagus, but excludes those with post-cricoid tumours. The primary must be considered resectable and metastatic disease (including cervical lymphadenopathy) excluded. Randomisation is to two cycles of 5FU and cisplatin before surgery or to surgery alone.

Combined chemotherapy, radiotherapy, and surgery

Because of the doubts about the benefit of preoperative chemotherapy and the fact that, despite a good response rate, chemoradiation alone does not always eradicate the tumour, a number of investigators are now employing a regimen of neoadjuvant chemoradiation before surgery.

Coia et al found that of 57 patients treated with chemoradiation for localised disease, local failure occurred in 14 (25%).[40] Five patients had local failure only. Two of these were salvaged by oesophagectomy, of whom one was a long term survivor.

Early experience with this multimodality approach to treatment was published in 1984 by the Wayne State University group.[46] The impetus had been the encouraging results that the group had experienced with a similar regimen in the treatment of anal carcinoma. The initial chemotherapy was a regimen of mitomycin and 5FU but a second study substituted cisplatin for mitomycin (see above). Concurrent radiation was given to a dose of 30 Gy in 15 fractions. If at surgery there was evidence of residual disease, further chemotherapy was given, with postoperative radiotherapy to a total dose of 50 Gy in 25 fractions. These were two small pilot studies and little can be concluded regarding survival, but the toxicity of the regimen is clear. Of a total of 42 patients undergoing surgery, 12 (29%) died without leaving hospital; 11 (26%) had a complete response to chemoradiation and this was found to be the best predictor of long term survival. The value of surgery in complete responders was doubtful, and as the operative mortality was unacceptable, the subsequent trial reserved surgery only for those patients who failed to achieve a complete response to chemoradiation.

The largest series has been reported by Poplin et al.[47]

This Radiotherapy Oncology Group and Southwest Oncology Group study enrolled 113 patients to a regimen of 5FU and cisplatin combined with radiotherapy. This trial was a follow on from the Wayne State trial and again allocated surgery after two cycles of chemotherapy and a radiation dose of 30 Gy. Chemoradiation was continued postoperatively if there was evidence of residual disease histologically.

Almost one third (32%) of patients had no operation, and only a half (49%) had the tumour resected. Complete eradication of the tumour was achieved in 18 (17%) of the 106 evaluable patients. In 28% of the original population, disease progression was documented before, or at, surgery. The median survival was 12 months and the two and three year survival was 28% and 16% respectively; operative mortality was 11%. A complete response to chemoradiation was again the most influential prognostic indicator, and the additional benefit of surgery in this group was doubtful.

The one study to have shown a potential survival advantage for surgery after chemoradiation was published by Forastiere et al.[48] A median survival of 29 months and a one, two, and five year survival of 65, 55, and 34% respectively were observed in a series of 43 patients treated with a regimen of 5FU, cisplatin, and vindesine combined with twice daily radiotherapy (37·5 Gy in 15 daily fractions or 45 Gy in 20 fractions treating twice daily), administered over 21 days. Transhiatal oesophagectomy was performed on day 42. In contrast to other studies there were some long term survivors among patients who did not achieve a complete response to chemoradiation. Of the 41 undergoing surgery (there were two deaths due to chemoradiation), 36 were considered to have had a potentially curative operation. Of these, 26 had microscopic residual disease in the resected specimen. The median survival in this group was 26 months, and the five year survival 32%. The corresponding results in the 10 patients with a pathological complete response were a median survival of 70 months and a five year survival of 60%. The operative mortality was much more acceptable than in previous studies, with only one postoperative death recorded.

In 1984 Anderson et al reported a randomised trial comparing preoperative radiotherapy alone or combined with bleomycin.[49] The results were equally poor in both arms. Bleomycin is no longer regarded as the most active drug in the treatment of oesophageal carcinoma, and the radiation dose was low (30 Gy with bleomycin and 35 Gy in the control arm). One further study has compared sequential chemotherapy and radiotherapy with radiotherapy alone preoperatively.[50] No survival advantage was demonstrated for the combined treatment. No randomised trial comparing preoperative chemoradiation with surgery alone has yet been published but Forastiere's group has now commenced such a trial.

Palliative treatment

Earlam and Cunha-Melo's data suggest that at initial diagnosis approximately 50% of patients with oesophageal cancer will be incurable.[26 27]

A few will present in the terminal stages of disease when nothing more than supportive care would be appropriate, but the majority will be symptomatic, yet well enough to be considered for palliative treatment. This section considers non-surgical palliation of symptoms peculiar to oesophageal cancer, particularly dysphagia, and nutrition. Surgical and endoscopic methods are dealt with by Bancewicz and Osugi earlier in this chapter.

Many patients manage a soft diet or liquid feeds but some develop complete dysphagia. In general, nasogastric or gastrostomy feeding of terminally ill patients cannot be recommended, but with oesophageal cancer the loss of weight and poor nutritional state is often out of proportion to the extent of disease. The quality of life of such patients is significantly improved by enabling them to take some form of diet. A fine bore nasogastric tube is often acceptable in the short term—for example, during radiotherapy—but it is not always possible to pass a tube through a tight stricture. In this situation, or for longer term feeding, a gastrostomy should be considered. It is not possible to be dogmatic regarding the best approach and the patient's wishes should be the major consideration. The optimal palliative management of oesophageal cancer remains uncertain. A variety of options is available (see box).

> ## Palliative therapies for oesophageal cancer
>
> - Surgery
>   Resection
>   Bypass
>
> - Endoscopic techniques
>   Dilatation
>   Intubation
>   Laser
>   Diathermy
>   Photodynamic therapy
>   Injection of alcohol
>
> - Radiotherapy
>   External beam
>   Brachytherapy
>
> - Chemotherapy

Dysphagia is a major symptom in the majority of patients, and improving swallowing function is one of the main aims of palliative treatment. A retrospective analysis of 537 patients with unresectable oesophageal carcinoma has reported that surgical bypass is very effective in relieving dysphagia and that the median survival was longer and the hospital mortality lower than for patients treated with radiotherapy.[51] It is probable that these results are biased by patient selection and we agree with the surgical authors that resection or bypass should not be considered as routine palliative procedures.

Palliative radiotherapy

External beam radiation

The advantage of radiotherapy over other palliative modalities is that it can cause tumour regression. Although symptoms may take longer to improve, the response may be more prolonged. Intraluminal therapy is reported to produce more rapid symptomatic relief than external beam therapy, but the latter will also control disease in the mediastinum and is more likely to produce relief of the pain that these patients often experience.

The optimal dose of external beam irradiation is uncertain. In many American series doses as high as 50–60 Gy are employed for palliation, even in patients with distant metastatic disease. The British philosophy is somewhat different and most British oncologists would consider this dose excessive. The aim is not to eradicate the disease but simply to improve symptoms for the duration of the patient's survival.

A retrospective analysis of the effect of radiotherapy on dysphagia and survival has been reported by Caspers et al.[52] Fourteen potential prognostic factors were considered. The authors measured swallowing ability at presentation on a semiquantitative scale, which was termed the PASS score. Although radiation dose was found to be an independent prognostic factor in the full analysis, it had no effect on disease free survival or overall survival in patients with a PASS score of less than 2 (unable to swallow semisolid or solid food). The authors concluded that this group were equally palliated with a lower dose of radiation; however, in this study low dose was considered to be less than the equivalent of 50 Gy in 25 fractions over five weeks. A similar retrospective analysis has been reported by Albertsson et al,[53] but in this study the prescribed dose for palliative treatment was usually 40–44 Gy at 2 Gy/fraction, and for radical treatment 56–64 Gy, again at 2 Gy/fraction. Eighty one patients had treatment with palliative intent and 68 with curative intent. Before treatment all patients complained of dysphagia but at two months after completion of treatment 41% (of those remaining alive) had subjectively normal swallowing, and a further 44%, although not achieving completely normal swallowing, were able to eat normal food. The figures for those treated palliatively were 45 and 33% respectively, and for radical treatment 35 and 63% respectively. Interestingly, at this time only 43 patients (63%) who had received curative treatment were still alive, compared with 67 (83%) of those treated palliatively. Although both studies concluded that there is a survival advantage with a higher dose of radiation, which has been suggested by other authors, this is based on retrospective data and hence is naturally biased by patient selection.

Brachytherapy

The value of intraluminal therapy as a palliative treatment has already been mentioned; however, an advantage over external beam therapy alone has not been demonstrated in a randomised trial. Most investigators have combined intraluminal therapy with external beam therapy, but there are reports of intraluminal therapy alone achieving good palliation. The scheduling of treatment is probably less important than when considering curative therapy but it may be advantageous to employ intraluminal therapy before external beam therapy. It is reported that relief of dysphagia is achieved more rapidly after intraluminal therapy but this may be the result, at least in part, of dilatation of the oesophagus during the procedure, although this is less of an effect with some of the newer machines that employ a catheter of much finer bore.

Pagliero and Rowland have reported on the palliative value of intraluminal therapy alone.[54] It was reported that good palliation was achieved with a single treatment of 15 Gy (prescribed 1 cm from the source) with a response rate of 70% for squamous carcinoma and 60% for adenocarcinoma, measured at six weeks after treatment. In many patients this was sustained. If there was initially a good response but a subsequent relapse, the procedure was repeated.

Dawes *et al* employed a regimen of intraluminal therapy combined with external beam therapy.[55] Patients treated palliatively received 30 Gy in 10 fractions by external beam and then a subsequent insertion delivering 10 Gy at a distance of 1 cm from the source (dose rate 6·4 Gy per hour). Excellent palliation was reported (although this was not quantified) and the procedure was straightforward. Radiotherapy can, therefore, effectively palliate dysphagia, and high doses are not necessary to achieve this. The median survival of patients with advanced disease is in the region of six months and the disruption and toxicity of a prolonged course of treatment are not justified. A dose of 30 Gy delivered in 10 fractions over two weeks by parallel opposed anterior and posterior fields is well tolerated and effectively controls symptoms in the majority of patients. Dawes *et al* reported that at endoscopy after this dose there was invariably complete or almost complete regression of the tumour.[55] If intraluminal therapy is available locally it may offer an improvement in local control at acceptable cost in terms of discomfort to the patient, but this remains uncertain.

Combined radiotherapy and endoscopic techniques

As endoscopic techniques such as laser therapy or intubation offer rapid relief of dysphagia but do nothing to prevent tumour progression, whereas radiation therapy, although taking longer, produces a more durable response, it seems reasonable to consider that a combined approach may offer optimal palliation. Two prospective randomised trials and one retrospective study that have considered this have been published. Although the number of patients is small the results suggest that the addition of radiotherapy to endoscopic techniques has no positive effect on survival.

Reed *et al* randomised 27 patients to one of three possible treatment arms:[56] intubation with an Atkinson tube; intubation plus radiotherapy; or laser therapy followed by irradiation. The radiation dose was 45 Gy in 25 fractions in the second and third arms. There was no significant difference in improvement in symptoms or median survival (119, 72, and 169 days respectively) between the three groups. The authors comment that the addition of radiation to laser therapy proved advantageous, in terms of duration of response, when compared with data available from other series which report a significant rate of recurrence of dysphagia. This approach was preferable to intubation, as the complication rate was significantly lower.

Schmid *et al* conducted a randomised trial comparing intubation alone with intubation in conjunction with subsequent chemotherapy or radiotherapy;[57] 127 patients with advanced inoperable oesophageal cancer were entered. Patients in the group treated by intubation alone were observed to have the longest median survival at 15 weeks, compared with 9 and 11 weeks for those receiving radiotherapy and chemotherapy respectively. The difference was not statistically significant. This trial may be criticised because the radiation dose and fractionation was unusual—20 Gy in five fractions over one week, repeated after a five week gap. Also a variety of chemotherapy regimens was employed but none included cisplatin, which is considered by most investigators to be the most active drug in oesophageal cancer.

The results of these two trials are supported by a study published by Oliver *et al.*[58] The authors retrospectively analysed the results of the treatment of oesophageal cancer in Nottingham. Thirty two patients were treated by endoscopic intubation alone, six received radical radiotherapy and 21 intubation plus radical radiotherapy. An unspecified number received a palliative dose of radiation after intubation. The populations of the different groups were not equivalent. Those treated by intubation alone were significantly older and more likely to have metastatic disease. Most patients were initially intubated and then a decision made as to further treatment. As might be expected, the median survival for the group treated by

151

intubation alone was less than for the irradiated group—75 days compared with 188 days; however, this was clearly biased by patient selection. Eleven (34%) of the patients intubated died within 30 days of diagnosis, whereas none of those irradiated died in this period. If these 11 patients are excluded, there is no significant difference in survival between the two groups. Also of note is that the average time spent in hospital was 46 days for the irradiated group, compared with only 23 days for the intubated group (again excluding those dying within 30 days).

Palliative chemotherapy

Many American studies investigating chemoradiation (see above) have included patients with locally advanced and metastatic disease. Despite good local control of disease these patients usually die within a few months. We believe this aggressive approach should only be considered for patients with a realistic chance of cure.

Palliative chemotherapy is not routinely considered for oesophageal cancer because of the disappointing response rate, even with modern combination regimens, and the associated toxicity in patients who are often elderly and of poor performance status. Local control is achieved more effectively and with less toxicity with other treatment modalities and to date there is little evidence that chemotherapy significantly improves systemic symptoms or survival. There are, however, reports of phase II trials now appearing in the literature.

Stahl et al have reported the results of a regimen of 5FU, folinic acid, etoposide, and cisplatin given to 38 patients, 12 of whom were known to have metastatic disease.[59] Similarly, Allen et al have published the results achieved with a regimen of mitomycin, ifosfamide, and cisplatin (MIC) in 45 patients, of whom 20 were considered incurable because they were unfit for surgery or had extensive disease.[60] Of the 12 patients in Stahl's series, two achieved a complete response, and three a partial response, giving an overall response rate (complete plus partial) of 42%. The median survival was six months, but this increased to 15 months in those who responded. Of the 20 inoperable patients receiving MIC chemotherapy, one achieved a complete response and a further four a partial response, giving an overall response rate of 25%. Again, a survival benefit was observed in the responding group. The one patient with a complete response was alive and disease free 29 months from the start of treatment, the four achieving partial response dying at 4, 9, 12, and 26 months. This was in contrast to a median survival of six months in those in whom disease remained static during treatment, and three months for those with progressive disease.

A phase II study of 5FU, adriamycin, and mitomycin (FAM) in adenocarcinoma of the oesophagus and gastro-oesophageal junction has been reported.[61] The rationale for the use of FAM was the experience with the regimen in the treatment of gastric adenocarcinoma. The overall response rate (all partial) was 37% (6 of 16 patients). The authors suggest that this is similar to the response seen in gastric carcinoma.

These studies suggest that, although only a minority of patients respond to treatment, there is a potential survival advantage for this group. Toxicity was considered acceptable and there were no treatment related deaths.

Further studies are required to try to determine which patients are most likely to benefit from palliative chemotherapy and which is the most active regimen. There are no trials comparing chemotherapy with best supportive care in patients with oesophageal cancer. At present, therefore, palliative chemotherapy remains experimental and should only be considered in the context of a clinical trial.

Future developments

With the more widespread availability of endo-oesophageal ultrasonography the staging of oesophageal carcinoma may be improved. This modality has been demonstrated to be superior to CT in determining the depth of oesophageal wall invasion and the presence of mediastinal node involvement. With more accurate staging it should be possible to select more appropriately those patients who may benefit from aggressive treatment regimens. Early diagnosis is important but the disease is usually advanced by the time that symptoms have developed. Dysphagia does not normally occur until the lumen of the oesophagus is at least 50% occluded. In China, where there is a very high incidence of oesophageal carcinoma, screening programmes have been successful in improving survival figures; however, in the West oesophageal cancer is less common and routine screening is not practical.

Delivering a higher dose of radiation to the tumour may increase local control rates but is unlikely to have a big impact on the overall mortality. This has been demonstrated with intraluminal therapy, which does produce a change in the pattern of disease relapse, with less local failures and a greater proportion of distant failures, but has not been conclusively shown to improve overall survival. Modern techniques, such as conformal therapy and three dimensional or "beam's eye view" planning, may enable a higher dose of radiation to be delivered by external beam therapy but, again, whether this is advantageous remains to be seen.

The response to chemotherapy remains disappointing, and the optimal regimen remains uncertain. It is always hoped that the next cytotoxic agent to be discovered will be the "magic bullet" (originally used by Ehrlich in relation to antibiotic therapy), but experience suggests otherwise. More recent developments, such as immunotherapy and biological modulators, have not as yet found a role in the treatment of oesophageal carcinoma.

Whether or not adenocarcinoma and squamous carcinomas should be treated differently remains controversial. Some trials of chemotherapy or radiotherapy exclude adenocarcinoma. Others do include adenocarcinoma, but the numbers are often small and subgroup analysis is not possible.

It is clear that many questions regarding the treatment of oesophageal carcinoma remain unanswered, and that further trials are necessary. This is true of both radical and palliative treatment. Recent data suggest that there may be a survival advantage for combined modality regimens but most of this data comes from phase II studies and comparison with historical controls. At present it is only concurrent chemoradiation that has been demonstrated to achieve this in a randomised controlled trial, and this is at the expense of a significantly increased toxicity. Patient selection is therefore important and this approach can only be recommended for the minority of patients of good performance status with localised disease, in whom there is a realistic chance of cure.

References

19 Dobbs J, Barrett A, Ash D. *Practical radiotherapy planning*. London: Edward Arnold, 1992.
20 O'Rourke IC, Tiver K, Bull C, *et al.* Swallowing performance after radiation therapy for carcinoma of the esophagus. *Cancer* 1988;**61**:2022–6.
21 Mendenhall WM, Sombeck MD, Parsons JT, *et al.* Management of cervical esophageal carcinoma. *Semin Radiat Oncol* 1994;**4**:179–91.
22 Earlam R, Cunha-Melo JR. Oesophageal squamous cell carcinoma: I. A critical review of surgery. *Br J Surg* 1980;**67**:381–90.
23 Earlam R, Cunha-Melo JR. Oesophageal squamous cell carcinoma: II. A critical review of radiotherapy. *Br J Surg* 1980;**67**:457–61.
24 Oliver SE, Robertson CS, Logan RF. Oesophageal cancer: a population based study of survival after treatment. *Br J Surg* 1992;**79**:1321–5.
25 Sagar PM, Gauperaa T, Sue-Ling H, *et al.* An audit of the treatment of cancer of the oesophagus. *Gut* 1994;**35**:941–5.
26 Newaishy GA, Read GA, Duncan W, *et al.* Results of radical radiotherapy of squamous cell carcinoma of the oesophagus. *Clin Radiol* 1982;**33**:347–52.
27 Flores AD, Nelems B, Evans K, *et al.* Impact of new radiotherapy modalities on surgical management of cancer of the esophagus and cardia. *Int J Radiat Oncol Biol Phys* 1989;**17**:937–44.
28 Hishikawa Y, Kurisu K, Taniguchi M, *et al.* High-dose-rate intraluminal brachytherapy for esophageal cancer: 10 years experience in Hyogo college of medicine. *Radiother Oncol* 1991;**21**:107–14.
29 Hareyama M, Nishio M, Kagami Y, *et al.* Intracavitary brachytherapy combined with external-beam irradiation for squamous cell carcinoma of the thoracic esophagus. *Int J Radiat Oncol Biol Phys* 1992;**24**:235–40.
30 Yin W. Brachytherapy of carcinoma of the oesophagus in China. *Brachytherapy 2: Proceedings of the 5th international SELECTRON user's meeting*, 1988. Leersum: Nucletron International, 1989:439–41.
31 Launois B, Delarve D. Campion JP, *et al.* Preoperative radiotherapy for carcinoma of the esophagus. *Surg Gynecol Obstet* 1981;**153**:690–2.

32 Gignoux M, Roussel A, Paillot B, *et al.* The value of preoperative radiotherapy in esophageal cancer: results of a study of the EORTC. *World J Surg* 1987;**11**:426–32.

33 Arnott SJ, Duncan W, Kerr GR, *et al.* Low dose preoperative radiotherapy for carcinoma of the oesophagus: results of a randomised clinical trial. *Radiother Oncol* 1992;**24**:108–13.

34 Wang L, Huang G. Combined preoperative irradiation and surgery versus surgery alone for carcinoma of the midthoracic esophagus [abstract]. *Proceedings of the fourth world congress of international society for diseases of the esophagus*; 1989:63.

35 Kelson D. Chemotherapy of esophageal cancer. *Semin Oncol* 1984;**11**:159–68.

36 Kelson DP. The role of chemotherapy in the treatment of esophageal cancer. *Chest Surg Clin North Am* 1994;**4**:173–84.

37 Valerdi JJ, Tejedor M, Illarramendi JJ, *et al.* Neoadjuvant chemotherapy and radiotherapy in locally advanced esophagus carcinoma: long term results. *Int J Radiat Oncol Biol Phys* 1993;**27**:843–7.

38 Stewart FM, Harkins BJ, Hahn SS, *et al.* Cisplatin, 5-fluorouracil, mitomycin c, and concurrent radiation therapy with and without esophogectomy for esophageal carcinoma. *Cancer* 1989;**64**:622–8.

39 Poplin EA, Khanuja PS, Kraut MJ, *et al.* Chemoradiotherapy of esophageal carcinoma. *Cancer* 1994;**74**:1217–24.

40 Coia LR, Engstrom PF, Paul AR, *et al.* Long-term results of infusional 5-FU, mitomycin-c, and radiation as primary management of esophageal carcinoma. *Int J Radiat Oncol Biol Phys* 1991;**20**:29–36.

41 Sischy B, Ryan L, Haller D. Interim report of EST 1282 phase III protocol for the evaluation of combined modalities in the treatment of patients with carcinoma of the esophagus, stage I and II [abstract]. *Proc Am Soc Clin Oncol* 1990;**9**:105.

42 Herskovic A, Martz K, Al-Sarraf M, *et al.* Combined chemotherapy and radiotherapy compared with radiotherapy alone in patients with cancer of the esophagus. *N Engl J Med* 1992;**326**:1593–8.

43 Arauja CMM, Souhami L, Gil RA, *et al.* A randomised trial comparing radiation therapy versus concomitant radiation therapy and chemotherapy in carcinoma of the thoracic esophagus. *Cancer* 1991;**67**:2258–61.

44 Roth JA, Pass HI, Flanagan MM, *et al.* Randomized clinical trial of preoperative and postoperative adjuvant chemotherapy with cisplatin, vindesine, and bleomycin for carcinoma of the esophagus. *J Thorac Cardiovasc Surg* 1989;**96**:242–8.

45 Schlag PM. Randomised trial of preoperative chemotherapy for squamous cancer of the esophagus. *Arch Surg* 1992;**127**:1446–50.

46 Leichman L, Steiger Z, Seydel HG, *et al.* Combined preoperative chemotherapy and radiation therapy for cancer of the esophagus: the Wayne State University, Southwest oncology group and radiation oncology group experience. *Semin Oncol* 1984;**11**:178–85.

47 Poplin E, Fleming T, Leichman L, *et al.* Combined therapies for squamous-cell carcinoma of the esophagus, a southwest oncology group study (SWOG-8037). *J Clin Oncol* 1987;**5**:622–628.

48 Forastiere AA, Orringer MB, Perez-Tamayo C, *et al.* Preoperative chemoradiation followed by transhiatal esophagectomy for carcinoma of the esophagus: final report. *J Clin Oncol* 1993;**11**:1118–23.

49 Anderson AP, Berdal P, Edsmyer F, *et al.* Irradiation, chemotherapy and surgery in esophageal cancer: a randomised clinical trial. *Radiother Oncol* 1984;**2**:179–88.

50 Le Prise E, Etienne PL, Meunier B, *et al.* A randomised study of chemotherapy, radiation therapy, and surgery versus surgery for localised squamous cell carcinoma of the esophagus. *Cancer* 1994;**73**:1779–84.

51 Sawant D, Moghassi K. Management of unresectable oesophageal cancer: a review of 537 patients. *Eur J Cardiothorac Surg* 1994;**8**:113–17.

52 Caspers RJL, Welvaart K, Verkes RJ, *et al.* The effect of radiotherapy on dysphagia and survival in patients with esophageal cancer. *Radiother Oncol* 1988;**12**:15–23.

53 Albertsson M, Ewers SB, Widmark H, *et al.* Evaluation of the palliative effect of radiotherapy for esophageal carcinoma. *Acta Oncol* 1989;**28**:267–70.

54 Pagliero KM, Rowland CG. The place of brachytherapy in the treatment of carcinoma of the esophagus. Brachytherapy HDR and LDR. *Proceedings of a brachytherapy meeting:*

Remote afterloading; state of the art; 1989. Columbia: Nucletron Corporation, 1990:44–51.

55 Dawes PJDK, Clague MB, Dean EM. Combined external beam and intracavitary radiotherapy for carcinoma of the oesophagus. *Brachytherapy 2: Proceedings of the 5th international SELECTRON user's meeting*; 1988. Leersum: Nucletron International, 1989: 442–4.

56 Reed CE, Marsh WH, Carlson LS, *et al.* Prospective, randomized trial of palliative treatment for unresectable cancer of the esophagus. *Ann Thorac Surg* 1991;**51**:552–6.

57 Schmid EU, Alberts AS, Greeff F, *et al.* The value of radiotherapy or chemotherapy after intubation for advanced esophageal carcinoma: a prospective randomised trial. *Radiother Oncol* 1993;**28**:27–30.

58 Oliver SE, Robertson CS, Logan RFA, *et al.* What does radiotherapy add to survival over endoscopic palliation alone in inoperable squamous cell oesophageal cancer? *Gut* 1990; **31**:750–2.

59 Stahl M, Wilke H, Meyer HJ, *et al.* 5-Fluorouracil, folinic acid, etoposide and cisplatin chemotherapy for locally advanced or metastatic carcinoma of the oesophagus. *Eur J Cancer* 1994;**30A**:325–8.

60 Allen SM, Duffy JP, Walker SJ, *et al.* A phase II study of mitomycin, ifosfamide and cisplatin in operable and inoperable squamous cell carcinoma of the oesophagus. *Clin Oncol R Coll Radiol* 1994;**6**:91–5.

61 Khansur T, Allred C, Tavassoli M. 5-Fluorouracil, adriamycin, and mitomycin-c in adenocarcinoma of the esophagus or gastroesophageal junction. *Am J Clin Oncol* 1994; **17**:506–8.

6: Stomach

Tumour biology, investigation, and surgical management

PETER McCULLOCH and MITSURU SASAKO

Epidemiology

Gastric cancer remains the leading cause of death from malignant disease in the world. This fact is often forgotten in Western countries where its incidence has declined, and it has become principally a disease of the elderly. A global review shows that the incidence is highest in the Far East, most notably Japan but also in China, the Philippines, and South East Asia. Other areas of particularly high incidence are in the Andean countries of South America and in eastern Europe. Amongst the lowest incidences recorded are those from Australia and the USA, where the disease has declined dramatically over the last 30 or 40 years. The decline in the United Kingdom and western Europe has been less stark, and here gastric cancer still ranks about fourth or fifth in the causes of cancer death amongst adults. There are interesting variations within countries—for instance, in the United Kingdom. Here the disease is most common in the north and west and has declined very significantly in the south east. A number of genetic and environmental factors have been identified which can partly account for the described variations in incidence, and for the changes in incidence over the last few decades. Probably the most important of these is the association of gastric cancer with diet. A comparison of high and low incidence areas reveals a rather consistent association between particular dietary features and a high incidence of gastric cancer. These include a high consumption of complex carbohydrates—for example, rice or potatoes—associated with a low intake of vitamin C. The role of salt in particular, and of food additives in general, may also be important.[1] These epidemiological findings have been supported by experimental work showing that these combinations of factors promote the production of nitrosamines in the stomach. The dramatic reduction in gastric cancer incidence in the USA and Australia has been attributed by some to marked changes in the dietary habits of these countries, associated with increasing affluence, and with the change to refrigeration as opposed to other methods of food preservation.

Dietary factors alone are not sufficient to account for observed variations in gastric cancer incidence. Another factor that has been of great interest lately is infection with *Helicobacter pylori*. Population studies have shown a strong association between *H. pylori* antibodies and the incidence of gastric cancer. It has been estimated that this is equivalent to a fivefold variation in incidence between a population with a zero infection rate and one with an infection rate of 100%.[2] *H. pylori* infection appears to be acquired in childhood, and is thought to predispose to cancer by initiating the sequence of events that progresses via chronic gastritis through metaplasia and dysplasia to ultimate neoplasia. There are interesting variations in the relationship between *H. pylori* and gastric cancers. In Northern Nigeria, for instance, *H. pylori* infection is endemic but the gastric cancer incidence is low. There is relatively little evidence to suggest gastric cancer has a strong genetic predisposition. In most countries, the male incidence is approximately twice that of the female: this has been attributed by some to environmental factors. There is compelling evidence for such an influence in certain defined industrial groups, such as coal miners. Histologically, gastric cancer is conveniently classified into intestinal and diffuse types; the intestinal type appears to be more common in areas of high endemicity, and it is for this type that a plausible aetiological hypothesis has been constructed.[3] The groups at highest risk for gastric cancer are relatively small and easily defined. These are patients with autoimmune atrophic gastritis associated with pernicious anaemia and those with previous gastric surgery for benign disease. In the latter case there is an increased incidence of up to 20-fold which develops approximately 20–30 years after the original operation. This finding is one of the principal arguments in support of the importance of bile reflux in gastric carcinogenesis. The marked variation in stage at diagnosis between the countries is a source of current controversy. The diagnosis of gastric cancer at a pathologically early stage (primary tumour confined to the mucosa or submucosa) has increased dramatically in Japan, from less than 10% to nearly 50% over a 30 year period. Early gastric cancer was rarely described outside Japan before the 1980s, but during this period a rise in incidence has also been noted in European countries, from a baseline of around 1%. Many recent European series record an incidence of 10–15%. The lack of prospective controlled studies has led to dispute as to whether these changes indicate an alteration in the natural history of the disease (particularly in Japan) or whether they can be entirely attributed to more efficient efforts to achieve early diagnosis—for example, the Japanese screening programmes. On the basis of consistent Japanese reports of improved survival after curative surgery, together with their unusually high incidence, early age at diagnosis, and high incidence of early cancer, some authors have suggested that gastric cancer in Japan is a fundamentally different disease from that seen in the West. Preliminary studies on the molecular biology of the disease have, however, failed to support this view.[4]

Clinical presentation and diagnosis

The symptoms and signs of advanced gastric cancer are well documented, easy to recognise, and of low clinical value, because their presence indicates incurability and a very short median survival. Early gastric cancer, on the other hand, has no signs, and symptoms may be absent or relatively mild. This had led to considerable delay in diagnosis in the average case. The traditional reputation of gastric cancer as "captain of the men of death" has been due to the traditional perception that diagnosis is usually not possible until the condition is incurable. Amongst the signs of advanced disease are Virchow's node, acanthosis nigricans, Blumer's shelf, ascites, gross cachexia, a palpable abdominal mass, and jaundice. The principal symptoms are anorexia and dyspepsia. The abdominal discomfort is usually relatively mild and is often associated with belching. Vomiting is not a particularly frequent feature and is probably related to pyloric outlet obstruction. A high proportion of tumours of the cardia cause dysphagia when they reach an advanced stage. Because of the difficulty in differentiating these symptoms from those of other diseases, and particularly because of the relatively mild and non-specific nature of the symptoms in early cancer, it is necessary to suspect gastric cancer in any patient over 40 with new dyspeptic symptoms, and particularly anorexia. There is relatively little evidence on the natural history of early gastric cancer. Much of this derives from Japan. Existing evidence does, however, suggest that between 50 and 80% of patients with early gastric cancer have associated dyspeptic symptoms.[5] The frequency with which symptoms are reported is undoubtedly related to the degree of education and concern of the population with regard to gastric cancer. This represents a major difference between the Japanese population and those of Western countries and partly explains the Japanese success in early diagnosis.

Population screening may be appropriate in countries like Japan where gastric cancer is sufficiently common to be given priority as a public health problem, and the economy and technological infrastructure are sufficiently strong to justify the use of health expenditure in this way. Even in these circumstances, screening by gastroscopy or barium meal poses problems because it conforms poorly to the World Health Organisation's criteria for a satisfactory screening test. Both tests are technologically rather demanding and expensive, somewhat invasive, and have a significant false negative rate. The use of vital dye spray to show up irregularities of the gastric mucosa, and of random biopsy at endoscopy, has been suggested to improve sensitivity (Figure 6.1). Serum and saliva tests for pepsinogens have been used to identify a population of patients with gastric atrophy who are more likely to develop gastric cancer. None of these methods has found wide favour and the value of regular surveillance has been questioned, even for the relatively small high risk groups which can be identified in Western populations—for example, long term survivors of peptic ulcer surgery, patients with pernicious anaemia, and those with known type II intestinal metaplasia. In the individual patient the onset of new dyspeptic symptoms over the age of 40, and particularly over the age of 50, indicates gastroscopy with biopsy of any abnormal areas. It may be useful to test for Helicobacter infection, although it is not known whether eradication of the organism in middle age has any influence on gastric carcinogenesis. Further endoscopic surveillance may be worthwhile in patients with any degree of dysplasia, and perhaps in those with intestinal metaplasia type II or atrophic gastritis (Figure 6.2). Early gastric cancer, as opposed to advanced disease, is a relatively subtle phenomenon that may easily be missed on a cursory inspection either by gastroscopy or contrast meal. Certain common diagnostic difficulties may interfere with the diagnosis even of advanced gastric cancer on endoscopy. Proximal lesions, particularly those on the lesser curve or on the posterior surface, are sometimes difficult to visualise, requiring a good J manoeuvre in a well distended stomach. Linitis plastica often presents as a non-distensible stomach, and biopsies often fail to take a deep enough bite to identify the carcinoma cells. Fine needle aspiration cytology via a needle passed down the biopsy channel has been used to overcome this problem. Finally, the diagnostic dilemma of the large, non-healing gastric ulcer in the elderly person continues to cause problems. Repeated biopsies often show necrotic slough unless taken from the inrolled edges of the ulcer, but even when correctly taken it sometimes requires several repeat examinations with multiple biopsies to demonstrate carcinoma, if present.

Diagnosis and staging

In the absence of proven or generally accepted adjuvant treatments for stomach cancer, the main purpose of careful staging is to plan appropriate surgery. In Britain and other Western countries this commonly involves studies aimed at the detection of incurable disease, which would render

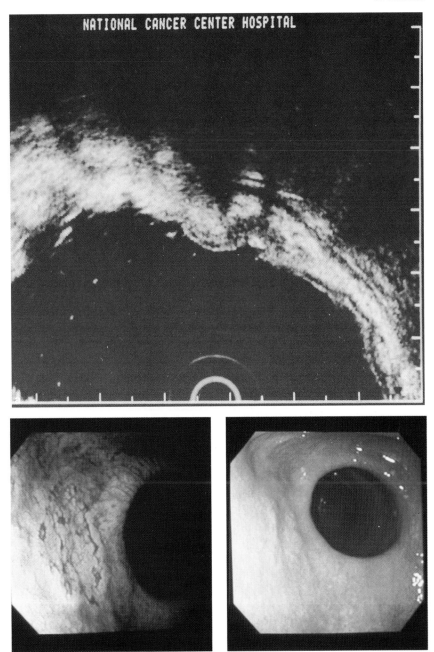

FIGURE 6.1—*Early gastric cancer type IIb and IIc; endoscopic pictures with (left) and without (right) indigo-carmine dye spray; note the subtlety of the lesion and the enhanced definition provided by the dye spray; ultrasound (above) and conventional endoscopic (below).*

161

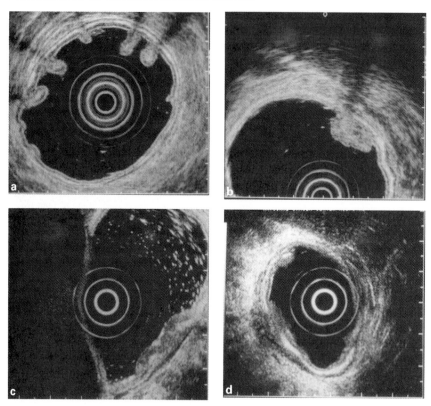

FIGURE 6.2—*Endoscopic ultrasound pictures of the stomach showing: (a) normal stomach with prominent folds (b) early gastric cancer type IIa, invading submucosa (c) gastric cancer invading (slightly) into muscularis propria (d) cancer invading through serosa; note the five-layered appearance of the normal stomach, which is disrupted by progressive invasion by the tumour.*

radical surgery inappropriate. In the case of early gastric cancer, however, the aim is to determine whether limited surgery or endoscopic local resection can be safely used.

Endoscopy

Experienced Japanese endoscopists are frequently able to differentiate mucosal from submucosal invasion levels by endoscopic inspection. Biopsy is of some value in assisting in this differentiation, but often does not provide sufficient submucosal material. The differentiation may be of value, because the incidence of lymph node metastasis in mucosal disease is around 2–3%, whereas it is 5–6 times higher in submucosal disease.[6] The argument for extended lymphadenectomy is therefore considerably stronger if the disease can be proven to be submucosal. Gastroscopy alone cannot determine inoperability in advanced disease, although extension into the duodenum and oesophagus, together with very extensive disease, clearly makes curative resection less likely.

Radiology

Computed tomography (CT) is commonly carried out for staging in gastric cancer but is a relatively inaccurate and insensitive test. Its main value is in the detection of liver metastases and of gross distant lymphadenopathy. It can also help by providing firm evidence of direct invasion of other organs, but is often particularly misleading in this aspect and a CT diagnosis of local invasion should not be used alone to determine operability unless invasion is particularly gross. Posterior invasion of the pancreas and the omental bursa are particularly difficult to determine. Several recent studies have suggested that a prone position with the stomach full of water may help to delineate local invasion better, particularly in the posterior gastric bed.

Endoluminal ultrasonography

This technique has rapidly gained popularity as available reports suggest that it is substantially more accurate than any other available technique in judging the T stage of the gastric tumour preoperatively. Local invasion may also be better demonstrated. Lymphadenopathy is frequently detected, but, as with other imaging techniques, endoscopic ultrasonography is not sufficiently specific to be relied upon in the diagnosis of lymph node metastasis. Recent studies have suggested that the accuracy of endoscopic ultrasonography for T stage approaches 90%.

Laparoscopy

Aided by the rapid rise of minimal access surgery in general, laparoscopic staging for gastrointestinal cancer has rapidly gained popularity. It is particularly useful in gastric cancer because of its high sensitivity for peritoneal dissemination, which cannot adequately be detected using any other technique. Peritoneal lavage can be carried out at the time of laparoscopy, and the fluid aspirated for cytology. The prognostic significance of positive peritoneal cytology at open operation is grave, and it seems certain that this will be reproduced when the technique is used laparoscopically. Laparoscopy is also useful in assessing the extent of local invasion. It is particularly valuable in assessing the left lobe of the liver, the hepatoduodenal ligament, the mesocolon and transverse colon, and the diaphragmatic hiatus. Like CT, it has a weak spot in assessing posterior invasion. This can be improved somewhat by opening the lesser sac, but this converts the procedure to a rather lengthy operation without a major concomitant increase in diagnostic certainty. Contact ultrasonography via the laparoscope may improve the scope and specificity of the technique in the future; preliminary results are encouraging.

Computer program

Maruyama and colleagues have designed and validated a predictive computer program based on the large and exhaustive database at the National Cancer Centre in Tokyo.[7] This uses seven preoperative variables to predict the extent of lymph node metastases, and can be used for planning surgery. It has been validated in European patients with good results. Recent evidence, however, suggests that its accuracy is inadequate in predicting distant nodal metastases in patients with T3 and T4 tumours. The original database contained relatively few cases in which a D3 dissection had been carried out in the presence of such a tumour. It is hoped that further work may correct this defect.

Intraoperative staging

Intraoperative peritoneal cytology with immediate reporting has been used in a number of Japanese centres to determine whether to proceed with radical lymphadenectomy. A lymph node biopsy from the infrarenal para-aortic nodal group (Japanese lymph node station 16B) has been used by some Western authorities in the same way. The planning of surgery, and in particular the selection of patients for radical surgery with curative intent, remains an area of judgment in which individual cases may often cause difficulties. Widespread liver or peritoneal metastases are absolute contraindications to this kind of surgery, but in less extreme cases the decision is often influenced, particularly in Western countries, by the age and fitness of the patient. The remarkable achievements of Japanese surgeons in performing radical surgery with extremely low mortality rates are partly attributed to their technical expertise, but are also partly due to the differences in cardiorespiratory physiology between racial groups. In particular, the low incidence of atherosclerosis, obesity, and thromboembolic disease in Japan is of undoubted benefit to the Japanese surgeon.

Surgical therapy

Surgical resection is currently the only modality that is able to offer the potential for curing gastric cancer (with the possible exception of endoscopic

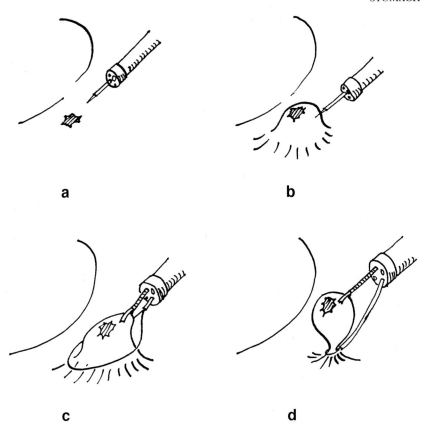

FIGURE 6.3—*The technique of endoscopic mucosal resection (strip biopsy) for early gastric cancer: (a) the lesion (b) the lesion after marking with diathermy and submucosal injection of saline and adrenaline (c) gasping of the lesion with forceps and placement of a diathermy snare around the base (d) diathermy resection of the lesion leaving bone muscularis propria.*

strip biopsy for intramucosal cancer, see Figures 6.3 and 6.4). The most controversial aspect of the management of gastric cancer relates to the surgical approach to be adopted. Proponents of radical lymphadenectomy point to the excellent survival rates obtained in retrospective series using this technique. Opponents point to the evidence for increased morbidity and mortality in several reports of the use of this type of surgery in Western patients. The Japanese, with an enormous experience of gastric cancer surgery, have developed an aggressive approach to lymphadenectomy en bloc with the gastric resection. Their claims of considerable improvements in survival related to the use of this approach have met with considerable scepticism in Western countries. As in most forms of surgery, the evidence in this debate has largely been based on uncontrolled retrospective series,

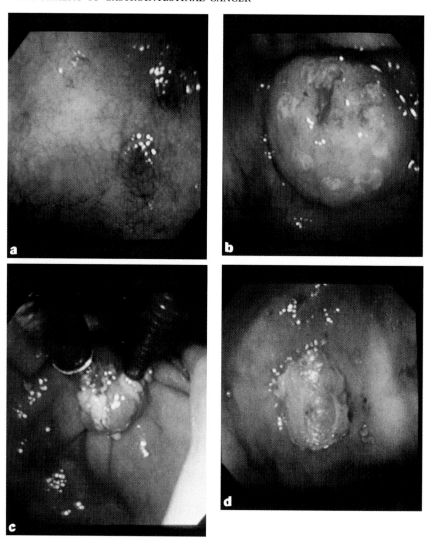

FIGURE 6.4—*Endoscopic pictures of strip biopsy in action: (a) the lesion after dye spray (b) the lesion after submucosal injection of saline and mucosal marking (c) the lesion being grasped (left instrument) and the diathermy loop used to excise it (right instrument) (d) bare muscularis propria after excision of lesion. (Figures 6.3, 6.4 reproduced with permission from* Japanese Research Society for Gastric Cancer, *Japanese Classification of Gastric Carcinoma.* Tokyo: Kanehara, 1995. 8–9.)

with all the problems of comparability that this brings. Two major trials have recently been completed, in Britain and the Netherlands, both of which aim to compare Western and Japanese surgical methods for the curative resection of gastric cancer. Both have shown a doubling of postoperative mortality with the more radical approach, but this may partly be a "learning curve" phenomenon. Survival results are awaited with interest. In discussing this East–West debate it may be useful to provide a summary of the Japanese approach, which is often misunderstood in the West.

Japanese surgical philosophy

The philosophical approach to cancer surgery, particularly of the gastrointestinal tract, differs somewhat between East and West. Western surgical thinking has been profoundly influenced by the revolution in the understanding of breast cancer that occurred in the 1950s and 60s. The demonstration that, in this disease, radical surgery with regional lymphadenectomy conferred no survival benefits when compared with less radical surgery has been adopted by many as a general principle for all cancer surgery. It has frequently been stated by Western authors that cancer should be considered a systemic disease, and the logical inference drawn that the role of surgery is limited to excision of all obvious disease at the site of the primary. The Japanese, on the other hand, have been more influenced by studies carried out in their own country, showing that lymphatic metastases from gastric cancer generally follow a pattern defined by the lymphatic flow along the gastric vasculature. These studies defined a series of concentric circles of nodal groups around the stomach and showed that it was unusual for metastases to skip from an inner to an outer circle without involving an intervening one. A uniform policy of radical resection, adopted on a national basis from an early date, resulted in the accumulation of convincing evidence to show that (except in the case of pathologically early gastric cancer) metastasis to nodes unlikely to be removed by Western style surgery was rather frequent. In essence, therefore, the difference between the two approaches lies in the significance attributed to the resected nodal metastases. In the traditional Western view, these are irrelevant to survival because they are an indicator of disseminated and surgically incurable disease elsewhere. In the Japanese view, they are essentially an extension of the local growth of the primary tumour and do not exclude curative resection provided they themselves are resected. The Japanese system groups the nodes into a number of stations (Figures 6.5 and 6.6) and these are allocated to one of the concentric rings mentioned above, depending somewhat on the site of the gastric tumour. The concentric circles are designated N1, N2, N3, and so on. The Japanese approach has been to excise all nodes in the circle that is likely (from past experience) to be involved, together with all nodes in the circle beyond this. In the majority of resectable cases of non-early cancer this has meant removing the N1 and N2 circles, and this has led to the designation

167

LN No.		AMC MAC MCA CMA	A AM AD	MA M MC	C CM	Additional LN when tumour invades the oesophagus
1	rt cardial		N2			
2	lt cardial		N3	N2		
3	lesser curve					
4sa	short gastric			N1		
4sb	lt gastroepipl					
4d	rt gastroepipl					
5	suprapyloric					
6	infrapyloric					
7	lt gastr a			N2		
8a	ant hept a					
8p	post hept a			N3		
9	coeliac					
10	spenic hilum			N2		
11	splenic a					
12	hept duod lig			N3		
13	retropanc					
14A	sup mesent a			N4		
14V	sup mesent v			N3		
15	mid colic					
16a2, b1	paraaorta			N4		
16a1, b2	paraaorta					
17	ant panc			N3		
18	inf panc					
19	infradiaphr		N4			N2
20	oesoph hiatus	N3			N2	N1
105	upper oesoph					
106	tracheal					N4
107	trach bifurc					
108	middle oesoph					N3
109	pulmon hilum					N4
110	lower oesoph	N3			N3	N2
111	supradiaphr					
112	post mediast					N3

FIGURE 6.5—*The classification of the different stations depending on the site of the primary tumour; to qualify as a D2 resection, an operation must remove all the stations designated as N1 or N2 for a tumour at the affected site.*

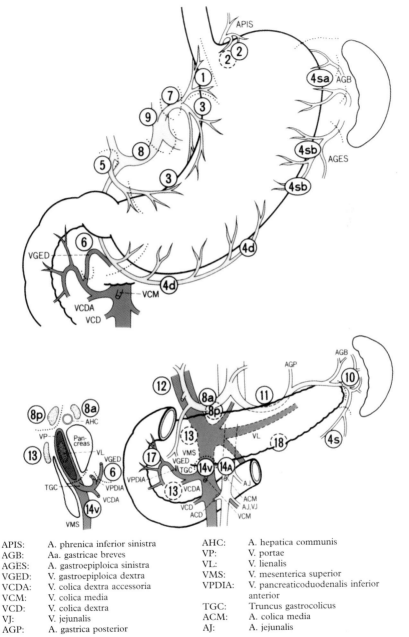

APIS: A. phrenica inferior sinistra
AGB: Aa. gastricae breves
AGES: A. gastroepiploica sinistra
VGED: V. gastroepiploica dextra
VCDA: V. colica dextra accessoria
VCM: V. colica media
VCD: V. colica dextra
VJ: V. jejunalis
AGP: A. gastrica posterior

AHC: A. hepatica communis
VP: V. portae
VL: V. lienalis
VMS: V. mesenterica superior
VPDIA: V. pancreaticoduodenalis inferior
         anterior
TGC: Truncus gastrocolicus
ACM: A. colica media
AJ: A. jejunalis

FIGURE 6.6—*Lymph node "stations" in the Japanese classification, and their boundaries.*

R2 gastrectomy.[8] The normal extent of radical gastrectomy for a cancer performed in the West would be described by the Japanese as R1. (The terms R1, R2, and R3 resection have recently been changed to D1, D2, and D3 following the decision of the International Union against Cancer (UICC) to adopt a modification of the tumour, node, metastases (TNM) system for tumour staging, which confusingly designates complete resection of cancer of any kind R0, and progressively more incomplete resections R1 and R2.) The logical corollary of the lymphadenectomy required by the Japanese approach is that splenectomy and distal pancreatectomy are carried out in cases of total gastrectomy because this ensures removal of the nodes at the splenic hilum (station 10) and along the entire length of the splenic artery (station 11). This has been the standard practice in Japan, although modifications that sometimes avoid these extra procedures have been introduced with the passage of time (see below). The conclusion of the surgical debate is clearly some way off, and, indeed, may not be settled by the national trials whose results we await. One of these has been significantly criticised on the basis of the inadequate training in the D2 technique received by the surgeons involved, while the other (which made diligent efforts to avoid this weakness) has recently published data to show that these efforts were only partially successful.[9] This and other problems reported by the trial participants underline the enormous difficulty of conducting multicentre controlled trials of something as innately variable as a major surgical operation. While the debate continues, however, it is important that it should be conducted on a factual basis. There are a number of common Western misconceptions of the Japanese position and data, which only serve to confuse the argument.

Japanese results are better because they detect the disease earlier

This is undoubtedly true, and greatly affects the overall survival rates reported by Japanese surgeons. It is clearly not the complete explanation for the superiority of the Japanese figures. If one analyses the figures by stage as accurately as possible, by grouping node positive and serosa positive patients against the node and serosa negative cases, it is clear that Japanese reports show consistently superior survival in advanced cases with positive nodes and serosa (Table 6.1). The remarkable achievement of the Japanese in detecting between 30 and 50% of cases when the tumour has penetrated only the mucosa or submucosa is therefore not sufficient to explain their excellent results. The converse argument is of case selection—that is, that the results are good because doubtful cases do not receive surgery (see below).

The natural history of gastric cancer is more favourable in Japan

This has been suggested by several Western authors but there is no positive evidence for this belief, and the evidence that is available suggests

TABLE 6.1—*Five year survival figures from Western and Japanese source. Reproduced with permission from* GI Cancer.[20] *Results of surgery for gastric cancer*

Author	5 year survival rates (%) for curative resections								
	%CR	Overall	N0	N+	S0	S+	n1	n2	n3
Clarke	39	9	—	—	—	—	—	—	—
Brookes	26	18·4	—	—	—	—	—	—	—
Gilbertsen	49	24·5	38	15	—	—	—	—	—
Cantrell	*	21	46	14·6	—	—	—	—	—
Hoerr	46	42·6	88	21	84	35	—	—	—
White	*	18·6	38	8	—	—	—	—	—
Cassel	46	19	—	—	—	—	—	—	—
Serlin	*	24	—	—	—	—	—	—	—
DuPont	22·5	14·6	—	—	—	—	—	—	—
Adashek	26	32	44	23	44	15	—	—	—
Yap	50·5	36	—	—	—	—	—	—	—
Bizer	48	20·5	—	—	—	—	—	—	—
Faivre	40	29	—	21·7	—	—	—	—	—
Yan	45	36·2	—	—	—	—	—	—	—
Gall	57	51·8	—	—	—	—	—	—	—
Scott	37	15	—	—	—	—	—	—	—
Gennari	*	50	67	28	—	—	—	—	—
Sjostedt	30	25·5	—	—	—	—	—	—	—
Burmeister	*	45·5	80	32	76	32	47	20	10
Cunningham	39	24	31	17	47	13	—	—	—
Shiu	24	30	56	13	—	—	16	3	—
Lindahl	48	35	—	—	—	—	—	—	—
Irvin	30	43	60	18	—	—	—	—	—
Elias	63	54	—	—	—	—	—	—	—
Msika	55	44	75	18	—	—	27	7	—
Gouzi	*	48	69	18	74	16	—	—	—
Pacelli	*	65	—	—	—	—	—	—	—
Sue-Ling	42	60	88	35	—	—	—	—	—
Mine	56	27·5	50	17·3	65	14·5	—	—	—
Koga	84	86	—	—	—	—	—	—	—
Soga	73	43·5	50	33·5	74·5	38·5	44	25	22@
Kajitani	*	46	85	38	82	30	60	25	11#
Kodama	*	58	81	39	88	41	60	31	21
Maruyama	75	75	85	36	86	31	61	31	10

*=deals only with curative resection group.
@=results from subgroup with advanced (non-early) cancer.
#=results from period 1966–1970 only.
Overall survival is for curatively resected patients only.
%CR=% of all patients who received curative resection.
N0=node negative patients amongst curative resections.
N+=node positive patients amongst curative resections.
S0=serosa negative patients amongst curative resections.
S+=serosa positive patients amongst curative resections.
n1, n2, n3=patients with involved nodes in tiers 1, 2 and 3 according to the JRSGC classification.

that it is incorrect. Gastric cancer occurs in earlier age groups in Japan than in the West and there is a somewhat higher incidence of intestinal type cancer. The pattern of metastases remains the same, however, and untreated disease and advanced inoperable cancer have the same dismal prognosis. A recent comparison of the molecular biology of matched cancers from Britain and Japan showed no differences in the underlying genetic abnormalities.

Reported Japanese series are highly selected

The basis for the Japanese claims of improved prognosis come either from unselected hospital populations or from the reports of the national organisation that has been set up to monitor gastric cancer treatment. Efforts to gain a global picture of the disease in Japan have been somewhat frustrated by the concentration of all of these reports on patients undergoing curative resections. It is clear from other reports, however, that the percentage of patients who do undergo a curative resection is higher than in Western series. This seems likely because the Japanese believe strongly in the benefits of even palliative resection, and have less need for concern than the Western surgeon over the associated morbidity and mortality. The stage distribution of the cases reported from Japanese centres of excellence do not suggest that the populations studied differ greatly from those in other Japanese series in terms of stage, and an analysis of the referral patterns in such centres confirms this.

While we can dismiss these factors from our discussions, there are a number of unanswered questions about the differences between Japanese and British practice. Perhaps the thorniest question is that of the magnitude of the stage migration effect. This effect occurs when new methods lead to improved staging of a cancer. Generally speaking, more cases are then attributed to higher stages than before, leading to an apparent improvement in the results of treatments in these stages.[10] It is quite clear that the extended lymphadenectomy performed in Japan does provide much better staging than the more limited surgery performed in the West. The nature of this question makes it extremely difficult to determine the extent to which this influences the apparent results. Recent studies from Germany and Japan have come to opposite conclusions on this.[11 12] Another factor which should be taken into consideration is the common Japanese practice of carrying out perioperative chemotherapy, often combined with various forms of immunotherapy. The drugs used are usually mitomycin C and/or 5-fluorouracil or its derivative tegafur. These have been studied in a number of Western adjuvant trials and have shown no benefit whatsoever, with the exception of the findings of the Gastrointestinal Tumour Study Group (GITSG) trial and the Spanish group.[13] It remains possible that the difference in timing between Japan (where the chemotherapy is often given within one week of the operation) and the West (where the normal delay is at least three weeks) is of importance. The overall evidence in favour of perioperative adjuvant chemotherapy for cancer is, however, less than overwhelming.

Morbidity and mortality concerns

Apart from scepticism over the results claimed, the main concern of Western surgeons over extended lymphadenectomy has related to the potential increase in morbidity and mortality. Initial reports on radical surgery from Gilbertsen in the USA in the 1960s showed a great increase in both morbidity and mortality, with no survival benefit.[14] In retrospect these results were predictable, given the high surgical morbidity and mortality "radical gastrectomy" of the Western type in that era, and the evidence from Gilbertsen's papers showing that the majority of his patients had very advanced disease that was unlikely to be cured surgically, whatever technique was used. More worryingly, both the national trials of D1 versus D2 gastrectomy have now reported that morbidity and mortality are increased by the increased extent of surgery.[15 16] By contrast, a number of Western centres with a special interest have reported excellent figures for both five year survival and operative mortality while carrying out D2 gastrectomy. Although there have been no formal comparisons of surgical morbidity and mortality in Japan and Western countries, and these would be difficult to arrange, it is very clear from the striking contrast between reports from the two populations that a major difference exists. Analysing the extensive database at the National Cancer Centre Hospital in Tokyo, we have found that the incidence of serious technical complications (anastomotic leakage and pancreatic fistula) is comparable with that of several Western reports on gastric cancer surgery. The mortality in this population is, however, less than in any comparable Western series by a factor of 5 or 10. This dramatically demonstrates the more robust physiology of the Japanese patient undergoing gastric cancer surgery. There is a significant age related element, in that the Japanese patient is, on average, 5–10 years younger, but a substantial part of the Japanese advantage must be related to their very low incidence of atherosclerotic cardiovascular disease and venous thromboembolism. Analysis of the causes of morbidity in Tokyo shows that neither myocardial infarction, progressive cardiac failure nor pulmonary embolus feature in the list of causes of postoperative death during a five year period, whereas these are very frequently reported in Western series. It therefore appears rational to suggest that radical lymphadenectomy for gastric cancer should be restricted, in a Western setting, to specialist centres performing a substantial number of procedures per year, and that patient selection for this procedure should give great attention to the fitness of the patient for major surgery.

Splenic and pancreatic preservation

The potential morbidity of the Japanese approach continues to daunt many surgeons in other countries, despite impressive series from single centres showing good results with acceptable operative mortality rates.[17 18] The resection of the non-involved spleen and distal pancreas has attracted particular attention. It is undeniable that each of these procedures individually carries well recognised risks, and therefore logical that addition of these to another major operation is likely to produce additional morbidity. The general increase in susceptibility to infection after splenectomy is well recognised, but is less marked in mature and elderly adults than in the young. There are few well documented cases of overwhelming pneumococcal infection in patients over 40, but preoperative vaccination is still recommended. Occasional patients also have problems with thrombocytosis. Resection of the normal pancreatic tail is perhaps more problematic still. The risk of creating a pancreatic fistula is significant, even in the most skilled hands, and if infection then supervenes the situation quickly becomes life threatening. The Japanese literature documents the occurrence of mild to moderate leakage of pancreatic juice in up to 10% of patients after distal pancreatectomy. This stops spontaneously after a few days in most cases, but even where it remains uninfected can be a potent cause of morbidity and delayed discharge from hospital. There has been controversy over the possible role of the spleen in orchestrating immune defences against stomach cancer, with some laboratory evidence to support the view that splenectomy may be deleterious in this regard. Retrospective studies have suggested that splenectomy does not improve survival, and may even be deleterious, but the selection of patients for different procedures may have been important in producing this result. A number of Western authors have followed the lead of Maruyama in Japan, and perform a pancreas preserving lymphadenectomy, stripping the nodes along the splenic artery. Japanese authors with experience of Western patients regard this approach with some suspicion because of the greater technical difficulty of the procedure in the fatter Western patients, but Western surgeons report less risk of pancreatic leakage than with transection. The recent reported experience from Leeds shows what can be achieved in the West by a combination of surgical skill and experience and improved case finding with earlier stage at diagnosis.[18] There are no prospective comparative data on which to base a choice of splenic preservation or splenectomy in patients with tumour of the upper stomach. The Maruyama computer program will predict a high incidence of positive nodes in the splenic hilum in patients with more advanced tumours in this region. This has been validated for use in

Europe, but T3 and T4 tumours with extensive lymphadenectomy are underrepresented in the database used to create the program, and the predictions concerning outcome for these groups must be treated with caution.

Total gastrectomy de principe

The idea that total extirpation of the stomach was more likely to prevent recurrence and promote cure dates from the 1940s, when this procedure first began to achieve mortality rates considered acceptable by the standards of the day. The spreading submucosal pattern of linitis plastica, and the marked tendency for diffuse type cancer to microscopic infiltration well beyond the macroscopic boundaries of the tumour, provided the rationale for this approach. Total gastrectomy de principe has not been shown to have any advantage provided strict criteria for resection margins are observed, and the importance of lymphatic and transperitoneal spread in gastric cancer suggests that attention to these aspects of the disease is more likely to prove fruitful. The increased postoperative risks associated with an oesophageal anastomosis and the greatly increased long term morbidity from nutritional and motility problems make it hard to justify excision of the proximal stomach where it is not strictly necessary to eradicate mural disease. Extended lymphadenectomy implies total gastrectomy in all patients in whom the splenic artery is ligated at its root, as this renders the remaining blood supply to the fundus from the oesophageal vessels too precarious for safe healing.

Carcinoma of the cardia

Adenocarcinoma arising at or very close to the epithelial transition zone in the cardia has become a more frequent problem in recent years. It poses a difficult problem for the surgeon because of its position, which requires major manoeuvres to ensure adequate exposure. The results of surgery are generally poorer than for more distal tumours. Tumours in this area often metastasise to mediastinal nodes, as well as posteriorly via the "bare area" directly to nodes on the left side of the aorta and around the left renal vessels. This poses difficulties in obtaining adequate lymphadenectomy. Japanese authors have claimed improved survival from extended surgery removing these nodes, but there is no trial evidence to support the claims. The higher incidence of diffuse or poorly differentiated tumours in this region compared with the distal stomach may also be important. Such tumours are prone to extensive proximal submucosal spread, often with "skipping" of extensive segments of normal oesophagus.

175

Quality of life after gastrectomy

The nutritional and symptomatic problems associated with gastrectomy are well known, although still incompletely understood. Distal gastrectomy guarantees a degree of biliary reflux gastritis, although this may often be relatively asymptomatic. Dumping, diarrhoea, and late nutritional deficiencies can also occur, but functional disturbance, with post-prandial pain and vomiting that is not obviously related to gastritis, is the most common major problem interfering with the postoperative quality of life. This is occasionally due to afferent loop obstruction in patients with a Billroth II anastomosis. Subjectively, it often appears that patients who drink or eat faster suffer more; often no precise cause can be found. Satisfactory treatment is difficult; prokinetic agents and mucosal protectants such as sucralfate may play a role, and some patients benefit from conversion of the simple Billroth II anastomosis into a Roux-en-Y arrangement. Supplementation of the diet with vitamin C and calcium, and regular injections of vitamin B_{12}, should be arranged, although major nutritional problems are much commoner after total gastrectomy. A variety of pouch procedures have been designed to substitute for the reservoir function of the stomach, but none has found widespread favour, the Hunt–Lawrence pouch being the most common variant used in Western countries. As in other situations where there is no widely accepted surgical solution, the candidates all suffer from one drawback or another. Many experienced surgeons reject them all in favour of the standard end to side oesophagojejunostomy with a 40 cm Roux loop. While sometimes alleviating nutritional problems, the pouches have a higher risk of leakage and other postoperative complications, and predispose more than the simple anastomosis to reflux symptoms.

Conservative surgery: laparoscopic and endoscopic surgery

The locoregional aggressiveness of gastric cancer limits the potential of minimally invasive surgical approaches. They have their principal uses in staging, in the treatment of early cancer, and in palliation of the symptoms of advanced disease. In certain situations it may be safe to excise early gastric cancers endoscopically, using the "strip biopsy" technique (Figures 6.3 and 6.4).[19] This is particularly suitable for the frail elderly patient who is unlikely to withstand major surgery. The risk of leaving possible lymph node metastasis unresected should be carefully evaluated and balanced against the risks of major surgery. Recent reports suggest that early cancers of types I and IIa or IIb may be suitable, provided they are small (less than 2 cm diameter), non-ulcerated, and confirmed as completely excised mucosal lesions by histology. The 20% risk of lymph node metastasis in tumours that have definitely invaded the submucosa is a contraindication to endoscopic removal unless the fitness of the patient precludes any other approach. Endoscopic laser ablation may also be used for early cancer, but has the disadvantage of greater difficulty in accurately assessing the risk of recurrence.

Laser therapy is useful for the treatment of malignant dysphagia caused by tumours at the cardia. It has been compared with intubation techniques in a number of studies, although these are mainly concerned with oesophageal cancer. Laser produces somewhat better quality swallowing but requires fairly frequent repeat sessions, and the risk of complications is at least as high. The choice of treatment in this situation is therefore determined largely by local availability. Expanding mesh stents have recently been in vogue for the palliation of dysphagia. They are certainly easier to place than Celestin or Atkinson tubes, and seem less likely to dislodge, but it remains to be seen whether their advantages are significant enough to outweigh their high cost. Laser has not proved particularly effective in relieving functional obstruction in the stomach or pylorus. This is usually caused either by massive tumour replacement of the stomach or by the linitis pattern of spread, which reduces the compliance of the stomach. In both of these situations it seems that loss of peristalsis and distensibility are more important than mechanical blockage in producing the dysfunction.

Isolated reports of laparoscopic surgery for gastric cancer treatment have appeared. Palliative gastroenterostomy may be possible using this approach, provided there is an easily accessible portion of uninvolved stomach anteriorly. Wedge resection of a segment of the greater curve around a small tumour has been described. This may have value in the treatment of the frail elderly with small symptomatic lesions not suitable for strip biopsy. The temptation to carry out a distal gastrectomy through the laparoscope has already produced at least one report. Current caution about the use of laparoscopic approaches for radical cancer surgery is certainly justified in the case of gastrectomy, particularly if extended lymphadenectomy is carried out. The distinction between operations that are possible and those that are desirable is gradually beginning to be applied to laparoscopic surgery, and it seems unlikely that laparoscopic resection will find a place in the foreseeable future.

Surgical palliation techniques and their efficacy

The ability of surgeons to provide useful palliation of symptoms remains sadly limited in cases where the primary tumour cannot be removed. It is worth emphasising that resection, as in most solid tumours, provides the best palliation, even when gross residual disease is left in place. It is now well accepted that even total gastrectomy is worth performing as a palliative procedure in a suitable symptomatic patient. Bypass procedures, on the

177

other hand, are of limited value. They do not greatly enhance the duration of survival, and their success in improving its quality is very variable. Bypass operations do not prevent bleeding, which is common, frequently lethal, and distressing. In many cases the advanced primary tumour causes sufficient damage to the function either of the gut or of its nerve supply to prevent effective peristalsis. In this situation the provision of a mechanical bypass of a blocked channel is remarkably ineffective. Cases with widespread peritoneal involvement are particularly difficult in this respect, as it is usually impossible to restore any effective function of the gut tube. The resulting distress for the patient and relatives is sufficiently unpleasant to persuade many clinicians that death from electrolyte imbalance should be allowed to occur with as little interference as possible consistent with comfort. The standard gastrojejunal bypass may in theory be made more effective by transecting the stomach above an inoperable distal tumour and making the anastomosis to the proximal remnant, the so called Devine exclusion technique. Unfortunately, tumours large enough to be unresectable usually invade extensively up the lesser curve, making the transection an uncomfortable business through gross tumour tissue. Another variant which may be of more value is an oesophagojejunal bypass for tumours involving too much proximal stomach to make gastrojejunostomy feasible. In this situation a satisfactory bypass can sometimes be achieved by opening the hiatus and mobilising the oesophagus sufficiently to allow a side to side stapled anastomosis, which can then be closed with one or two sutures.

Plan

Staging of gastric carcinoma should be by endoscopy, CT scan, and in advanced cases by laparoscopy (see algorithm). Endoscopic and laparoscopic ultrasonography are of great value when available. Resection is the only therapy that can offer a reasonable prospect of cure in gastric cancer. The logical case for extended lymphadenectomy appears strong because: (a) we know that lymph nodes more distant than the perigastric group are frequently involved; and (b) resection of such involved distant nodes can be associated with prolonged survival, but this hardly ever happens when residual nodal disease is noted and left in situ. The risks of extended resection must be carefully balanced against the potential benefits, particularly in frail patients with advanced tumours. Adjuvant chemotherapy is of no proven value and should not therefore be given outside trial settings. The same can be said of immunotherapy. Resection of the pancreas may be substituted by systematic lymphadenectomy along the splenic vessels, provided there are no obvious large nodes adhering to the pancreatic substance. This may be preferred because the risk of a pancreatic fistula

The management of gastric cancer

STAGING

Gastroscopy and biopsy
CT scan and/or endoscopic ultrasound

obvious early cancer   *others*

laparoscopy
$+/-$ cytology, biopsy

ASSESSMENT OF FITNESS FOR RADICAL SURGERY

Previous cardiorespiratory problems
exercise tolerance
ECG and CXR

Where indicated:
echocardiogram, pulmonary function tests, 24 hour ECG tape

DECISION

fit and potentially curable   *others*

Gastrectomy and D2 lymphadenectomy   Palliative gastrectomy[a]
+ para-aortic node biopsy   or bypass
                                                                 or no surgery

                                                                 consider endoscopic
Splenectomy with total gastrectomy[b]   stent or laser in
Pancreas preservation if possible   "no surgery" group

Combined resection of other organs   consider chemotherapy[c]
if necessary

Notes
a. The decision on which of these should be selected is based on the principles that resection is the best palliation, but that incurable patients should be subjected to minimum morbidity. Gastrectomy is therefore preferred where technically feasible and likely to relieve symptoms, unless the patient is too unfit.
b. Splenectomy is controversial in the West, because of the evidence that it increases morbidity. It should be undertaken when the surgeon has reason to believe there is a high risk of nodal involvement at the splenic hilum. The Maruyama computer program may be used to estimate this risk.[7]
c. Palliative chemotherapy using the ECF (Epirubicin, cisplatin, infusional 5-fluorouracil) regimen has shown encouraging initial results. Neoadjuvant chemotherapy and resection for Stage IV tumours should be restricted to clinical trials.

appears to be less. Resection of the spleen is another unresolved question. In the absence of prospective data convincingly showing that splenectomy is harmful, it seems logical to carry it out in proximal cancers, where invasion of the nodes at the splenic hilum may be expected in 10–20% of cases. Further research into the role of the spleen in gastric cancer immunology and the effect of its removal is, however, needed. Where curative resection is not possible, palliative resection without lymphadenectomy should be performed if possible. A bypass may be of symptomatic benefit for a proportion of the remainder, but minimally invasive means of palliation should be preferred where possible. Palliative chemotherapy may be useful in prolonging quality survival. In the occasional patient with an excellent response, resection should be carried out after downstaging of the tumour by neoadjuvant chemotherapy.

References

1 Buiatti E, Palli D, DeCarli A, *et al*. A case–control study of gastric cancer and diet in Italy. *Int J Cancer* 1989;**44**:611–6.
2 Eurogast Study Group. An international association between *Helicobacter pylori* infection and gastric cancer. *Lancet* 1993;**341**:1359–62.
3 Correa P. The new era of cancer epidemiology. *Cancer Epid Biomarkers Prev* 1991;**1**:5–11.
4 McCulloch P, Ochiai A, O'Dowd G, *et al*. Comparison of the molecular genetics of stomach cancers in Britain and Japan: c-erbB2 and p53. *Cancer* 1995;**75**:920–5.
5 Kaibara N, Kawaguchi H, Nishidoi H, *et al*. Significance of mass survey for gastric cancer from standpoint of surgery. *Am J Surg* 1981;**142**:543–5.
6 Maehara Y, Orita H, Okuyama T, *et al*. Predictors of lymph node metastasis in early gastric cancer. *Br J Surg* 1992;**79**:245–7.
7 Kampschoer GHM, Maruyama K, van de Velde CJH, *et al*. Computer analysis in making preoperative decisions: a rational approach to lymph node dissection in gastric cancer patients. *Br J Surg* 1989;**76**:905–8.
8 Kajitani T, for the Japanese Research Society for Gastric Cancer. The general rules for the gastric cancer study in surgery and pathology. *Jpn J Surg* 1981;**11**:127–39.
9 Bunt TMG, Bonenkamp JJ, Hermans J, *et al*. Factors influencing noncompliance and contamination in a randomized trial of "Western" (R1) versus "Japanese" (R2) type surgery in gastric cancer. *Cancer* 1994;**73**:1544–51.
10 Feinstein AR, Sosin DM, Wells CK. The Will Rogers phenomenon. Stage migration and new diagnostic techniques as a source of misleading statistics for survival in cancer. *N Engl J Med* 1985;**312**:1604–8.
11 Sasako M, McCulloch P, Kinoshita T, *et al*. New method to evaluate the therapeutic value of lymph node dissection for gastric cancer. *Br J Surg* 1995;**82**:346–51.
12 Fass J, Hungs M, Nachtkanp J, *et al*. On the role of upstaging in R1/R2 lymphadenectomy studies for gastric carcinoma. *Br J Surg* 1994;**81**(suppl 1):51.
13 Bleiberg H, Gerard B, Deguiral P. Adjuvant therapy in resectable gastric cancer. *Br J Cancer* 1992;**66**:987–91.
14 Gilbertsen VA. Results of treatment of stomach cancer. *Cancer* 1969;**23**:1305–8.
15 da Silva F, Fielding JWL, Craven J, *et al*. MRC trial of gastric cancer: morbidity and mortality after R1 and R2 resections. *Br J Surg* 1991;**78**:1501.
16 Bonenkamp JJ, Songun I, Hermans J, *et al*. Randomised comparison of morbidity after D1 and D2 dissection for gastric cancer in 996 Dutch patients. *Lancet* 1995;**345**:745–8.
17 Pacelli F, Doglietto GB, Bellantone R, *et al*. Extensive versus limited lymph node dissection for gastric cancer: a comparative study of 320 patients. *Br J Surg* 1993;**80**:1153–6.
18 Sue-Ling HM, Johnston D, Martin IG, *et al*. Gastric cancer: a curable disease in Britain. *BMJ* 1993;**307**:591–6.
19 Okazaki Y, Tada M. Endoscopic treatment of early gastric cancer. *Semin Surg Oncol* 1991; 7:351–5.

Chemotherapy, radiotherapy, palliative care and new approaches

HAN J BONENKAMP, I SONGUN, H I KEIZER,
J HERMANS, and C J H VAN DE VELDE

Gastric cancer has a dismal prognosis. The majority of the patients, except those with so called early gastric cancer, die from a combination of locoregional recurrence and metastatic disease. Resection may offer cure for more than 90% of patients with early gastric cancers, but for those with locally advanced tumours or established metastases, resection at most alleviates symptoms, with only limited impact on survival. The quest for adjuvant treatment is therefore strong.

Reduction of locoregional recurrence rates is attempted in various ways. The hypothesis that extended lymph node dissection will result in better local and regional control, with a subsequent improved survival for patients deemed curative, is currently being tested in two prospective randomised controlled trials, in the Netherlands and in Britain. Improvement of local control has also been attempted by using intraoperative or postoperative regional radiotherapy or intraperitoneal chemotherapy.[20–22]

In autopsy series, metastases are often found, although they are mostly combined with local recurrences; gastric cancer is, therefore, often viewed as a systemic disease for which multimodality treatment is indicated. Unfortunately, randomised trials of adjuvant chemotherapy after potentially curative surgery have not generally shown encouraging results, partly because the cytotoxic regimens used in early trials had rather limited efficacy in advanced disease. Recently, interest in multimodality therapy for primary cancer has been restimulated by the development of more potent cytotoxic regimens and preoperative chemotherapy. This section of the chapter reviews the historical development of chemotherapy until 1990, and provides a meta-analysis of randomised trials of adjuvant chemotherapy between 1980 and the mid-1990s.[23] Currently studied regimens and prospects for future research are then discussed.

Chemotherapy regimens since 1980

Adjuvant chemotherapy for gastric cancer was studied in the 1960s, but until 1980 there were virtually no effective chemotherapy regimens.[24] New research in this field was initiated after MacDonald et al reported encouraging results using a combination of fluorouracil, doxorubicin (Adriamycin) and mitomycin C (FAM).[25] FAM has been used extensively, both as primary treatment and as adjuvant treatment in gastric cancer, and is often considered the standard with which other regimens should be compared. New regimens for the adjuvant setting are selected depending on their activity in advanced disease, and a brief review of the development of the currently applied regimens is required. Because of the different pattern, prognosis, and treatment of gastric cancer in Japan, the Japanese experience will be discussed separately.

Chemotherapy regimens in advanced disease

The results of studies with FAM and FAM related regimens are listed in Table 6.2. Monotreatment with mitomycin C and fluorouracil induced responses in approximately 20% of treated patients.[26] Addition of doxorubicin, which is less effective as a single agent in gastric cancer, was attempted in advanced gastric cancer by MacDonald et al.[25] With this

TABLE 6.2—*Western studies of FAM in advanced gastric cancer*

Author	Regimen	No of patients	Trial Phase	Stage	Response %	Conclusion
MacDonald *Cancer* 1979	FAM	36	II	advanced	50	effective for palliation
MacDonald *Ann Int Med* 1980	FAM	62	II	advanced	42	effective
Woolley *Cancer* 1979	Ftorafur +AM	15	II	advanced	20	no advantage over FAM
Gisselbrecht *Cancer* 1983	FAM + chlorozotocin	23	II	advanced	26	no advantage over FAM
Gill *Aus NZ J Surg* 1983	FAM	28	II	metastatic	57	effective
Cunningham *BJS* 1984	FAM	84	II	advanced	35 5 CR	effective

F: fluorouracil; A: doxorubicin; M: mitomycin C; CR: complete response.

regimen, FAM, they achieved 50% response initially and 42% response in a second study, although without complete responders. Median duration of response was nine months and median survival for responding patients was 12·5 months, but the overall survival was only 5·5 months. The same group has tested doxorubicin, mitomycin C, and ftorafur (FAM II), but this combination was associated with serious haematologic toxicity without exhibiting therapeutic advantage over FAM. They also rejected the use of chlorozotocin, a nitrosurea, in addition to the FAM regimen. The Australian group of Gill *et al* obtained a response rate of 57% in 28 patients with inoperable or metastatic gastric cancer using FAM.[27] In 81 evaluable patients, Cunningham *et al* reported 28 (35%) responses, of which 4 (5%) had a complete remission.[28]

Adjuvant chemotherapy in Western randomised trials

The superior response rates to FAM in advanced gastric cancer, combined with the disappointing results of surgical treatment, stimulated interest in adjuvant therapy and resulted in a number of randomised trials (Table 6.3).

The Eastern Cooperative Oncology Group (ECOG) confirmed the efficacy of FAM in a trial of FAM versus doxorubicin and mitomycin C (AM) versus fluorouracil, doxorubicin and semustine (methyl-CCNU) (FAMe) versus fluorouracil and methyl-CCNU (FMe).[29] FAM induced a response in 39% of the patients with advanced disease, and proved to be the least toxic regimen.

In an International Collaborative Cancer Group (ICCG) trial, FAM was moderately well tolerated in most patients, although three possible treatment related deaths were noted.[30] The patients who received chemotherapy did not benefit in terms of disease free or overall survival.

MacDonald *et al* have tested adjuvant FAM in a randomised trial, initiated in 1978.[31] To accrue the required 200 patients took more than 13 years, and after a median follow up of 9·5 years, 63 patients in the FAM group and 71 in the control group died, a non-significant difference. This trial also failed to detect a difference in disease free survival.

In the second British Stomach Cancer Group trial, survival after adjuvant therapy with FAM or radiotherapy was compared with that of a control group undergoing surgery only.[32] After five years of follow up, the survival curves of the three groups showed no significant differences, and in all groups locally recurrent cancer was the most common cause of death (88%).

A number of trials compared cytotoxic combinations based on fluorouracil and the nitrosureas. Hattori *et al* examined the addition of mitomycin C to fluorouracil over single agent therapy.[33] In this randomised

TABLE 6.3—*Western randomised studies of adjuvant chemotherapy for gastric cancer*

Author	Regimen	Number	Stage	Conclusion
Douglas *JCO* 1984	FAM F-A-Me AM	183	advanced	more effective than FAMe; suitable for adjuvant therapy
Coombes *JCO* 1990	FAM control	315	operable	no advantage for chemotherapy
MacDonald *ASCO* 1992	FAM control	193	curative resected	FAM not effective
Hallissey *Lancet* 1994	FAM radiation control	436	resected	no advantage for chemo- or radiotherapy
Hattori *Jpn J Surg* 1986	FM M F	2873	resected	no survival difference
Douglass *Cancer* 1982	FMe control	142	curative resected	survival advantage for FMe
Higgins *Cancer* 1983	FMe control	134	curative resected	no survival or time to recurrence difference
Engstrom *Cancer* 1985	FAMe control	180	resected	too toxic; no survival advantage
Bonfanti *Br J Surg* 1988	FMe-lev control	213	curative resected	no effect on survival
Allum *Lancet* 1989	FM FM-ind control	411	resected	no advantage for chemotherapy
Krook *Cancer* 1991	FA control	125	curative resected	no advantage for chemotherapy
Estape *Ann Surg* 1991	M control	70	resected	survival advantage for mitomycin C

RCT: randomised controlled trial; F: fluorouracil; A: doxorubicin; M: mitomycin C; Me: methyl-CCNU; lev: levamisole; ind: induction with fluorouracil, vincristine, cyclophosphamide and methotrexate.

trial of 2873 resected patients, they could not detect a survival difference among the studied groups, although subset analysis revealed a beneficial effect of the FM regimen for patients with serosal invasion and lymph node metastases. Four randomised trials tested the combination of fluorouracil and methyl-CCNU after resected gastric cancer.[34-37] In the Gastrointestinal Tumour Study Group (GITSG) trial, surgical procedures were specified accurately in order to define which patients indeed underwent curative resection.[34] Five year survival was 45% for FMe and 32% for controls (p = 0·06), but this difference did not become apparent until two years after surgery. All subgroups benefited from chemotherapy, but the best results were obtained in the subgroups without lymph node metastases or having distal subtotal gastrectomy. Liver metastases occurred less frequently in the treated patients, but the overall incidence of distant metastases was equal in both groups; almost all deaths were associated with recurrence.

This suggests that the benefit of chemotherapy was attributable to better local control after resection. Such a delayed survival benefit has, however, also been suggested from extended lymph node dissection and it might be that inapparent differences in surgical approaches between the groups have occurred. This is suggested from the large survival difference in patients who were treated with total gastrectomy, a procedure more susceptible to surgical variations than distal subtotal gastrectomy.

Fluorouracil and semustine were also tested by the Veterans Administration group.[35] This study included "curative" and non-curative resections as well as unresectable patients. Of the 134 eligible patients who had curative resections, 36 in each group had died at the time of evaluation. There was no survival difference after 3·5 years and no reduction in the risk of recurrence was noted.

Like the Veterans Administration group, the ECOG could not reproduce the results of the GITSG.[36] Five year survival rates were 27% for chemotherapy (FMe) and 34% for controls, and chemotherapy had no influence on the occurrence of liver metastases. Furthermore, they found clinically important haematological complications and two of the 91 treated patients (2%) died of bone marrow failure.

The Italian Gastrointestinal Tumour Study group evaluated FMe and the immunomodulative effect of levamisole in an adjuvant setting.[37] They could not detect an effect on survival of FMe and patients did not benefit from additional levamisole. The British Stomach Cancer Group conducted a three arm randomised controlled trial comparing induction chemotherapy (fluorouracil, vincristine, cyclophosphamide, and methotrexate) followed by fluorouracil and mitomycin C (FM) with a group receiving fluorouracil and mitomycin C only.[38] Patients in a third arm had surgery only. Four hundred and eleven patients were entered, and after at least 5·5 years' follow up no survival advantage was detected for FM, with or without induction treatment.

The combination of fluorouracil and doxorubicin (FA) failed to improve survival in patients who had undergone potentially curative resection for gastric cancer.[39] There was no significant difference in time to recurrence, and the five year survival rates were similar.

Apart from the GITSG study using FMe, only one randomised study in the Western world has demonstrated a survival benefit for adjuvant chemotherapy.[40] This study compared adjuvant mitomycin C treatment after resection for locally advanced gastric cancer with resection only. There were only 70 patients entered between 1975 and 1979; five years after surgery there was a significant survival advantage for the patients treated with mitomycin C. After 10 years the survival advantage persisted and was not compromised by late toxicity or the occurrence of new malignancies.

Adjuvant chemotherapy in Japan

In most aspects of diagnosis and treatment of gastric cancer the Japanese experience has developed differently from that in the West. Screening and early detection in Japan have been associated with an increased incidence of early gastric cancer, whereas in Western countries screening is not considered cost effective because of the lower incidence of the disease. Surgical treatment with curative intent in Japan includes dissection of lymph node echelons outside the perigastric area and, if necessary, part of the upper abdominal organs (see McCulloch and Sasako above). The Japanese also have different opinions concerning adjuvant chemotherapy. The high incidence of gastric cancer and its impact on general mortality in Japan have stimulated a large number of randomised trials by various research groups. The National Hospital Group, with seven randomised trials between 1959 and 1978, the University Hospital Group, with six randomised controlled trials between 1961 and 1980, and the Gastric Cancer Adjuvant Chemotherapy Group (two trials) are the most important of these, but a number of other cooperative groups have also studied adjuvant chemotherapy.[41]

Among the agents tested, combinations of mitomycin C, fluorouracil, and oral fluorouracil derivates like futraful and dry syrup 5FU (5FUds) were the most important. Various routes of administration (intra-arterial, intraperitoneal) and timing (perioperative, postoperative) have been studied. Trials with a significant improvement of survival after resection utilised combined intraperitoneal and intravenous mitomycin C, or sequential mitomycin C and fluorouracil.[41]

In the early 1980s biological response modifiers were introduced into clinical trials. PSK (krestin), OK-432 (picibanil) and BCG strains have been used in the belief that they may inhibit tumour growth by stimulation of the immunological system. The combination of surgery, immunomodulation, and chemotherapy resulted in a new research field (immunochemosurgery). So far, trial evidence of benefit from immunochemosurgery has been confined to the rather small study of Kim[42] and a recent Japanese comparison with adjuvant chemotherapy.[43] In our overview of randomised controlled trials (see "Meta-analysis", below), only one was retrieved from a Japanese journal (see Table 6.4).[23 44] At least 11 other randomised controlled studies were reported in Japanese journals between 1980 and 1990, but most were beyond the scope of our overview because they investigated advanced disease.

Although the Japanese have gained enormous experience from their studies, there is reluctance among Western clinicians to implement their recommendations. Japanese researchers are able to enter a high proportion of their patients into clinical trials. For example, between 1960 and 1980 the Cancer Institute Hospital in Tokyo treated 4425 patients, of whom 3014 had curative resections. Of these, 969 (32%) were entered in various trials. If one lesson can be learned from the Japanese experience, it may be that even in their relatively large trials statistical differences are often not found. This indicates that if a survival advantage of adjuvant chemotherapy exists it is likely to be very small.

Discrepancy of results in advanced disease and in adjuvant trials

There are several possible explanations for the discrepancy between the positive results in phase II trials and the obvious lack of benefit in randomised trials of adjuvant chemotherapy. A comparison of results with historical control groups is hampered by differences in diagnostic accuracy. Detection and preoperative staging of gastric cancer is notoriously difficult. Advances in diagnostic techniques such as endoscopic ultrasonography and CT have only recently become readily available. In the 1980s most phase II studies relied on CT and ultrasonography for evaluation of response. Diagnosis of liver metastases by ultrasonography is quite accurate, but early detection of peritoneal seeding is difficult, even with CT. The absence of accurate methods of measuring abdominal tumour deposits in the 1980s has certainly limited accurate response evaluation. Some investigators now argue that randomised trials of chemotherapy should concentrate on response rather than on survival. The background to this viewpoint is that only regimens of proven efficacy will have an effect on survival, but that such regimens have not yet been identified. For example, responses to FAM have almost exclusively been partial; only in one trial were any complete responses observed. It is currently believed that chemotherapeutic agents for the adjuvant setting should be selected on the basis of the number of complete responders in phase II trials. If the complete response rate is less than 10%, a beneficial effect on survival seems unlikely.

The discrepancy between efficacy in advanced disease and in patients undergoing potentially curative resection may also be related to the inability to administer the planned dose of chemotherapy. Although FAM was well tolerated, in the ICCG trial more than 50% of patients required dose reduction because of drug related side effects.[30] In many Western trials chemotherapy is postponed until one month after surgery to allow the patient to recover, and this may explain the apparent lack of efficacy. On the other hand, it is likely that the early starters with the better outcome in the British study had better performance status, which is itself associated with improved outcome.[38] It should be recognised that, if dose reduction is frequently required for patients in a randomised trial, it is unlikely that it will prove feasible to deliver the planned dose outside trials. Variations in the ability of surgeons to achieve radical clearance of the primary tumour

187

are a major contributor to the failure of adjuvant chemotherapy. The GITSG trial required accurate documentation of staging and uniform surgical procedures, and only well documented, potentially curative cases were eligible.[34] Patients who have curative resections usually have a better performance status and a higher chance of receiving the planned chemotherapy dose.

Failure to demonstrate the efficacy of chemotherapy in randomised trials is doubtless contributed to by the inability to enrol sufficient numbers of patients. For example, given a 10% five year survival in the control group, around 2000 patients would be needed to detect a 5% survival difference. Even in Japan, not many studies have collected so many patients individually. Therefore we have to rely on overviews of results, obtained by meta-analysis, in order to increase our understanding of treatment benefits.

Meta-analysis of randomised trials of adjuvant therapy for gastric cancer[23]

Of the randomised controlled studies of adjuvant chemotherapy after resection for gastric cancer, only the studies of the GITSG[34] (fluorouracil and semustin) and of Estape *et al*[40] (mitomycin C) have shown significant survival advantage for the chemotherapy group. One must conclude that there is currently no individual cytotoxic regimen that could be used as standard therapy in the adjuvant setting. If a small overall influence on survival exists, however, a large number of patients would have to be studied to detect this. In order to evaluate the overall benefit of adjuvant chemotherapy in this situation, a meta-analysis is the best tool. We therefore performed a Medline search, updated to October 1994. This yielded 125 english abstracts published since 1980, of which 64 (40 in English and 24 in Japanese) were considered possibly relevant and retrieved. The search was restricted to trials published from 1980, because studies before that time had utilised regimens that failed to produce sufficient response in gastric cancer. Combination of evidence from randomised trials is only useful if these trials have one treatment in common. Surgical resection without adjuvant treatment is the standard treatment and therefore we only considered prospective trials with a no-treatment control arm.

The statistical method applied is described by Buyse *et al.*[45] For each treatment arm the crude mortality odds were calculated, and the odds of death for the treatment arm divided by the odds of death for the control arm to produce an odds ratio. For three arm trials, two odds ratios can thus be calculated. The odds ratios were tested for homogeneity, and combined using the Mantel–Haenszel new alinea. The Japanese reports included one relevant clinical trial and the Western reports 13. Of these, two Western articles and the Japanese paper did provide the data needed to calculate the odds ratio. Scanning the references of the retrieved reports did not yield unknown relevant studies, but direct communications resulted in inclusion of two further unpublished trials. The relevant

TABLE 6.4—*Randomised trials included in the meta-analysis*

Author	Regimen	Number per arm	Deaths per arm	Odds ratio	Authors' conclusion
Hallissey[32]	FAM	119	95	1·04	no advantage for
1994	radioth	129	111	1·62	chemo- or radiotherapy
	control	125	99		
MacDonald[31]	FAM	93	63	0·86	FAM not effective
1992	control	100	71		
Cirera[64]	M-Tegrafur	76	27	0·52	no significant
1992	control	72	37		differences in survival
Krook[39]	FA	61	42	0·93	no substantial benefit
1991	control	64	45		
Coombes[30]	FAM	133	73	0·76	not indicated as routine
1990	control	148	91		
Estape[40]	M	33	7	0·16	adjuvant therapy useful
1990	control	37	23		
Schiessel[65]	CDDP ip	33	26	1·14	no significant
1989	control	34	26		difference
Allum[20]	FM	140	127	1·47	no advantage for
1989	FM + ind	141	126	1·26	adjuvant FM
	control	130	113		
Bonfanti[37]	FMe + lev	69	38	1·12	no effect on survival
1988	FMe	75	35	0·80	
	control	69	36		
Kim[42]	P-Me-Fu/	74	42	0·40	significant
1988	P-FM-Ara-Fu	64	49		advantage for
	control				immunochemosurgery
Jakesz[66]	FM-Ara	53	29	0·50	no survival benefit
1988	control	34	24		
Yamamura[44]	FM-Ok	33	8	0·52	chemoimmunotherapy
1986	FM	32	10	0·73	may be effective
	control	34	13		
Engstrom[36]	FMe	91	57	1·25	no survival advantage
1985	control	89	51		
Nakajima[41]	FM-Ara + F	73	23	0·51	no proof for statistical
1984	F'M-Ara + F'	76	28	0·64	significance
	control	74	35		
Higgins[35]	FMe	66	36	1·07	improvement in
1983	control	68	36		survival
Douglass[34]	FMe	71	29	0·54	survival advantage
1982	control	71	40		
Schlag[67]	F-BCNU	42	17	0·71	no influence on
1982	control	53	26		survival

F: fluorouracil; A: doxorubicin; M: mitomycin C; CDDP ip: intraperitoneal cisplatin; ind: induction with fluorouracil, vincristine, cyclophosphamide and methotrexate; Me: methyl-CCNU; lev: levamisole; P: picibanil; Fu: futraful; Ara: cytarabine; Ok: OK-432; F': ftorafur.

trials and their odds ratios are listed in Table 6.4. Five trials compared 2 treatments to surgical controls and provided 2 odds ratios, all other trials provided one odds ratio and in total 21 odds ratios could be compared. In view of the survival benefit of mitomycin C-containing regimens reported from Japan, and the positive study of single agent mitomycin C, we repeated the combination procedure using only the odds ratios of the mitomycin C trials. The odds ratios and their 95% confidence intervals, calculated from the 21 comparisons of adjuvant chemotherapy with surgery alone, are depicted in Figure 6.7. In two cases the odds ratio was significantly in support of chemotherapy.[40][42] The homogeneity test did not point out any study to be significantly different to the others and all odds ratios could be used in the combination procedure. Combination of the 21 odds ratios yielded a common value of 0·77, with a 95% confidence interval of 0·65 to 0·88, significantly in favour of adjuvant chemotherapy (Figure 6.7).

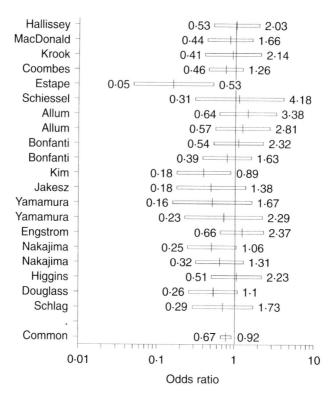

FIGURE 6.7—*Comparison of all odds ratios (randomised controlled trials 1980–1994) with their 95% confidence intervals.*

Combination of the odds ratios of the mitomycin based studies yielded an overall value of 0·75, with a 95% confidence interval of 0·6 to 0·93, also in favour of adjuvant treatment, but not significantly different from the common value of all regimens (Figure 6.8).

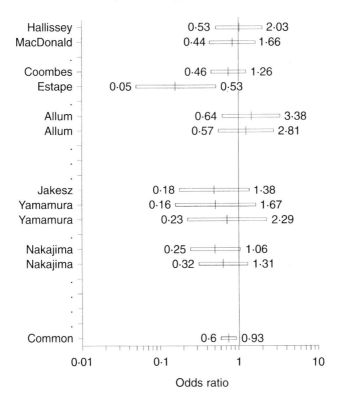

FIGURE 6.8—*Comparison of odds ratios of mitomycin combinations (randomised trials) with their 95% confidence intervals.*

This constitutes statistical evidence that adjuvant chemotherapy after curative resection provides a survival benefit. In a sense, this underlines the importance of large numbers of patients when studying treatments that are likely to have only limited impact on survival. On the other hand, the danger of publication bias becomes more important because trials with a negative outcome have a higher chance of not being published.

There is still not enough evidence to identify one regimen that could serve as a standard for treatment. The only reliable way of detecting regimens that could improve the outcome of gastric cancer patients is by increasing the number of patients in randomised controlled trials of adjuvant chemotherapy.

Future perspectives

Second generation regimens in advanced gastric cancer

The ability of future chemotherapy regimens to improve survival after resection for gastric cancer depends on the results of current phase I and phase II trials, which will therefore be discussed briefly. Active combinations using doxorubicin, methotrexate, cisplatin, and etoposide have recently emerged from phase II studies in advanced gastric cancer. The response rates of these regimens seem to be superior to those achieved with the older combinations, and the newer regimens are referred to as the second generation.

In the FAMTX regimen, methotrexate is substituted for mitomycin C. Doxorubicin is administered on day 15, in order to achieve maximal cytotoxic effect when a high percentage of the tumour cells are beginning the reproduction phase. Klein described the results of a prolonged follow up after the administration of FAMTX in 126 patients with advanced gastric cancer and reported a clinical response percentage of almost 60%, with 14 complete remissions.[46] The EORTC group conducted a randomised trial in which FAMTX was compared with FAM. FAMTX gave statistically higher response rates (41 versus 9%, p<0·001) and a longer survival (42 versus 29 weeks, p<0·0001).[47]

In FEMTX, epidoxorubicin is substituted for doxorubicin. This is reportedly less toxic and allows higher doses. Further study of this combination has led to FEMTX-P, in which the synergistic effect of cisplatin and fluorouracil is used. In a phase II trial this combination gave an objective tumour response of 47% and the primary tumour responded in 68%. FEMTX and FEMTX-P are now being compared in a randomised trial of the ICCG.

Using the combination EAP (etoposide, doxorubicin, and cisplatin), more than 60% of the patients showed a clinical response.[48] When applied at the original dosages, this combination is very myelotoxic; 64% of the patients developed grade 3–4 myelotoxicity and in one trial 2 of 10 patients died of septicaemia. EAP and FAMTX have been compared in a randomised trial. The efficacy of both combinations was comparable, but the EAP regimen showed unacceptably high toxicity.[49]

In a trial at the Royal Marsden Hospital (UK) a very high response rate was found (82%, with 8% complete remission) with ECF, a combination of fluorouracil as continuous infusion, cisplatin, and epirubicin.[50] Reports on continuous infusion of fluorouracil have suggested higher activity than fluorouracil given as conventional bolus injection. Cisplatin is moderately active as a single agent in gastric cancer and shows synergism with fluorouracil. In the ECF trial myelotoxicity was mild, and symptoms improved remarkably during the treatment. Practical use of the schedule may be impaired because of the venous access device needed to administer the fluorouracil, but Findlay *et al* demonstrated that the initial results could be reproduced in a larger series and the ECF regimen is now considered one of the most effective available.[51] Poorter *et al* studied fluorouracil, cisplatin, and doxorubicia but they used intermittent infusion of fluorouracil.[52] All of their nine patients experienced some form of toxicity and in seven patients progressive disease was seen during therapy. One more argument for the synergism between fluorouracil and cisplatin is found in a study of Rougier *et al*.[53] They administered fluorouracil as continuous infusion for five days and added cisplatin on day 2. Of the 83 evaluable patients, there were four complete (5%) and 32 partial responders (response rate 43%); however, 13 patients had progressive disease during chemotherapy and this was seen more frequently in patients with low performance status and a linitis plastica type of tumour. Haematological toxicity (neutropenia grade 3–4 in 22%) resulted in death from sepsis in three patients. Combined fluorouracil and cisplatin may be effective but, so far, toxicity limits its application in postoperative patients.

The efficacy of fluorouracil may be increased by adding leucovorin, and combination chemotherapy with epirubicin, leucovorin, and fluorouracil induced responses in 38% of 37 patients with advanced gastric cancer.[54]

The latest developments in cytotoxic agents involve agents like gemcitabine, a pyrimidine analogue and successor of Ara-C, and the taxones. Gemcitabine had no detectable antitumour effect in advanced gastric cancer, in a study executed by the EORTC.[55]

Preoperative chemotherapy

Subset analysis of the first British Stomach Cancer Group trial suggested a survival advantage if the chemotherapy was started within one month after surgery.[38] In the Japanese experience high dose mitomycin C immediately after surgery resulted in a higher survival rate than in control patients.[41] Even more interesting results have been obtained when chemotherapy was administered before surgery. For urinary bladder carcinoma, nephroblastoma, and breast cancer, preoperative chemotherapy has increased the rate of curative resectability. If complete remission is achieved, an increase in survival has been noted.[56 57] Preoperative chemotherapy for gastric cancer has been tested in phase II studies using etoposide and cisplatin. Wilke *et al* used preoperative EAP for advanced gastric cancer.[58] In 5 of 34 (14%) patients complete remission was achieved, and in 15 patients curative resection was possible. Ajani *et al* demonstrated that EFP (fluorouracil, etoposide and cisplatin) permitted curative resections in 18 of 25 studied patients (72%).[59] The recently published preliminary experience of the Memorial Sloan Kettering Hospital with preoperative chemotherapy reported that curative resections were possible in 16 of 23 patients (70%).[60] When preoperative endoultrasound staging was compared with the operative findings, downstaging was demonstrated in 33% of the patients. Rougier *et al* studied preoperative continuous infusion of fluorouracil and bolus cisplatin in locally advanced gastric cancer.[61] They had one complete and 14 partial responders in 30 treated patients (relative risk 56%); none of the patients had progressive disease during chemotherapy. Haematologic toxicity was seen in 13 patients and one of these patients died of sepsis. On the other hand, they found a rather high resectability rate (82%). Twenty three of the 28 patients who underwent surgery had macroscopically complete resections, while five had microscopically positive margins. The tumour was resectable in all patients with an objective response on chemotherapy, whereas it could be resected in only 8 of 12 non-responders. These results suggest that preoperative chemotherapy may influence resectability.

Conclusion

Adjuvant chemotherapy may have an impact on survival, although the survival advantage is small. The second generation regimens seem to be capable of inducing verifiable complete responses in around 10% of patients, and this is an important prerequisite for success in future trials. Results of studies applying preoperative chemotherapy suggest that resectability can be influenced. Preoperative administration is feasible and randomised trials in this field are warranted. There are currently (1995) two randomised controlled trials of preoperative chemotherapy, one from Britain using ECF and one from the Netherlands using FAMTX.

Radiotherapy

The place of radiotherapy in gastric cancer treatment is very limited. A rational case for adjuvant therapy to the gastric bed was made by Gunderson and Sosin in a study of recurrence sites (although the Japanese would suggest that more radical surgery would be more appropriate).[62] The argument attracted few supporters: the two main difficulties are that treatment planning must avoid unacceptable dosage to the adjacent liver, and that gastric cancer, like other gastrointestinal adenocarcinomas, is well known to be relatively radioresistant. This combination of factors effectively rules out external beam radiotherapy for bulk disease. The British Stomach Cancer Group trial studied adjuvant postoperative radiotherapy and showed no benefit, and there have been no convincing reports to the contrary.[32]

Some more promising results of pilot studies of intraoperative radiotherapy from Japan have not been developed into large studies.[63] The logistic difficulties of the approach are sufficient to prevent its widespread adoption unless convincing evidence of a major benefit can be demonstrated. The small amount of research activity going on in this area suggests that this is unlikely to be produced in the near future.

References

20 Allum WH, Hallissey MT, Ward LC, *et al.* A controlled, prospective, randomised trial of adjuvant chemotherapy or radiotherapy in resectable gastric cancer interim report. British Stomach Cancer Group. *Br J Cancer* 1989;**60**:739–44.

21 Sindelar WF. Intraoperative radiotherapy in carcinoma of the stomach and pancreas. *Recent Results Cancer Res* 1988;**110**:226–43.

22 Nakajima T, Nishi M. Adjuvant chemotherapy, immunochemotherapy and neoadjuvant therapy for gastric cancer in Japan. In: *Contemporary issues in clinical oncology (8): Gastric cancer. 125–145* Harold O. Douglass, Editor. Churchill Livingstone 1988.

23 Hermans J, Bonenkamp JJ, Ban MC, *et al.* Adjuvant therapy after curative resection for gastric cancer: meta-analysis of randomized trials. *J Clin Oncol* 1993;**11**:1441–7.

24 Serlin O, Keehn RJ, Higgins GA Jr, *et al.* Factors related to survival after resection for gastric carcinoma: an analysis of 903 cases. *Cancer* 1977;**40**:1318–29.

25 MacDonald JS, Wooley PV, Smythe T, *et al.* 5-fluoro-uracil, adriamycin and mitomycin C (FAM) combination chemotherapy in the treatment of advanced gastric cancer. *Cancer* 1979;**44**:42–7.

26 Schnall S, MacDonald JS. Mitomycin C therapy in gastric cancer. *Oncology* 1993;**50**: 70–7.

27 Gill PG, Jones AM, Abbott R. Chemotherapy of advanced gastric cancer. *Aust NZ J Surg* 1983;**53**:237–40.

28 Cunningham D, Soukop M, McArdle CS, *et al.* Advanced gastric cancer: experience in Scotland using FAM. *Br J Surg* 1984;**71**:673–6.

29 Douglass HO, Lavin PT, Goudsmit A, *et al.* An Eastern Cooperative Oncology Group evaluation of methyl-CCNU, mitomycin C, adriamycin and 5-fluoro-uracil in advanced measurable gastric cancer. *J Clin Oncol* 1984;**2**:1372–81.

30 Coombes RC, Schein PS, Chilvers CE, *et al.* A randomized trial comparing adjuvant 5-fluoro-uracil, doxorubicin and mitomycin C with no treatment in operable gastric cancer. International Collaborative Cancer Group. *J Clin Oncol* 1990;**8**:1362–9.

31 Cunningham D, Mansi J, Ford HT *et al.* Epirubicin, Cisplatin and 5-Fluorouracil (ECF) is highly effective in advanced gastric cancer. *Proc ASCO* 1991;**10**:412.

32 Hallissey MT, Dunn JA, Ward LC, *et al.* The second British Stomach Cancer Group trial of adjuvant radiotherapy or chemotherapy in resectable gastric cancer: five year follow-up. *Lancet* 1994;**343**:1309–12.

33 Hattori T, Inokuchi K, Taguchi T, *et al.* Postoperative adjuvant chemotherapy for gastric cancer: the second report. Analysis of data on 2873 patients followed for 5 years. *Jpn J Surg* 1986;**16**:175–80.

34 Douglass HO, Stabelein DM, Bruckner HM, *et al.* Controlled trial of adjuvant chemotherapy following curative resection for gastric cancer. The Gastrointestinal Tumour Study Group. *Cancer* 1982;**49**:1116–22.

35 Higgins GA, Amadeo JH, Smith DE, *et al.* Efficacy of prolonged intermittent therapy with combined 5-FU and methyl-CCNU following resection for gastric carcinoma. A Veterans Administration Surgical Oncology Group Report. *Cancer* 1983;**52**:1105–12.

36 Engstrom PF, Lavin PT, Douglass HO, *et al.* Postoperative adjuvant 5-fluorouracil and methyl-CCNU therapy for gastric cancer patients. Eastern Cooperative Oncology Group study. *Cancer* 1985;**55**:1868–73.

37 Bonfanti G, Gennari L, Bozzetti F, *et al*. Adjuvant treatments following curative resection for gastric cancer. The Italian Gastrointestinal Tumour Study Group. *Br J Surg* 1988;**75**: 1100–4.

38 Allum WH, Hallissey MT, Kelly KA. Adjuvant chemotherapy in operable gastric cancer. 5 year follow-up of first British Stomach Cancer Group trial. *Lancet* 1989;**18**:571–4.

39 Krook JE, O'Connell MJ, Wieand HS, *et al*. A prospective randomised evaluation of intensive-course 5-fluoro-uracil plus doxorubicin as surgical adjuvant therapy for resected gastric cancer. *Cancer* 1991;**67**:2454–8.

40 Estape J, Grau JJ, Lcobendas F, *et al*. Mitomycin C as an adjuvant treatment to resected gastric cancer. A ten year follow-up. *Ann Surg* 1991;**213**:219–21.

41 Nakajima T, Nishi M. Adjuvant chemotherapy, immunochemotherapy and neoadjuvant therapy for gastric cancer in Japan. In: *Contemporary issues in clinical oncology (8): gastric cancer*. Edinburgh, Churchill Livingstone: 1988.

42 Kim JP. Immunochemosurgery as a new approach to reasonable treatment of advanced cancer. *Ann Acad Med Singapore* 1988;**17**:48–54.

43 Nakazato H, Koike A, Saji S, *et al*. Efficacy of immunochemotherapy as adjuvant therapy after curative resection for gastric cancer. *Lancet* 1994;**343**:1122–6.

44 Yamamura Y, Nishimura M, Sakamoto J, *et al*. A randomised controlled trial of surgical adjuvant therapy with mitomycin C, 5-fluorouracil and OK432 in patients with gastric cancer. *Gan To Kakagu Ryoho* 1986;**13**:2134–40.

45 Buyse M, Zeleniuch-Jacquotte A, Chalmers TC. Adjuvant therapy of colorectal cancer: why we still don't know. *JAMA* 1988;**259**:3571–8.

46 Klein HO. Long-term results with FAMTX in advanced gastric cancer. *Anticancer Res* 1989;**9**:1025–6.

47 Wils JA, Klein HO, Wagener DJT, *et al*. Sequential high-dose methotrexate and fluorouracil combined with doxorubicin: a step ahead in the treatment of gastric cancer. A trial of the EORTC group. *J Clin Oncol* 1991;**5**:827–31.

48 Preusser P, Wilke H, Achterrath W, *et al*. Phase II study with the combination etoposide, doxorubicin and cis-platin in advanced measurable gastric cancer. *J Clin Oncol* 1989;**7**: 1310–7.

49 Kelsen D. FAMTX versus etoposide, doxorubicin and cisplatin: a random assignment trial in gastric cancer. *J Clin Oncol* 1992;**10**:541–8.

50 Cunningham D, *et al*. Epirubicin, Cisplatin and 5FU (ECF) is highly effective in advanced gastric cancer. *Proc ASCO* 1991;**10**:412.

51 Findlay M, Cunningham D, Norman A, *et al*. A phase I study in advanced gastro-oesophageal cancer using epirubicin and cisplatin in combination with continuous infusion 5-fluorouracil (ECF). *Ann Oncol* 1994;**5**:609–16.

52 Poorter PL, Bakker PJM, Taat CW, *et al*. Epirubicin, cisplatin and intermittent continuous infusion 5-fluorouracil (ECF) in advanced gastric cancer: an effective regimen? *Eur J Cancer* 1994;**9**:1404.

53 Rougier PH, Ducreux M, Mahjoubi M, *et al*. Efficacy of combined 5-fluorouracil and cisplatin in advanced gastric carcinomas. A phase II trial with prognostic factor analysis. *Eur J Cancer* 1994;**9**:1263–9.

54 Kornek G, Schulz F, Depisch D, *et al*. A phase I–II study of 5 FU, epirubicin and leucovorin in advanced adenocarcinoma of the stomach. *Cancer* 1993;**71**:2177–80.

55 Sessa C, Aamdal S, Wolff I, *et al*. Gemcitabane in patients with advanced malignant melanoma or gastric cancer: phase II studies of the EORTC Early Clinical Trials Group. *Ann Oncol* 1994;**5**:471–2.

56 Zuppan CW, Bechwith JB, Weeks DA, *et al*. The effect of preoperative chemotherapy on the histological features of Wilms' tumour. *Cancer* 1990;**68**:385–94.

57 Kurtz JM. Should surgery remain the initial treatment of "operable" breast cancer? *Eur J Cancer* 1991;**27**:1539–42.

58 Wilke H, Preusser P, Fink U, *et al*. Preoperative chemotherapy in locally advanced and nonresectable gastric cancer: a phase II study with etoposide, doxorubicin and cisplatin. *J Clin Oncol* 1989;**7**:1318–26.

59 Ajani JA, Ota DM, Jessup JM, *et al*. Resectable gastric carcinoma: an evaluation of preoperative and postoperative chemotherapy. *Cancer* 1991;**68**:1501–6.

60 Schwartz G, Kelsen D, Christman K, *et al.* A phase II study of neoadjuvant FAMTX and postoperative intraperitoneal 5-FU and cisplatin in high risk patients with gastric cancer. *Proc ASCO* 1993;**572**:195.

61 Rougier PH, Mahjoubi M, Lasser PH, *et al.* Neoadjuvant chemotherapy in locally advanced gastric carcinoma. A phase II trial with combined continuous intravenous 5 fluorouracil and bolus cisplatin. *Eur J Cancer* 1994;**9**:1269–75.

62 Gunderson LL, Sosin H. Adenocarcinoma of the stomach: areas of failure in reoperation series (second or symptomatic look) clinicopathologic correlation and implications for adjuvant therapy. *Int J Radiat Oncol Biol* 1981;**8**:1–11.

63 Abe M, Takahashi M, Yabumoto E, *et al.* Techniques, indications and results of intraoperative radiotherapy of advanced cancers. *Radiology* 1975;**116**:693–701.

64 Cirera L, Cardona T, Batiste E, *et al.* Randomised trial of adjuvant chemotherapy vs. control in stage III gastric cancer. *Proc Am Soc Clin Oncol* 1992;**11**:160 (abstract 454).

65 Schiessel R, Funovics J, Schick B, *et al.* Adjuvant intraperitoneal cisplatin therapy in patients with operated gastric carcinoma: results of a randomised trial. *Acta Med Aust* 1989;**16**:68–9.

66 Jakesz R, Dittrich C, Funovics J, *et al.* The effect of adjuvant chemotherapy in gastric carcinoma is dependent on tumor histology: 5-year results of a prospective randomized trial. *Rec Res Cancer Res* 1988;**110**:44–51.

67 Schlag P, Schrengl W, Gaus W, *et al.* Adjuvant 5-fluorouracil and BCNU chemotherapy in gastric cancer: 3-year results. *Rec Res Cancer Res* 1982;**80**:277–83.

197

7: Pancreas

Tumour biology, investigation, and surgical management

ANDREW KINGSNORTH

Pancreatic carcinoma is the fifth most frequent cause of cancer death and accounts for over 7000 deaths in England and Wales each year. Recent advances include improvements in operative morbidity and mortality and refinements in chemotherapy for advanced disease. These achievements have not been paralleled by earlier diagnosis, improved resectability, or significant advances in adjuvant treatment. Progress has been made in the ability to stage pancreatic cancer accurately, and in surgical and non-surgical approaches to palliative treatment.

Incidence

An incidence of 1 in 10 000 in the United Kingdom is approximately the same as that in the USA.[1] Although the UK incidence is approximately twice that of Japan, the rate in that country has risen sharply over the last 20 years, with a threefold increase in incidence. Environmental and genetic factors probably play a part.

Aetiology and risk factors

The overall prognosis is poor, with a less than 1% survival at five years. In some centres, however, presumably with careful case selection, a post-resection 20% actuarial survival at five years can be achieved. There is support for an association between cigarette smoking and pancreatic cancer but no evidence for an aetiological role for alcohol, coffee drinking, diabetes mellitus, gall stones, or previous gastric surgery. The results of numerous epidemiological studies are inconsistent. There is a weak association with pernicious anaemia, which may be a consequence of increased plasma gastrin and cholecystokinin levels. The high fat, high protein intake in westernised countries has been implicated, although the epidemiological data are inconsistent. A nearly fivefold increased risk has been discovered in chemical workers exposed to dichlorodiphenyltrichloroethane (DDT).[2] A small risk factor of the order of a twofold increase can be expected in patients with chronic pancreatitis, but this condition may only account for 0·1% of pancreatic cancer annually.[3] Of interest in the search for genetic markers are extended families with hereditary pancreatic cancer who may represent up to 3–5% of the total incidence.[4]

Tumour biology

Around 75% of pancreatic neoplasms show activating mutations in the Ki-ras oncogene at codons 12, 13, and 61. This oncogene encodes for a 21 kDa cell membrane protein (p21) involved in the signal transduction cascade. In its normal state this protein is activated by the binding of GTP; inactivation of this complex requires the binding of a second protein, called GAP, which then catalyses the dephosphorylation of GTP to GDP. The mutated p21 protein, on the other hand, has lost the ability to bind GAP and therefore is unable to be inactivated in the normal fashion, leading to an increased drive to the tumour cell to grow and divide.

The frequency of this oncogene mutation in pancreatic cancer has led to hopes that it may be an effective target for treatment strategies in the future. Several strategies could theoretically be employed.

- Antibodies against the abnormal protein could be utilised in either targeting cytotoxic therapy or as a means of augmenting the host response against the tumour.
- Drugs may be developed which bind to the abnormal protein, either deactivating it or allowing it to bind to GAP so that normal deactivation may occur. In vitro studies have been performed in which antibodies, raised against the abnormal p21 protein, have been injected into transformed cells expressing transformed p21. When the abnormal protein is deactivated in this manner the cells express a non-transformed phenotype, but revert back to the transformed phenotype when the antibodies are metabolised.
- The mutated ras oncogene may in the future be able to be directly replaced by its non-mutated counterpart. With the current state of knowledge this approach verges on science fiction; however, given the recent rapid advancement of knowledge in the field of molecular biology, a useful therapeutic tool may be only a few years away.

199

In clinical practice, however, the amazing progress in the field of molecular biology has, so far, made little impact on the management of pancreatic cancer.[5]

Tumour, node, metastases (TNM) Classification

Early carcinomas (T1aN0M0) occur in less than 5% of patients; in even these early cancers, lymphatic spread is present in 40% and there is an

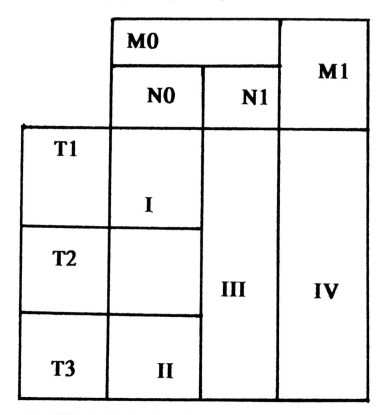

FIGURE 7.1—*TNM classification of exocrine pancreatic cancer.*

incidence of lymph node metastases in more than 30%. It is important to examine a resection specimen in the dorsal direction to detect lymphatic invasion into the retroperitoneum. This defines a further classification (R) for residual tumour after surgical treatment. R0, with no residual tumour found in the histopathological examination, occurs in only 60–70% of cases that were thought to be curative resections at the time of operation. In the remaining 30%, either R1 (microscopic residual tumour) or R2 (macroscopic residual tumour) will indicate a non-curative operation. An understanding of the detailed lymphatic drainage of the head of the pancreas provides a rationale for extended lymphadenectomy in the surgical treatment of the condition (Figure 7.2). Thus the prognosis after resection depends on the TNM stage and the R classification.[6]

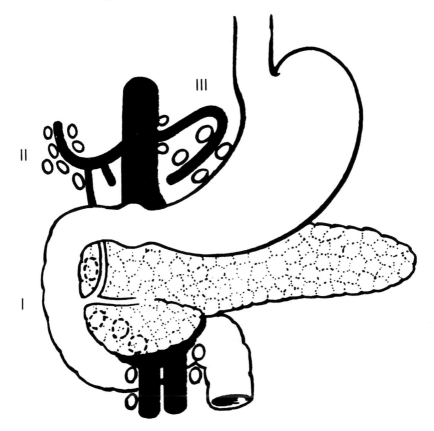

FIGURE 7.2—*Lymph nodes susceptible to invasion.*

Cost–benefit analysis

There is little doubt that resection is indicated for cancers of the duodenum, ampulla, and distal common bile duct, but many clinicians believe that resection for pancreatic carcinoma is not justifiable. Since these four primary periampullary carcinomas cannot always be differentiated accurately before resection, units with low operative mortality should attempt resection in all early tumours. Case selection is crucial: even an uncomplicated resection results in at least a fivefold increase in cost over palliative bypass surgery. Resection should therefore only be considered for physiologically young patients with small localised lesions.[7]

Investigation

Tumour markers

Tumour markers may have potential for the early detection of cancer or for use as screening tools. Unfortunately their use in pancreatic cancer has proved problematic. Carcinoembryonic antigen (CEA), CA 50, and CA 125, although often raised, are non-specific and of little use as screening tools, but they may have a role in assessing the response of the tumour to treatment if raised at presentation. Studies of the newer tumour markers, CA 19-9 and CA 242, have shown encouraging results. A recent study has shown that CA 242 has a specificity of 91% and a sensitivity of 74% in the detection of pancreatic cancer in a trial cohort of patients known to have pancreatic cancer compared with a comparable group of patients with benign pancreatic disease. CA 19-9, on the other hand, was 81% specific and 83% sensitive for detecting pancreatic cancer in the same cohort of patients. Several factors need to be remembered when considering these results.[8]

- The specificity and sensitivity for an assay depend on what value is used as a cut off point. Moving the cut off point to increase specificity in this situation will decrease the sensitivity of the assay.
- The most clinically useful parameter for a proposed screening test is the predictive value. This depends on the prevalence of the object disease in the population under study. For the trial quoted above, the predictive value for the test is high because of the artificially high prevalence of the disease in the study population. These markers, although promising, require much more widespread testing before their role in diagnostic and screening tests can be established.
- Tumour markers are most useful as a screening tool in those groups at highest risk of disease, and until such groups can be more accurately defined for pancreatic cancer the markers discussed above will be of limited use.

For practical purposes, therefore, no screening test has yet been devised that is sensitive enough to detect curable carcinoma of the pancreas sufficiently reliably to distinguish between pancreatic cancer and other causes of biliary obstruction. Even CA 19-9 is insufficiently sensitive to be useful for postoperative surveillance to detect early treatable recurrence.[9] Thus, for the present, no screening tests are useful in the management of this disease.

Symptoms and signs

In 70% of cases the classic presentation is with painless jaundice, and up to 50% of patients will have experienced some degree of mild epigastric discomfort or back pain. When jaundice appears, most patients have lost weight, which in some cases may amount to more than 10% of total body weight. Occasionally patients present with acute pancreatitis or hyperamylasaemia associated with discomfort. Carcinoma of the body and tail of the pancreas is associated with persistent back pain, anorexia, and weight loss. Thrombophlebitis migrans can be associated with carcinoma of the pancreas but is non-specific. The onset of diabetes mellitus in an individual of normal body weight and without a hereditary predisposition for diabetes mellitus is suspicious of the diagnosis.

Laboratory investigations

Biliary obstruction results in elevation of bilirubin and alkaline phosphatase, with a less marked elevation of γ-glutaryl transferase. Serological markers, such as CA 19-9, CA 50, and CEA, are often elevated once the tumour exceeds 2–3 cm in size.

Ultrasonography

The sensitivity and specificity of ultrasonography is now such that, in the hands of an experienced observer, when sonographic visualisation of the pancreas is adequate, a confident diagnosis can be made in up to 70% of patients. A dilated biliary system and the presence or absence of liver metastasis can also be verified. Thus in at least two thirds of patients, ultrasonography is the prelude to endoscopic retrograde cholangiopancreatography (ERCP) for diagnostic confirmation, with computed tomography (CT) being reserved for patients in whom surgery is contemplated and for those in whom ultrasonography was technically unsatisfactory, or when ERCP gave insufficient information. Ultra-sonography is usually incapable of diagnosing an ampullary carcinoma, although this should be visualised adequately at duodenoscopy. Findings at ultrasonography include the presence of a hypoechoic mass, dilatation of the pancreatic duct or atrophy of parenchyma surrounding the obstructed duct, and the presence of enlarged peripancreatic lymph nodes. At least 70% will be found to have an inoperable tumour on the basis of this examination alone.

Computed tomography

The current generation of computed tomographic scanners is capable of dynamic scanning with the use of an intravenous bolus injection of 150–180 ml of contrast medium (cCT). This results in highly detailed images of the pancreas, the pancreatic and biliary ducts, and the peripancreatic vasculature. Using this technique the correct diagnosis of pancreatic cancer can be made in more than 95% of patients, and we can assess accurately resectability in approximately 80% on the basis of local invasion, contiguous organ invasion, vascular invasion, and distant

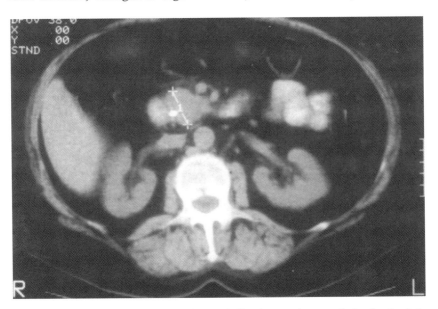

FIGURE 7.3—*Contrast-enhanced CT scan indicating carcinoma of the head of the pancreas.*

metastases (Figure 7.3). Vascular invasion is present in approximately 20% of patients and many surgeons managing the disease therefore supplement cCT with selective angiography. CT findings of pancreatic carcinoma can be mimicked by other disease processes, such as focal pancreatitis and occasionally secondary tumours and lymphoma. CT diagnosis can be confirmed by a guided fine needle aspiration (FNA) biopsy. If the CT findings are anything but typical, FNA guided biopsy should be mandatory.

Magnetic resonance imaging

Magnetic resonance imaging (MRI) of the pancreas has been used to only a limited extent.[10] It has not been found to have as high an overall accuracy as cCT, nor to offer any significant advantage over cCT. However, MRI technology is in a state of rapid evolution and further developments may improve the overall accuracy of this method of diagnosis.

Endoscopic retrograde cholangiopancreatography

ERCP allows visualisation and radiological assessment with the potential for cytological sampling and treatment of the obstructive process. The sensitivity of ERCP in the detection of pancreatic carcinoma is over 90% in most series. Visualisation of the periampullary region may reveal an ampullary tumour, a mass bulging into the duodenum, with compression or stenosis, or erosion of a mass into the gut lumen from the pancreatic head. Endoscopic pancreatography reveals either complete obstruction of the main duct or stenosis with upstream dilatation. The cholangiographic features include a block or stricture of the bile duct at the same level as the pancreatic duct obstruction, giving the appearance of the "double duct" sign, which is a reliable, although not pathognomonic, sign of pancreatic head carcinoma (Figure 7.4). Many of these features can be mimicked by chronic pancreatitis, particularly when focal. Tissue sampling can be performed at the time of ERCP, using brush cytology or aspiration of pancreatic or bile juice for subsequent cytological examination. The diagnostic yield for these tests is low, however, with positive rates of no more than 20–25%. The use of small brushes that can be placed directly into the pancreatic duct has improved the diagnostic yield somewhat, but a negative result does not exclude the diagnosis of carcinoma.

Angiography

Angiography has a small but well defined role in the evaluation of patients with pancreatic carcinoma. It can give a precise definition of the vascular anatomy and identification of vessel encasement or vessel occlusion in patients who were defined as candidates for pancreatic resection on the basis of preceding imaging investigations such as ERCP or cCT (Figure 7.5). In addition, angiography has a role in the localisation of functioning pancreatic islet cell tumours for portal venous sampling. On its own, there is a poor relationship between resectability and angiographic features. Vessel encasement or vessel occlusion, other than small end arteries in the pancreatic head, indicates irresectability. Angiography can identify

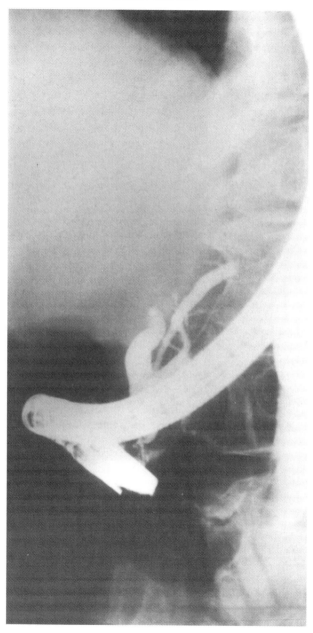

FIGURE 7.4—ERCP indicating "double duct" sign of pancreatic carcinoma.

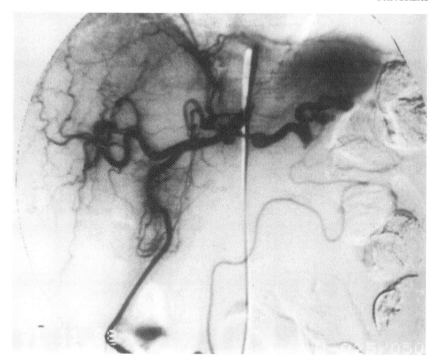

FIGURE 7.5—*Subtraction angiogram indicating encasement of coeliac axis.*

vascular anomalies such as origin of the right hepatic artery from the superior mesenteric artery, providing useful preoperative information to the surgeon (Figure 7.6).

Preoperative biopsy

A selective policy should be exercised in obtaining a percutaneous fine needle aspirate for cytology because of the small but real risk of needle track seeding of tumour cells. The tumour can be localised by ultrasonography or CT and a biopsy obtained through the anterior abdominal wall. There is thus potential for peritoneal as well as abdominal wall seeding, which has been documented in a small number of cases. This is a safe procedure with a very low complication rate but there are problems with interpretation of the aspirate. An experienced cytologist is therefore essential, although even in expert hands the false negative rate is high and it is difficult to obtain a diagnosis of the histological type of the tumour. Thus a positive result may be of clinical value for planning treatment, whereas a negative result does not exclude malignancy.[11] Aspiration cytology has equal sensitivity and specificity to fine bore needle (Tru-Cut) biopsy and is

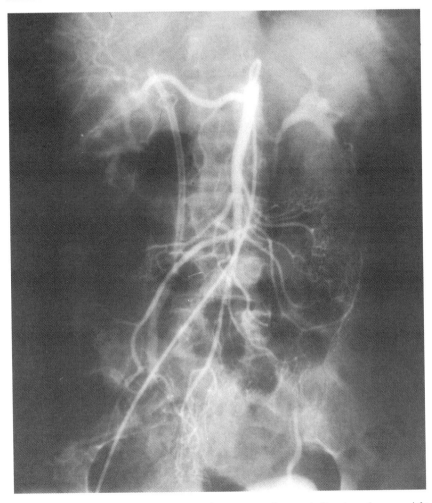

FIGURE 7.6—*Selective superior mesenteric artery angiogram indicating aberrant right hepatic artery.*

considerably safer. Because of the problem with needle track spread, the place of FNA cytology is better confined to those who are not candidates for surgery, in whom a tissue diagnosis would be helpful in planning exploratory palliative or non-radical treatment.

Intraoperative fine needle aspiration cytology

As with preoperative percutaneous FNA, the same pitfalls are apparent with the intraoperative technique. Although a positive predictive value of

100% is achievable, the negative predictor value is 75%, which means that the justification for pancreatic resection cannot always be based on cytological findings. The same concerns regarding peritoneal spread from needle tracks exists with this investigation. This method should always be used in preference to fine bore needle biopsy, in which accidental puncture of a distended pancreatic duct and subsequent fistula formation can result in considerable morbidity and mortality. Some groups claim a high degree of accuracy in the differentiation of pancreatic masses, both benign from malignant and in the diagnosis of specific histological types.[12]

Laparoscopy

The value of laparoscopy in assessing resectability as an adjunct to ultrasonography, ERCP, CT, and angiography is controversial. It has been argued that, in otherwise operable tumours, peritoneal seedlings have been found in a quarter of patients by laparoscopy,[13] and that this investigation, supplemented by contact ultrasonography to detect deep seated hepatic metastasis not otherwise detected on CT, will save a significant number of patients unnecessary laparotomy. It is unusual, however, for isolated peritoneal seedlings or small deep seated hepatic metastases to be the sole reasons for inoperability and most pancreatic surgeons would consider laparoscopy to be useful only in selected cases and would not use it routinely.

Endosonography

The value of this investigation lies in its ability to stage potentially resectable tumours. Endosonography cannot discriminate accurately between inflammation and tumour, nor can it detect metastases. Thus conventional ultrasonography and/or cCT is still required for complete staging. Endosonography can distinguish early stage tumours from advanced stage tumours in terms of local invasion but it cannot predict accurately whether enlarged lymph nodes are metastatic or non-metastatic. Splenic or portal vein occlusion is predicted accurately but other evidence of venous involvement by tumour cannot be detected. For the present, therefore, endosonography is operator dependent, expensive, and requires further evaluation.[14]

Endoscopic stenting

Palliation versus cure

A young fit patient, with a limited tumour mass, no metastases, and no evidence of lymph node involvement, should be given the best possible surgical treatment with curative intent; however, with increasing age and medical fitness, an operative mortality of 5% and five year survival of only 10–20% after curative resection, realism dictates that palliative treatment will be the best form of management in such patients. Obstructive jaundice being the presenting symptom in most patients means that endoscopic stenting will be the form of management selected. A full understanding of the effectiveness of this form of palliation and its complications is therefore required.

Symptom relief

Endoscopic stenting is not only effective in relieving jaundice and pruritus, which is a constant reminder to the patient of their underlying condition, but it also results in a rapid improvement in appetite and dyspepsia. Quality of life is also improved, with elevation of mood, physical health, and level of activity.[15] Because of these benefits, the placement, before investigation, of an endoscopic stent in all patients with obstructive jaundice has been advocated. Indeed, during a diagnostic ERCP the placement of a stent for therapeutic purposes does not greatly increase the timing, cost, or complications of the procedure; however, a high level of expertise is required, successful stent placement on the first attempt being successful in only two thirds of patients, with a 10 Fr stent. After a second or third attempt, 90% of patients will have effective biliary drainage, but at a cost of cholangitis in approximately 10% and pancreatitis in 5%. Duodenal narrowing prevents stent placement in approximately 7·5% of patients.[16] Median survival in operable patients after endoscopic stenting is approximately six months, with a low procedure related mortality of about 5%. Stent blockage may occur after three months and some would advocate routine stent change at this time, although others advocate an expectant policy in view of the short survival in these patients.

A more rational basis for the use of endoscopic stents versus palliation by surgery has recently been advocated, in which prognostic criteria, such as advanced age, male gender, liver metastasis, and large tumours, being judged as unfavourable, have been used to guide treatment options. In short term survivors, the higher rate morbidity after endoprosthesis is offset by the higher early morbidity rates and longer hospital stays after surgical bypass. The late morbidity rate can be higher in patients receiving an endoprosthesis. Thus the optimal palliation is endoprosthesis for patients predicted to be short term survivors (less than six months), and surgical biliary bypass for those predicted to survive more than six months.[17]

Metal stents

Because of the limited patency of polyethylene stents, self expanding metal stents are an alternative option. The stents can be placed either by endoscopic or percutaneous route, with low procedure related morbidity and mortality. In a randomised trial the patency of the first stent was more than double when expandable metallic prostheses were used, compared with polyethylene, resulting in a patency rate approaching nine months.[18] The cost of metal stents has been a disincentive in many units, where metallic prostheses are reserved for failed endoscopic attempts with a polyethylene stent. The metal stent is best placed by the percutaneous route. With time, tumour may permeate the meshwork of expandable metal stents, leading to recurrent biliary obstruction. This situation requires the placement of a polyethylene stent through the metal stent because removal of the metal stent is difficult.

Combined percutaneous and endoscopic procedures

It is possible to insert a 10 or 12 Fr stent endoscopically using a transhepatic guidewire provided by a radiologist, who need only make a 5 or 7 Fr track through the liver, thus avoiding the main complication of this procedure, which is biliary peritonitis. This strategy should be adopted in patients with an obstructed system that has been contaminated with contrast medium after unsuccessful endoscopic stent placement. Percutaneous drainage can then be provided within 24 hours, or, failing successful placement of a percutaneous stent, external drainage should be instituted for 48 hours, then a combined percutaneous and endoscopic procedure carried out. As outlined above, the best option in this situation is to place a metal stent after endoscopic stent failure. Expandable metal stents with an internal diameter of up to 30 Fr can be introduced through a transhepatic track of 7 Fr.[19] Procedure related morbidity and mortality are not increased with these approaches in skilled hands (Figure 7.7).

Experimental studies

Biliary decompression has a beneficial effect, not only on relief of obstructive jaundice but also on reticuloendothelial function of the liver. Theoretically this could decrease the incidence of sepsis and renal insufficiency in the early period after biliary surgery in jaundiced patients. Studies in mongrel dogs, however, have indicated that preoperative stent placement before surgical procedures on an obstructed biliary tree results in significant fibrosis and severe inflammatory changes in the bile duct, causing postoperative complications related to the hepaticojejunal anastomosis. To date there have been no controlled clinical trials in patients,

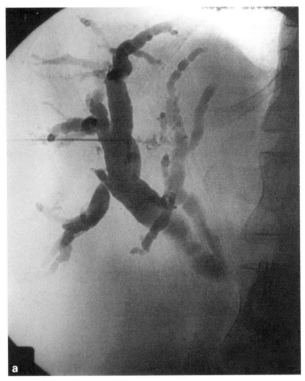

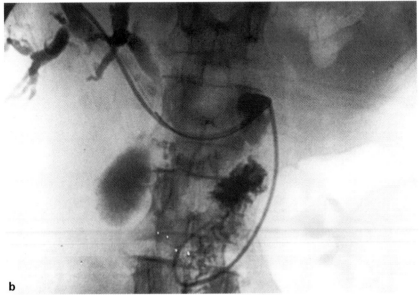

FIGURE 7.7

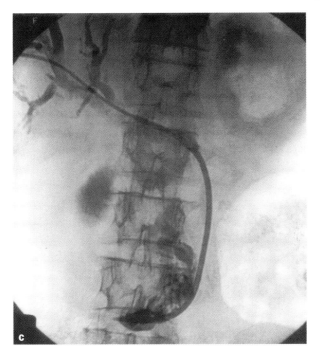

FIGURE 7.7—*Combined percutaneous endoscopic and radiological drainage of lower common bile duct stricture.*

randomising groups to preoperative stent placement or no preoperative stent. One small study carried out over a four year period in selected patients, with both high and low common bile duct obstruction, indicated similar morbidity and mortality in both treatment arms. There are advocates of preoperative stent placement by surgeons who claim a decrease in the complications of bleeding, sepsis, and renal insufficiency, while others are fearful of bacteriological contamination of bile after preoperative stent placement, resulting in complications at the biliary anastomosis.

Surgical bypass

A biliary bypass can be effected by joining the gall bladder or the bile duct to a jejunal loop in continuity or defunctioned. The choice of which palliative biliary procedure to perform should depend on the patency of the cystic duct or its proximity to the tumour mass. If the surgeon can be sure that the cystic duct will not soon be occluded by encroaching tumour, a cholecystenterostomy may be performed. In all other circumstances, a choledochal bypass procedure is the best option. After such a procedure,

213

jaundice should resolve within 3 weeks. Because duodenal obstruction from inoperable pancreatic carcinoma occurs in a minority of patients, perhaps less than 15%, prophylactic gastroenterostomy is not advisable because of the increased morbidity and mortality associated with this added procedure in frail patients; however, if duodenal obstruction is real or imminent, then gastroenterostomy can be performed concurrently with the biliary bypass. Other options for duodenal obstruction include a Roux loop anastomosed both to the anterior wall of the stomach and the bile duct. Procedures for surgical palliation in carcinoma of the pancreas carry a mortality of approximately 10%, even in the best hands, as well as the reduction in the quality of life for a finite period of time in a patient with limited survival. Other less invasive forms of palliation should therefore be explored before considering the surgical option.

Surgical resection

The first successful one stage radical pancreaticoduodenectomy was performed by Allen O Whipple in 1940. Kausch had performed a successful pancreaticoduodenectomy in 1909 for a primary biliary tumour, having first performed a defunctioning cholecystenterostomy to relieve jaundice. The operation lasted four hours and the patient lived for nine months. The Whipple operation carried a mortality of approximately 25% until the 1980s, when mortality from the operation fell dramatically (Table 7.1).

TABLE 7.1—*Recent operative morbidity and mortality for the Whipple procedure*

Author	No. of patients	Morbidity (%)	Mortality (%)
Grace (1986)	37	27	3
Braasch (1986)	87		3
McAfee (1989)	33	45	6
Pellegrini (1989)	36	27	2
Morel (1990)	33	24	0
Cameron (1991)	37		2
Roder (1992)	55	28	5

Specialised units worldwide now achieve a mortality rate of 5% or less, indicating careful selection of patients, operations performed by a limited number of surgeons, attention to surgical technique, particularly the pancreaticojejunal anastomosis, and intensive postoperative care with early intervention for complications, often with the assistance of interventional radiology.[8]

214

Risk factors

Age alone is no longer a bar to successful radical resection. Overall operative mortality below 10% can be achieved in carefully selected elderly patients and survival is related to tumour histology rather than comorbidity. Histological type is the most important factor predicting survival, with five year survival rates after successful resection for ampullary, lower common bile duct, duodenal, and pancreatic carcinoma, being approximately 40, 20, 30, and 5% respectively. Tumour size alone is not predictive of survival but lymph node status is an important factor; however, because spread to local lymph nodes cannot be predicted accurately preoperatively, the presence of enlarged nodes detected radiologically should not preclude resection in the absence of other negative factors. Histological grade further predicts survival, indicating that tumour biology is important. Weak determinants are perioperative blood loss and preoperative prodrome symptoms, such as weight loss, but management should not be governed by any one negative factor alone.

Radical resection

The pattern of surgical failure after successful surgical resection of pancreatic carcinoma is largely unknown. Anecdotal reports suggest that local recurrence is more important than distant metastases. For this reason, radical extended resections have been advocated. There are, however, no prospective controlled clinical data indicating that such an approach achieves better results.

Regional pancreatectomy, with regional lymphadenectomy, antrectomy, and sleeve resection of the portal vein, has been discarded because of unacceptably high postoperative mortality and morbidity, without apparent advantages in survival rates. The addition of a lymphadenectomy alone and connective tissue clearance around the para-aortic region has been advocated from centres in Japan.[20] Among patients with nodal involvement, retrospective comparison with patients having less radical resection has pointed towards an improvement in survival; however, the problem is defined by some as being retroperitoneal lymphatic rather than metastatic peripancreatic lymph node invasion. When resection specimens are carefully examined in the retroperitoneal region rather than the cut end of the pancreas, lymphatic invasion is found in a high percentage of patients and is probably responsible for the large number of patients with local recurrence. Whether this delicate network of lymphatics embolised with tumour cells can be effectively treated by surgery alone remains open to question.

Portal vein resection may become a necessity in some patients with a small area of infiltration on the right lateral wall of the vein discovered towards the end of the surgical resection when the neck of the pancreas has been cut. A reasonable survival is gained in these patients without compromising short term morbidity and mortality.

Preoperatively it is often impossible to distinguish between tumours of the duodenum, ampulla, head of pancreas, and distal bile duct. Histopathological differentiation may also be difficult. Prognosis of these four different periampullary tumours after resection is markedly different with the five year actuarial survivals being approximately 5% for pancreatic, 20% for duodenal, 30–40% for ampullary, and 30% for distal common bile duct. An incidence of multicentricity of pancreatic cancer of between 3 and 40% has been observed, reportedly higher in Japan.[21] For this reason, there are advocates of total pancreatectomy when a diagnosis of pancreatic cancer is certain.[22] This is a minority view and has been further marginalised because of the higher operative mortality and problems of long term morbidity with this procedure.

Reconstructive techniques

Three visceral ends remain after pancreaticoduodenectomy: the divided bile duct, the divided pancreas, and the divided gastric stump or duodenal stump. Continuity can be restored in a variety of ways and the success of each procedure is related to the anastomotic leak rate and the long term functional outcome. More than 50 reconstructive methods have been described but none has received a comparative study in the hands of the same group of surgeons. Thus it is difficult to recommend any particular reconstructive technique as superior to any other. The pancreatic anastomosis, with a leakage rate of around 10% in most series, has the greatest impact on morbidity and mortality. After such a leak, death occurs in one in four patients. The safety of this pancreatic anastomosis can be improved by using an isolated Roux loop or joining the pancreatic stump to the stomach. Some have also advocated a duct to mucosa anastomosis to unite the pancreatic duct to stomach or intestine, improving its integrity.

The pylorus preserving operation has proven to be an adequate oncological operation and avoids the morbidity associated with gastric resection. Because local infiltration occurs predominantly posteriorly, the first part of the duodenum is several centimetres distal from the primary in operable cancers and can be safely divided 1–2 cm from the pylorus with no risk of tumour infiltration. Patients receiving the pylorus preserving procedure tend to regain their premorbid weight, and survival rates are comparable to those of patients receiving the standard Whipple operation. Some centres have reported an increase in incidence of gastric stasis in the early postoperative period but reconstructive techniques have been devised that avoid this complication (Figure 7.8).

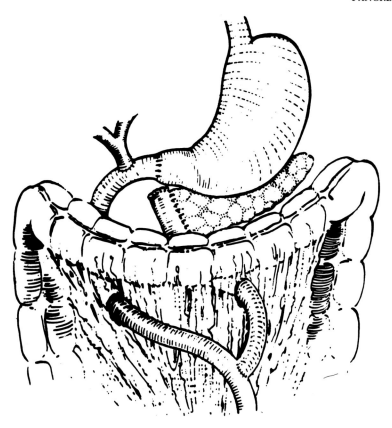

FIGURE 7.8—*A reconstructive technique after pancreaticoduodenectomy to achieve optimal functional outcome.*

Management of complications

The most frequent and most dangerous complications arise at and around the pancreaticoenteric anastomosis. A minor disruption can be treated successfully with percutaneous drainage, established either through a preoperative drain or radiological intervention, with the addition of octreotide to decrease the flow of pancreatic juice and enhance closure of the anastomotic leak. Major leaks require surgical intervention, with exteriorisation of the pancreatic stump or resection of the remaining pancreas. Aggressive surgical treatment is warranted because of the high mortality and septic complications should intra-abdominal sepsis intervene.

Biliary leaks are unusual and their management is also expectant, with established drainage and octreotide treatment, and surgery reserved for the prevention or treatment of established or related sepsis.

217

Postoperative haemorrhage is a common complication after the Whipple procedure, occurring in up to 10% of patients, and its early detection is essential during intensive surveillance in an intensive therapy unit. The usual source is small vessels around the portal or superior mesenteric vein.

The development of septic complications once again can be treated definitively by radiological intervention, or more complex abscesses should be drained by open surgical intervention.

The best management of complications is prevention and optimal preoperative and perioperative care. Standardised techniques can keep morbidity levels between 20 and 30% in the best units; however, compared with other abdominal procedures, this is a high figure and emphasises the need for close surveillance in the early postoperative period.

Surgical treatment of special histological types

Carcinoma of body or tail of pancreas

Although previously deemed to be a virtually inoperable and untreatable tumour, resection of this rare cancer achieves results not substantially different from pancreaticoduodenectomy for proximal carcinoma of the pancreas. Thus, in the absence of local infiltration demonstrated by vessel encasement on angiography or metastatic disease, patients should be offered resection, which is the only chance of long term cure. The operability rate is of the order of 10%.

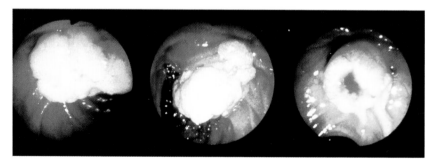

FIGURE 7.9—*Endoscopic appearance of an ampullary tumour.*

Ampullary carcinoma (Figure 7.9)

Most, if not all, ampullary carcinomas originate in ampullary adenomas. Thus the biopsy finding that an ampullary tumour is apparently an adenoma does not rule out the presence of invasive carcinoma. For this reason it is recommended that all ampullary tumours in fit patients should be treated

218

by radical resection. Initial local resection for apparent ampullary adenomas results in an unacceptably high incidence of later development of invasive carcinoma. Because ampullary tumours generally obstruct the pancreatic duct, resulting in dilatation and firm pancreatic parenchyma, the morbidity related to the pancreatic anastomosis is low, and thus overall morbidity is also low. Moreover, five year survival after resection of this tumour is approximately 40%; because of this favourable outcome, all efforts should be made to offer suitable patients an operation. Endoscopic ampullectomy for putative ampullary adenomas is not an option in patients otherwise fit for resection for what may be an invasive carcinoma.

Duodenal carcinoma

These tumours are usually found in the second part of the duodenum and the presenting symptoms are related to biliary tract obstruction, occult bleeding, or obstruction of the duodenum. Many appear to have originated in villous tumours and random biopsy may not reveal the infiltrating nature of an invasive carcinoma. These cancers are rare, representing only 0·35% of cancers of the digestive tract.[23] A recommended operation is the standard Whipple procedure for radical clearance. Prognosis is not as good as ampullary carcinoma but five year survival range is around 20%. There is a 9% incidence of associated gastrointestinal adenocarcinomas, warranting investigation and surveillance of the whole gastrointestinal tract.

References

1 Warshaw AL, Fernandez-del Castillo C. Pancreatic carcinoma. *N Engl J Med* 1992;**326**: 455–65.
2 U-M Reports. DDT can cause pancreas cancer in humans. *Mich Med* 1992;**91**:14–6.
3 Lowenfels AB, Cavallini PMG, Ammann RW, *et al.* Pancreatitis and the risk of pancreatic cancer. *N Engl J Med* 1993;**328**:1433–7.
4 Lynch HT. Genetics and pancreatic cancer. *Arch Surg* 1994;**129**:266–8.
5 Warshaw AL, Swanson RS. Pancreatic cancer in 1988—possibilities and probabilities. *Ann Surg* 1988;**208**:541–53.
6 Hermanek P. Staging of exocrine pancreatic carcinoma. *Eur J Surg Oncol* 1991;**17**:167–72.
7 Lea MS, Stahlgren LH. Is resection appropriate for adenocarcinoma of the pancreas: a cost–benefit analysis. *Ann Surg* 1987;**154**:651–4.
8 Haglund C, Lundin P, Kuusela P, *et al.* CA 242, a new tumour marker for pancreatic cancer: a comparison with CA 19-9, CA 50 and CEA. *Br J Cancer* 1994;**70**:487–92.
9 Parsons L, Palmer CH. How accurate is fine-needle biopsy in malignant neoplasia of the pancreas? *Ann Surg* 1989;**124**:681–3.
10 Freeny PC. Magnetic resonance imaging. In: Trede M, Carter DC, eds. *Surgery of the pancreas.* Edinburgh: Churchill Livingstone, 1993:73–5.
11 Glenhoj A, Sehested M, Torp-Pedersen S. Ultrasonically guided histological and cytological fine needle biopsies of the pancreas: reliability and reproducibility of diagnoses. *Gut* 1990; **31**:930–3.
12 Bodner E, Glaser K. Intraoperative needle aspiration and biopsy. In: Trede M, Carter DC, eds. *Surgery of the pancreas.* Edinburgh: Churchill Livingstone, 1993:153–8.

13 Warshaw AL, Gu Z, Wittenberg J, *et al.* Preoperative staging and assessment of resectability of pancreatic cancer. *Arch Surg* 1990;**125**:230–3.

14 Tio TL, Tytgat GNJ, Cikot RJLM, *et al.* Ampullopancreatic carcinoma: pre-operative TNM classification with endosonography. *Radiology* 1990;**175**:455–61.

15 Ballinger AB, McHugh M, Catnach SM, *et al.* Symptom relief and quality of life after stenting for malignant bile duct obstruction. *Gut* 1994;**35**:467–70.

16 Huibregtse K, Katin RM, Coene PP, *et al.* Endoscopically placed stents in the jaundiced patient with pancreatic cancer. *Gastrointest Endosc* 1986;**32**:334–8.

17 van den Bosch, van der Schelling, Klinkenbijl JHG, *et al.* Guidelines for the application of surgery and endoprostheses in the palliation of obstructive jaundice in advanced cancer of the pancreas. *Ann Surg* 1994;**219**:18–24.

18 Davids PHP, Groen AK, Rauws EAJ, *et al.* Randomised trial of self-expanding metal stents versus polyethylene stents for distal malignant biliary obstruction. *Lancet* 1992;**340**: 1488–92.

19 Martin DF. Combined percutaneous and endoscopic procedures for bile duct obstruction. *Gut* 1994;**35**:1011–2.

20 Ishikawa O, Ohhigashi H, Sasaki Y, *et al.* Practical usefulness of lymphatic and connective tissue clearance for the carcinoma of the pancreas head. *Ann Surg* 1988;**208**:215–20.

21 Nakao A, Ichihara T, Nonami T, *et al.* Clinicohistopathologic and immunohistochemical studies of intrapancreatic development of carcinoma of the head of the pancreas. *Ann Surg* 1989;**209**:181–7.

22 Brooks JR, Brooks DC, Levine JD. Total pancreatectomy for ductal cell carcinoma of the pancreas: an update. *Ann Surg* 1989;**209**:405–10.

23 Rotman N, Pezet D, Fagniez PL, *et al.* Adenocarcinoma of the duodenum: factors influencing survival. *Br J Surg* 1994;**74**:83–5.

Chemotherapy, radiotherapy, palliative care, and new approaches

MARTIN M EATOCK and MIKE SOUKOP

Advanced disease

Unfortunately, 50–60% of those undergoing "curative" resection relapse with local recurrence, and a similar percentage with distant disease. In addition, the majority of patients present with locally advanced or metastatic disease and are not candidates for surgical resection. Radiotherapy or chemotherapy can be offered to a selected group of these inoperable patients, or patients with recurrence, provided the stage of disease and physical health based on Karnofsky status are appropriate (Table 7.2).

Prognostic factors

Several prognostic factors have been described, the most important being the performance status of the patient at presentation, the mode of presentation, and the site of the tumour within the pancreas. Poor prognostic factors are: impaired performance status, tumour arising in the body or tail of the pancreas, male sex, advanced disease at presentation, and the presence of abdominal or back pain at presentation. In addition to these, elevation of the acute phase reactive protein, CRP, has recently been shown to be associated with rapidly progressive disease and a poor prognosis.

Clinical trials of chemotherapy and radiotherapy

The high rates of inoperability and postoperative relapse have naturally led to trials of the use of chemotherapy and radiotherapy in selected patients. Such trials however, present major logistic problems. Phase II

221

TABLE 7.2—*WHO and Karnofsky performance scores*

	Karnofsky	WHO
Normal, no impairment in activities	100	0
Normal activity, minor symptoms of disease	90	1 (Normal activity)
Normal activity with effort, some symptoms of disease	80	
Self caring, unable to carry on normal activity	70	2 (Impaired activity but active for >50% of the day)
Requires occasional assistance	60	
Requires considerable assistance and frequent medical care	50	3 (In bed or resting for >50% of the day)
Disabled, requires special care	40	
Severely disabled, hospitalisation required	30	4
Very sick, supportive treatment necessary	20	
Moribund	10	

studies define the activity of a particular drug or combination of drugs in terms of response rates but infrequently give information about duration of response, survival, or the palliation of symptoms, which are the clinical end points in managing patients with this disease. The selection of patients for entry into phase II clinical trials may also provide a source of bias for a number of reasons.

Firstly, by their very nature phase II studies demand the presence of measurable and quantifiable disease; however, quantification of the size of primary pancreatic tumours is difficult as they have an infiltrative growth pattern and are radiologically often difficult to distinguish from chronic pancreatitis, which may coexist in the same patient. For this reason many patients, who would be otherwise fit to receive chemotherapy, are excluded from trials.

Secondly, where measurable disease is present it is often in the form of distant metastases. The process of metastasis involves the invasion of tumour cells into blood vessels or lymphatics, development of the ability to survive in the circulation, and then the ability to invade and grow at the site of their arrest. Only a proportion of cells in a given tumour will undergo the necessary phenotypic changes to allow dissemination to occur, and therefore the behaviour of the metastases may differ biologically from that of the primary tumours. Bearing this in mind, it cannot be concluded that a regimen that is active against metastatic deposits will necessarily be active against the primary tumour.

The third problem in evaluating the role of chemotherapy or radiotherapy in the management of this disease is the fact that most patients who present with unresectable disease have a large disease burden and are physically debilitated. This makes them poor candidates for entry into clinical trials.

A fourth problem exists in interpreting the significance of stable disease in those who are receiving chemotherapy. Commonly, markers of disease such as CEA, CA 125, CA 19-9, or CA 50 are raised before the start of chemotherapy but fall progressively with treatment, despite a lack of radiological evidence of response; whether this predicts for increased length of survival remains to be determined.

In discussing the management of pancreatic cancer it is not possible to provide a definitive text as so many uncertainties exist. Where clinical trials have been performed they are mostly of small size and the results are therefore difficult to interpret and apply to clinical practice. Patients should, where possible, be treated in the context of large, well supervised clinical trials so that the value of treatments other than surgery can be fully assessed.

Chemotherapy in advanced disease

If the cure rate after surgical resection is to be increased then effective additional treatment needs to be established. Chemotherapeutic agents likely to be of use in the context of adjuvant or neoadjuvant treatment must first be shown to have some activity against locally advanced disease.

Single agent chemotherapy

5-Fluorouracil

The most commonly used drug in the management of pancreatic cancer is the pyrimidine analogue, 5-fluorouracil (5FU). This is metabolised to 5-fluorodeoxyuridine monophosphate (5FdUMP), which inhibits thymidylate synthetase, thereby reducing the pool of thymidine available for DNA synthesis (Figure 7.10), and 5-fluorouridine triphosphate, which is incorporated into RNA, rendering it inactive and thereby inhibiting protein synthesis. The relative importance of these two modes of cytotoxicity is uncertain but probably varies for the treatment of different tumours and for different normal tissues.

The primary site of metabolism of 5FU is the liver, and both normal tissue toxicity and tumour response to the drug can be shown to depend on the area under the concentration/time curve for a particular method of administration. The main toxicities encountered relate to the gastro-intestinal tract and include diarrhoea and mucositis. Myelosuppression, which is unusual with conventional doses, may become a problem with

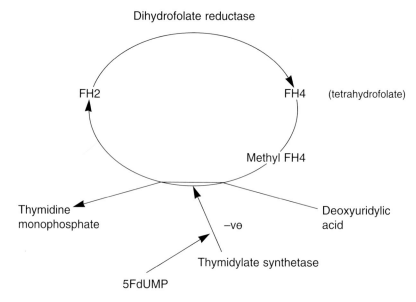

FIGURE 7.10—*The folate cycle and mechanism of action of 5FU.*

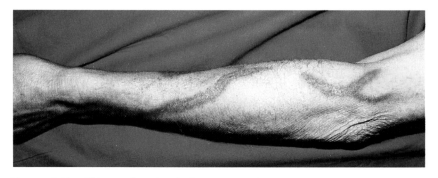

FIGURE 7.11—*Skin reaction after the intravenous administration of 5FU and folinic acid without extravasation.*

protracted treatment. Skin discolouration may be widespread or may occur locally at the site of administration (Figure 7.11).

In a widely cited article reviewing 212 patients Carter and Cornis found an overall response rate of 28%.[24] More recent trials have suggested this figure to be somewhat optimistic and a more realistic response rate of 15–20% is to be expected. The optimal schedule of administration for 5FU remains to be determined and some of the disappointing results quoted in the literature may be attributable to suboptimal methods of drug administration.

It is now appreciated that 5FU and its active metabolites have short half lives of around 20 minutes and that 5FU is a phase specific cytotoxic agent, preferentially exerting its effect on cells in S phase of the cell cycle. It can be shown experimentally that only around 5% of malignant cells in a tumour are in this phase at any given time, and these facts have led to the use of 5FU as a protracted infusion in the treatment of both gastro-intestinal and breast malignancies. It has been shown that doses up to $300 \, mg/m^2/day$ are well tolerated if 5FU is administered as a single agent.

This approach is still relatively untested in pancreatic cancer, although one study from Japan reports no complete or partial responses in 18 patients following a median treatment duration of 59 days (range 35–112 days), although 10 patients had stable disease for the duration of their treatment.[25] These results are difficult to interpret for two reasons: the small size of the trial, and the relatively low dose of 5FU employed by the investigators. The use of continuous 5FU with weekly cisplatin therapy to exploit the reported synergy between these drugs has also been evaluated and will be discussed later.

In addition to protracted administration of 5FU, attempts have been made to enhance the activity of 5FU in vivo by the concurrent administration of drugs that modify either its metabolism or its intracellular target.

Biochemical modulation of 5FU activity N-phosphonacetyl-L-aspartate (PALA) has been shown in vitro to enhance the activity of 5FU by reducing the intracellular concentration of the thymidylate synthetase substrates, uridine triphosphate and cytosine triphosphate. The combination of PALA and 5FU has been evaluated by the Southwest Oncology Group in the USA; however, their results are disappointing, with a response rate of 5% observed and a high incidence of serious toxicity.[26] These results must be interpreted with caution, however, as the study contained 27 patients entered from 21 different centres.

It has been shown in vitro that the addition of a source of reduced folate to 5FU enhances the binding of 5FU to thymidylate synthetase (Figure 7.10) and thereby enhances its activity. In colorectal carcinoma there seems to be a definite advantage in combining 5FU with folinic acid, although the optimum schedule remains to be determined. In pancreatic cancer this combination has been evaluated in a number of studies with conflicting results. All of these trials have included small numbers of patients and the results range from the wildly optimistic, with response rates of 50%, to unwarranted pessimism. This regimen is associated with a low incidence of serious toxicity. A complete lack of activity from this combination would be surprising, given the activity of 5FU as a single agent. The administration of folinic acid with 5FU still awaits evaluation in a phase III study.

Mitomycin C

This is an effective agent in advanced pancreatic cancer, with response rates quoted of around 20–30%. The main toxicity noted as myelosuppression, with the nadir white blood count being more prolonged and sustained beyond the usual 10–11 days for most other agents. For this reason the drug is often given in monthly or six weekly cycles. The phase II single agent data for mitomycin C are relatively sparse; however, it is one of the most commonly used drugs in combination regimens for the treatment of this disease.

Anthracyclines

The anthracycline derivatives doxorubicin and epirubicin have been evaluated in phase II studies. Of the two, the more active drug appears to be epirubicin, which was reported in a European Organisation for the Research and Treatment of Cancer (EORTC) trial of high dose treatment (90 mg/m^2 three weekly) to have an overall response rate of 24%, with a 5% complete response rate. In addition to this an increase in median survival time from five to nine months was observed in responders. The toxicity of epirubicin was low, the most frequently encountered problems being alopecia and vomiting.[27] This compares with a 13% response rate for doxorubicin reported by the Gastrointestinal Tumour Group (GITSG).[28] Both of these trials recruited small numbers of patients (39 and 13 respectively) but both these drugs have clinical activity.

In a phase III study epirubicin as a single agent has been compared with a combination regimen of 5FU, epirubicin, and mitomycin C;[29] the results in both treatment arms were disappointing with only 2 of 26 evaluable patients responding in the epirubicin alone arm, and 2 of 18 evaluable patients responding in the combination arm. Toxicity was similar in both arms of the trial and there was no significant difference in the median survival time between treatments. Such a result in a trial of small proportions is not surprising.

Alkylating agents

The alkylating agent ifosfamide is not extensively used in the treatment of pancreatic carcinoma; however, it has been reported to have activity, with response rates quoted of around 20%, ranging from 6 to 60%. The large range in reported activity may result from difficulties in objective response assessment and patient selection. Trials have used doses of ifosfamide ranging from 1·2 to 2 g/m^2/day administered over five consecutive days in each treatment cycle. In early studies there was a high incidence of haemorrhagic cystitis due to the metabolism of ifosfamide to acrolein; the concomitant use of thiol compounds such as mesna or N-acetylcysteine has been shown to ameliorate this and are now administered routinely with ifosfamide. This drug remains, despite these promising results, little used in combination regimens and further evaluation is necessary.

In the past, other alkylating agents have been used in the management of pancreatic cancer. There are anecdotal reports of response to cyclophosphamide, chlorambucil, and nitrogen mustard. Melphalan has been more rigorously tested by the Northwestern Gastrointestinal Tumour Group in England.[30] Two partial responses were seen in 15 patients treated with melphalan 1 mg/kg every 28 days. There was no improvement in median survival in the responders and the treatment was extremely toxic, resulting in one toxic death and life threatening toxicity in three other patients.

Other agents

Many chemotherapeutic agents have been evaluated in the treatment of pancreatic cancer; however, with the exception of the above mentioned drugs, few others show any objective evidence of activity. New agents recently tested in phase II studies that may be promising for further scrutiny are the taxoids and the antimetabolite, gemcitabine.

Paclitaxel and its semisynthetic sister compound, docetaxel, have both been evaluated in clinical trials and appear to have different activities. These drugs bind to intracellular microtubules and prevent microtubule disassembly; cellular microtubule formation becomes disorganised and when the affected cells attempt to enter mitosis the formation of mitotic spindles is prevented. The precise mechanism of cell death remains to be elucidated. The most commonly reported side effects in phase I studies of paclitaxel included myelosuppression, peripheral neuropathy, transient myalgia and arthralgia, and a hypersensitivity reaction, which appears to be less of a problem if the drug is administered over a 24 hour period and premedication with hydrocortisone is given.

In phase II studies, docetaxel has been reported to have a response rate of 28% in 18 patients with locoregional disease and hepatic metastases.[31] In the same study, two patients with exclusively locoregional disease were treated with docetaxel and local irradiation and were reported to be alive and well 10 and 12 months after completing treatment.

Paclitaxel, on the other hand, does not appear to be as promising. No patients achieved complete or partial remission in a study in the USA by the Southwest Oncology Group.[32]

Gemcitabine is an analogue of cytidine and has been shown to have a response rate of 13%, with minimal toxicity[33] and is now licensed for the treatment of pancreatic cancer in the USA.

In general the response of advanced pancreatic cancer to chemotherapeutic agents used on their own is disappointing (Table 7.3).

TABLE 7.3—*Combined response rates from reported trials of single agent chemotherapy**

Drug	Response rate (%)	95% CI (%)
5FU	25	20 to 30
Mitomycin C	24	14 to 34
CCNU	16	4 to 36
Ifosfamide	14	8 to 20
Epirubicin	12·5	8 to 17
Gemcitabine	13	3 to 23
Doxorubicin	8	2 to 24

* Conventionally, drugs with response rates of <10% are considered inactive.

This has led to the development of combination regimens and also to the investigation of novel agents and methods of circumventing cellular drug resistance to chemotherapy, which will be discussed later.

Combination chemotherapy

Ideally, any combination of drugs to treat any neoplasm should consist only of agents with demonstrated efficacy in the treatment of that disease. The analysis of trials conducted using multiple agent chemotherapy regimens in pancreatic cancer is complicated by the fact that many of them have used drugs that do not seem to have any activity when used alone. Since so few drugs have undisputed single agent activity, this approach may be justified to explore possible therapeutic synergy between agents, such as that seen with 5FU and cisplatin.

The early promise that combinations of chemotherapeutic agents would improve the response to treatment and prolong the survival of those with carcinoma of the pancreas has to be fulfilled. It remains to be shown decisively that combination chemotherapy has any advantages over single agent regimens. There are many studies using combinations of the previously mentioned drugs; however, reported response rates seldom exceed 20% and there are few randomised trials comparing single agent with multidrug regimens. Those trials that do exist show similar response rates at the expense of considerably increased toxicity in those treated with more than one agent. The existence of a wide variety of different regimens and schedules for their administration bears testimony to the lack of superiority of one regimen over another.

The first trial to suggest a significant increase in median survival in patients treated with chemotherapy was reported by Mallinson *et al* in 1980.[34] This was a randomised controlled trial and the group of patients treated with chemotherapy had a median survival of 44 weeks, compared with nine weeks in the control group. Although the number of patients enrolled in this trial was small (21 in the treatment arm, 19 in the control arm), the treated and the control groups appeared well matched for age, sex, duration of symptoms, and volume of disease present.

A similar increase in overall survival in patients receiving FAM (5FU, doxorubicin, and mitomycin C) has been reported by Palmer and colleagues. In this trial 46 patients were randomised to receive no chemotherapy or FAM. The median survival in the control arm was 15 weeks, compared with 33 weeks in the treatment arm. Toxicity associated with chemotherapy was generally mild, with only 3 of the 22 treated patients experiencing grade 3 or above side effects.[35] A number of other trials show a survival advantage in those responding to chemotherapy; however, when the treatment group is assessed as a whole, no overall increase in survival is seen. FAM is one of the most commonly used regimens in the treatment of pancreatic cancer. A number of different schedules have been used with variations in the dose intensity of mitomycin administered, which may explain the variation in response rates and survival. The response rates for a selection of these schedules are shown in Table 7.4.[35-37]

TABLE 7.4—*FAM chemotherapy in pancreatic cancer*

Regimen	Response rate (95% CI)	Median survival
Palmer *et al*[35] 5FU 600 mg/m^2 i.v. days 1+29 orally days 8+36 Doxorubicin 30 mg/m^2 i.v. days 1+29 Mitomycin C 10 mg/m^2 i.v. days 1+29 Repeated 8 weekly		33 weeks (versus 15 weeks in control arm)
Smith *et al*[36] 5FU 600 mg/m^2 i.v. days 1, 8, 29, 36 Doxorubicin 30 mg/m^2 days 1+29 Mitomycin C 10 mg/m^2 day 1 Repeated 8 weekly	37% (19 to 55%)	Responders = 12 months Non-responders = 3·5 months
Bitran *et al*[37] 5FU 500 mg/m^2 i.v. days 1, 8, 21, 28 Doxorubicin 30 mg/m^2 days 1+21 Mitomycin C 10 mg/m^2 day 1 Repeated 6 weekly	40% (19 to 67%)	Responders = >13 months Non-responders = 2·7 months

The most common severe toxicity seen with this regimen is myelosuppression, which may be life threatening (WHO grade 4) in around 10% of patients. Alopecia is almost invariable and some degree of mucositis occurs in around 40% of patients, although this is only severe enough to require hospital admission in around 5%. Emesis is usually well controlled by appropriate antiemetic therapy, particularly when a 5-hydroxytryptamine (5HT3) antagonist is administered.

Another regimen shown to have activity in pancreatic cancer is the combination of 5FU, streptozotocin, and mitomycin C (SMF) (Table 7.5).

TABLE 7.5—*A schedule for 5FU, streptozotocin, and mitomycin C combination therapy (repeated every 8 weeks)*

Drug	Day			
	1	1–4	5	29–33
5FU 500 mg/m^2		X	X	X
Streptozotocin 300 mg/m^2		X		X
Mitomycin C 10 mg/m^2	X			

As with FAM, a number of different schedules have been used but variations in the dose intensity of 5FU and streptozotocin rather than mitomycin are seen.

Response rates in phase II studies are of the order of 30–40%, but the initial promise of these early studies has not been borne out in the few phase III trials that have been performed. These suggest a much lower response rate of the order of 15–20%, which is comparable to many of the single agents discussed previously.

As with FAM, SMF is usually well tolerated. Most patients develop some degree of myelosuppression, although this is only life threatening in around 5%. Unlike FAM, mucositis with SMF is uncommon.

Studies of 5FU in combination with the nitrosureas, CCNU and methyl-CCNU, have also been performed. The results are disappointing, with response rates quoted for each combination of 7 and 10% respectively.

Regimens incorporating protracted infusion of 5FU

An area for future consideration in the development of new combination regimens is the use of protracted venous infusion of 5FU. The combination of continuous 5FU and weekly bolus cisplatin has been assessed by the Mid-Atlantic Oncology Program.[38] This regimen consisted of 20 mg/m^2 cisplatin given over 15 minutes once weekly, with a continuous infusion of 5FU 300 mg/m^2/day, and produced a response rate of 16% (95% confidence interval, 8 to 29%). This is comparable to a similar regimen that has been used in a phase II study at the Royal Marsden Hospital.[51]

Studies of a continuous infusion of 5FU with bolus doxorubicin and mitomycin C or with ifosfamide would be interesting as these would combine the optimal schedule for 5FU administration with the most active single agents. This approach does have its drawbacks as it requires the insertion of an indwelling central venous catheter. This has its own complications, the most common of which are sepsis and thrombosis. Hickman line infection is extremely difficult to eradicate and the majority of patients with this complication will require removal of the catheter.

The incidence of thrombosis can be reduced by low dose warfarin treatment for the duration of the chemotherapy. If thrombosis does occur, thrombolysis with either streptokinase or urokinase, followed by full anticoagulation, is the most effective method of treatment and often with this approach the line may be salvaged.

Protracted infusion of 5FU has a different side effect profile from bolus administration, the most notable feature being the hand–foot syndrome; conjunctivitis and increased skin pigmentation are also described.

Biological response modifiers in pancreatic cancer

Therapeutic synergy has been described between 5FU and interferon in the management of a number of neoplasms, including renal carcinoma and colorectal carcinoma, although the exact mechanism of this synergy is unclear. This approach has also been evaluated in pancreatic cancer, although the results of the trials reported so far do not suggest any benefit over the use of 5FU alone. The addition of folinic acid to the combination of 5FU and interferon has also been evaluated, again with the conclusion that there was no advantage in using this combination instead of 5FU alone.

Selection of patients with advanced disease for chemotherapy

The selection of patients with locally advanced and metastatic carcinoma of the pancreas for chemotherapy poses a difficult problem. Many clinicians feel that the role of chemotherapy in the management of this disease is negligible. In the past this view could be justified because of the toxicity of treatment and the poor prognosis that most patients could expect. As can be seen from the preceding paragraphs, the incidence of serious toxicity with many useful regimens is low. Emesis, a major problem in patients receiving chemotherapy, is less of a problem now than it was in the past, with the use of the 5HT3 inhibitors, which control nausea and vomiting in around 80% of patients. Recent clinical trials describe a survival advantage for patients who respond to chemotherapy and there is some evidence that, as a group, patients treated with chemotherapy survive longer than comparable patients not receiving chemotherapy.

Few trials published to date include a quality of life analysis; however, Palmer used the hospital anxiety and depression (HAD) questionnaire for both treatment and control groups and found that there was a significant reduction in depressive symptoms in the cohort of patients receiving chemotherapy, although the symptoms of anxiety experienced in the two groups were similar.[35] The reasons for these findings are unclear but one possible suggestion is that patients are likely to be more positive about their illnesses if they are receiving active treatment.

If these findings are confirmed in further studies, there are obvious implications for the treatment of advanced pancreatic cancer and it will be unacceptable to deny patients the offer of chemotherapy if they are considered well enough to tolerate this form of treatment. At present, where possible, patients should be entered into clinical trials aimed at answering some of the questions raised by the smaller studies already discussed. The two main questions requiring confirmation are the following:

- Does chemotherapy actually confer a survival advantage on those treated and, if there is a survival advantage, which patients are most likely to benefit from treatment?
- What are the optimal treatment regimens and schedules? There are very few phase III trials comparing different regimens in the literature and in view of the low response rates observed in trials to date new combinations of agents need to be assessed.

Outwith the context of a clinical trial, or where a patient declines entry into a trial, it is our practice to offer chemotherapy to palliate symptoms such as pain not controlled by simple measures, provided that:

- survival may be long enough to potentially benefit from treatment
- patients have no other serious underlying pathology, such as severe ischaemic heart disease
- patients have relatively normal liver function and do not have a raised bilirubin if the use of an anthracycline is being considered.

Full information about the likelihood of response and alternative treatments should be discussed with the patient and the final decision about the mode of treatment belongs to the patient. If the patient accepts the offer of chemotherapy then the response to treatment must be carefully evaluated and the decision about continuing or discontinuing treatment made depending on the presence or absence of disease progression and the presence or absence of significant toxicity.

The choice of treatment regimen is essentially at the discretion of the clinician. Review of current literature suggests the most active combination regimen is FAM; however, there is a significant overlap of the 95% confidence intervals for this regimen and for those for single agent 5FU and it is not unreasonable to suggest that, outwith the context of clinical trials, patients should be offered single agent treatment with 5FU, either as a continuous infusion or with folinic acid, as it is considerably less toxic than combination therapy.

Radiotherapy for advanced disease

As with chemotherapy, the aim of radiotherapy in advanced pancreatic cancer is improved quality of life and symptom control (see box). Radiotherapy, as it is a localised treatment, is only a suitable treatment option for those patients with advanced but localised, unresectable disease or those with localised symptoms related to either the primary tumour or a metastatic deposit, such as back pain. The major acute toxicities encountered with radiotherapy in the treatment of pancreatic cancer are nausea, vomiting, and anorexia. Where the large bowel has received a significant dose of radiation, diarrhoea may also occur. For these reasons patients with significant weight loss and cachexia should be considered unsuitable for this method of treatment. Late toxicity of radiation therapy includes stricture formation affecting the small bowel, the large bowel, and the biliary tree. Endocrine and exocrine pancreatic insufficiency is to be expected in the longer term and requires replacement therapy with pancreatic supplements and insulin. Paraparesis resulting from spinal cord irradiation is a possible but rather unusual late side effect of pancreatic irradiation.

Aims of therapy in advanced pancreatic cancer

- Palliation of pain
- Palliation of other symptoms related to tumour
- Improvement in performance status and quality of life
- Improvement in life expectancy

One problem to be considered in the planning of radiotherapy is defining the volume of tissue to be treated. The aim is to treat the primary tumour with sufficient margin to incorporate infiltrating disease not visualised radiologically, while at the same time minimising the volume of normal tissue incorporated into the radiotherapy field. It is often difficult to ascertain the extent of local disease in the pancreas radiologically and so it is difficult to be sure that an adequate volume of tissue has been irradiated.

Early studies of the treatment of pancreatic cancer with radiotherapy showed little effect on either symptom control or survival; however, they utilised relatively low doses of irradiation. Where the dose of treatment was raised to 50 Gy (using 2 Gy per fraction), improvement in back pain was reported in around 30% of patients. A further increase in total administered dose to 60 Gy resulted in improved symptom control of around 60%, indicating the existence of a dose-response relationship, at least for the palliation of symptoms related to pancreatic cancer.

The response to radiotherapy and, to a large extent, the acute and late toxicity related to treatment is determined by a number of factors, such as the dose per fraction, the total dose of radiation administered, the total duration of treatment, and the quality of radiation used. These regimens have all been varied and a number of different schedules and modes of treatment have been investigated.

The repair of radiation induced sublethal DNA damage in normal cells is almost complete around six hours after the dose is administered; tumour cells, on the other hand, appear to have a reduced capacity for such repair and it thus takes longer. This has led to trials of the use of hyperfractionated treatment regimens to exploit this difference and increase the therapeutic window for radiotherapy. Hyperfractionated regimens treat patients more frequently than once daily, the administered fractions being given 4–6 hours apart, hopefully after the repair process has been completed in normal cells but before this is the case for tumour cells. This treatment approach has been assessed in pancreatic cancer; however, it appears to be little better than conventional schedules.

The use of high linear energy transfer radiation, such as neutron beams, appears to result in increased normal tissue toxicity, with little evidence of improved local disease control or overall survival.

Intraoperative radiotherapy

Intraoperative radiotherapy uses an electron beam applied directly to the pancreatic tumour at laparotomy. This method of treatment requires the installation of a linear accelerator in the operation room and involves considerable initial capital expenditure if such a facility is to be established. In view of this expense this treatment modality would require to be significantly more effective than conventional radiotherapy and have a more acceptable toxicity profile. There are a number of theoretical advantages for this form of treatment.

- The treatment volume is defined at operation and is therefore more likely to be accurate than external beam therapy.
- The maximum range of electrons in tissue varies depending on their energy; however, the dose distribution is reasonably well suited to the treatment of localised disease.
- The dose to normal tissues can be minimised as they are removed from the treatment field.

- The spinal cord dose from this form of treatment is minimal and so late paraparesis is unlikely.

The National Cancer Institute reported a series of 85 patients with locally advanced intra-abdominal, retroperitoneal, and intrapelvic tumours in 1988.[39] This approach in conjunction with surgical debulking, although not specifically used in the treatment of pancreatic carcinoma, resulted in a median survival of 14 months and 34% of patients were projected to have local control of their disease at five years. A follow up report looked at autopsy findings in 13 patients with locally advanced pancreatic cancer treated with this modality. Residual or recurrent tumour was found in the majority of patients. Pancreatic fibrosis was commonly found and degenerative changes were seen in the primary tumour as a result of treatment.

The largest experience with the use of intraoperative radiotherapy as the sole treatment option for pancreatic cancer has been reported by the Japanese. One hundred and eight patients from 14 institutions were treated with electrons applied to the primary tumour at varying doses. The treatment was well tolerated; however, there was a 25% incidence of duodenal ulceration and haemorrhage in those patients in whom the duodenum was included in the treatment field. The median survival of patients treated in this fashion was six months and there was little obvious therapeutic gain.[40] Another Japanese study has reported a rapid relief of pain in 50% of patients receiving a dose to the pancreas in excess of 20 Gy.[41]

The Mayo Clinic also reported their experience of the use of intraoperative radiotherapy in 1988. Over a 10 year period they compared 122 patients with locally advanced pancreatic carcinoma treated with external beam therapy alone with 37 patients treated with a combination of external beam therapy and intraoperative radiotherapy. The majority of patients received 5FU in conjunction with radiotherapy. This was not a randomised trial and the results should be treated with caution; however, there was significant improvement in local control rates in the group of patients receiving intraoperative treatment at 12 and 24 months after the completion of treatment. Overall there was no difference in median survival in the two groups because of the incidence of distant metastases.[42]

Although the evidence suggests a limited role for intraoperative radiotherapy in the treatment of advanced pancreatic cancer, the suggestion of improved local control rates with this form of treatment has led to its investigation as an adjunct to definitive surgery. Trials of this approach reported to date are of small size and are therefore unlikely to be powerful enough to demonstrate a statistically significant difference in survival; however, there would appear to be decreased incidence of local disease recurrence in the patients receiving this treatment. Comparison with external beam therapy is required.

At present intraoperative radiotherapy is limited to a relatively small number of centres, where this approach to the treatment is still being evaluated, and it must still be considered an experimental tool that has no established role outwith the context of clinical trials.

Interstitial radiotherapy

The potential advantage of this modality is the provision of a relatively high local dose of radiation with a rapid fall off in dose with increasing distance from the radioactive source. The dose rate is much reduced in comparison with external beam therapy and when the growth kinetics of the tumour are taken into consideration this conveys a theoretical advantage over external beam treatment. Most studies of interstitial radiotherapy in the treatment of pancreatic cancer have employed the use of implanted iodine-125 seeds. Treatment complications include abscess formation, duodenal ulceration and perforation, pancreatitis, and the formation of pancreatic fistulas, although the incidence of these problems is relatively low and several American studies report low treatment related mortality and morbidity. Precise placement of the iodine seeds is required to give a dose distribution across the treatment volume approximating to the ideal dose distribution and this may be difficult to achieve.

No study to date has compared in a prospective manner this form of treatment with external beam therapy; however, comparisons between groups of patients treated with interstitial therapy and historical control groups treated with external beam therapy suggest only a small benefit not reaching statistical significance. Further randomised studies with larger numbers in both treatment arms are awaited.

Combined modality therapy

The relatively small improvement in survival for either chemotherapy or radiotherapy when used alone in the treatment of pancreatic cancer has led to the assessment of treatment regimens which combine both of these modalities.

The concurrent administration of chemotherapy with radiotherapy may potentiate the effects of radiotherapy. The most commonly used of these so called radiosensitisers are cisplatin, 5FU, and mitomycin C, and all of them have been used, singly or in combination, with radiotherapy, although the optimal regimen and schedule remains to be established.

The concomitant administration of 5FU and radiotherapy followed by weekly 5FU given until there was evidence of tumour progression has been compared with concomitant radiotherapy and doxorubicin treatment followed by seven pulses of doxorubicin administered 3–4 times a week. No survival difference was seen; however, the group of patients receiving doxorubicin experienced significantly worse toxicity.

There are a number of retrospective reports of the treatment of pancreatic cancer using combined modality treatments. One of the largest reports has been produced by the Thomas Jefferson University Hospital group, who report a series of 410 patients treated at this institution between 1975 and 1988.[43] This is an observational study and the results must be interpreted with caution. Ignoring for the time being the 23 patients who underwent surgical resection of their primary tumour, patients received chemotherapy alone, external beam radiotherapy alone, combined chemotherapy and external beam radiotherapy, combined interstitial radiotherapy and external beam radiotherapy, or combined interstitial and external beam radiotherapy in conjunction with chemotherapy (either 5FU alone, 5FU and CCNU, or 5FU and mitomycin C). The combination of chemotherapy with radiotherapy overall resulted in a two year survival rate of 20%; the median survival in the chemotherapy and external beam radiotherapy group was 10 months, compared with 13 months in the group of patients where all three modalities of treatment were employed. Although this survival difference was not significant, local control rates were higher in the latter group.

The GITSG have conducted several trials of combined radiotherapy and 5FU since 1974. The first of these trials compared radiotherapy alone with radiotherapy and 5FU followed by maintenance 5FU in patients with locally advanced unresectable pancreatic cancer. Accrual to the radiotherapy alone arm of the trial was discontinued after an interim analysis of the data showed a significant survival advantage in those treated with the combination regimen, with these patients surviving on average almost twice as long.

This group have also reported a randomised trial of combined treatment with 5FU and radiotherapy followed by SMF chemotherapy versus SMF alone in patients with locally unresectable pancreatic cancer.[44] Although a relatively small trial, with only a total of 43 patients entered into the study, a statistically significant survival difference is reported at one year in favour of the group of patients receiving the combined treatment (41 versus 19%). These results have led to the investigation of combined modality therapy as adjuvant therapy after definitive surgery.

Adjuvant treatment after resection of pancreatic cancer

Trials of postoperative radiotherapy alone in this situation failed to show any advantage over surgery alone because of the incidence of distant metastases. As a result, most recent trials of adjuvant treatment for pancreatic cancer have employed the use of combination therapy with external beam radiotherapy and 5FU, although some groups have used intraoperative radiotherapy to the pancreatic bed or interstitial radiotherapy in conjunction with chemotherapy.

Following their initial trial of combined radiotherapy and 5FU in the treatment of locally advanced disease, the GITSG conducted a trial of the same regimen in patients who had undergone radical surgery. This small trial randomised patients to receive treatment or observation and showed a significant improvement in the two year survival rate (43 versus 18%), median survival (21 versus 11 months), and disease free survival (11 versus 9 months).[45] Similar results have been produced in another small trial coordinated by the National Cancer Institute in the USA.[46]

Despite the promise of these results the relative role of chemotherapy and radiotherapy in the setting of adjuvant treatment remains unclear. It is likely that the way forward for the future will be trials of combined modality therapy; such a trial is underway in the United Kingdom at present. Before this form of treatment can be adopted as standard the results of the relatively small trials reported above will need to be validated in much larger multi-institutional studies.

Palliative care for those with advanced pancreatic carcinoma

Perhaps the most distressing problem encountered in advanced pancreatic cancer is the associated cachexia, and there are a number of reasons why this may occur. Patients' appetite may be poor owing to pain or to nausea, which may be related to opiate analgesia. Where possible a treatable cause should be excluded and rectified. Anorexia due to the tumour itself may respond to steroid administration, although this does not seem to produce any real increase in the body mass index in these patients. Recently it has been shown that progestagens such as megesterol acetate are useful, both in terms of stimulating appetite and encouraging some weight gain.

Pain is a common problem in those terminally ill with this disease and it is often difficult to achieve satisfactory levels of pain control with the use of opiate analgesia alone; coanalgesics, such as non-steroidal anti-inflammatory drugs, steroids, tricyclic antidepressants, or carbamazepine, may be useful in this situation. Even with these measures a significant number of patients will still experience pain. It is important to determine the site, character, frequency, and timing of the patient's pain as poor pain control may simply be a result of inappropriate intervals between analgesic dose.

Where patients describe lancinating pain it may be worth giving a test dose of lignocaine 100 mg by intravenous injection, cautiously. This is not a licensed indication for the use of this drug but a substantial proportion of patients report an improvement in their sensation of pain and, if this is the case, continued medication with oral flecainide or mexiletine may be helpful.

In those with intractable pain a coeliac plexus nerve block may provide good pain relief; however, this is only effective for around 1–2 months, limiting its use to those who are reaching the final stages of their illness.

Future directions in chemotherapy and radiotherapy

Despite the modest advances detailed previously, carcinoma of the pancreas remains a tumour with a poor prognosis. Methods to improve the prognosis of this disease are being directed at earlier detection, improving the response to standard chemotherapy and radiotherapy, and assessing the role of new treatment modalities such as immunotherapy. In addition to these three approaches, recent developments in the field of molecular biology have led to hopes of new treatment strategies for the treatment of this disease, such as the use of gene therapy or signal transduction modifiers.

The reason for the poor response of pancreatic carcinoma to standard chemotherapy remains unclear. It has been shown that normal pancreatic ductal cells and some human pancreatic cancer tumour cell lines express P glycoprotein on their cell surface, although the incidence of expression of this cell surface protein in human pancreatic cancer is unclear. This protein is associated with the multidrug resistance type 1 phenotype and, if expressed by pancreatic tumours, this would explain resistance to a number of compounds including the anthracycline analogues, etoposide, vincristine, and mitomycin C. P glycoprotein function in vitro can be modulated by a number of compounds, such as verapamil, quinine, and cyclosporin, and a number of clinical trials of modulation of type 1 multidrug resistance are under way.

The demonstration, in vitro at least, that pancreatic tumour cell growth and proliferation can be stimulated by a number of peptides, such as growth hormone, secretin, and cholecystokinin, has led to the investigation of the role of somatostatin and its analogues in the management of pancreatic cancer. A number of pancreatic tumours have been shown to express high affinity receptors for somatostatin and, as this hormone can suppress the secretion of some pituitary and gut hormones as well as exerting a negative effect on cell proliferation, it may be a useful treatment in pancreatic cancer. One such somatostatin analogue, somatuline, has been shown to provide symptomatic improvement in terms of pain control and improved performance status in 6 of 19 patients in one trial.[47] Only one patient in this study had radiological evidence of response; however, the further investigation of this group of drugs in the palliation of symptoms due to advanced disease is warranted.

Trials of immunotherapy techniques, such as antibody directed cell mediated cytotoxicity (ADCC) and antibody directed radiotherapy or chemotherapy, have been disappointing; however, this may be due to the lack of a suitable antibody rather than inherent problems with the technique. Further trials of this technique using different antigen targets are awaited.

In normal tissue, cells exist in an extracellular matrix composed of collagens, fibronectin, and elastin. The remodelling and turnover of these proteins is regulated by a family of enzymes known as the matrix metalloproteinases and by tissue specific inhibitors of these enzymes. Pancreatic cancer exhibits excessive production of these enzymes but only low levels of inhibitor production,[48] leading to the increased degradation of the extracellular matrix necessary for tumour cell invasion and metastasis, and for the process of tumour neovascularisation. Specific inhibitors of these metalloproteinases have been developed and in animal studies have shown inhibition of tumour progression and neovascularisation.[49 50] Phase I studies in humans have shown little toxicity and phase II studies in pancreatic cancer are currently being undertaken.

Summary

- Only a small percentage (probably less than 5%) of pancreatic cancers are resectable.
- Even early tumours (less than 2 cm in diameter with no nodal metastases) have a 40% incidence of lymphatic invasion.
- Tumour markers are not sufficiently sensitive or specific for use in routine clinical practice.
- A negative radiologically guided or operative biopsy does not exclude the diagnosis of carcinoma.
- Randomised trials are required to evaluate preoperative endoprostheses.
- The most effective single agent in pancreatic cancer is 5FU, with response rates of 15–20%. Doses up to 300 mg/m^2/day by continuous infusion are well tolerated but optimal methods of drug administration are yet to be determined.
- Adjuvant and neoadjuvant trials of chemotherapy and regimens for the treatment of advanced disease have been performed in small numbers of patients and are difficult to interpret in the context of routine clinical practice.

- Combination chemotherapy with FAM or single agent 5FU, either as a continuous infusion or in conjunction with folinic acid, are currently the most active regimens for selected patients with advanced disease.
- The benefits and optimal treatment schedules for external beam, intraoperative, and interstitial irradiation alone or in combination with chemotherapy have yet to be determined.

References

24 Carter SK, Cornis RL. Adenocarcinoma of the pancreas, prognostic variables and criteria of response. In: Stuquet MJ, ed. *Cancer therapy: prognostic factors and criteria of response.* New York: Raven Press, 1975:237–53.

25 Tajiri H, Yoshimori M, Okazaki N, *et al.* Phase II study of continuous venous infusion of 5-fluorouracil in advanced pancreatic cancer. *Oncology* 1991;**48**:18–21.

26 Morrell LM, Bach A, Rickman SP, *et al.* A phase III multiinstitutional study of low dose PALA and high dose 5-FU as a short term infusion in the treatment of adenocarcinoma of pancreas. *Cancer* 1991;**67**:363–6.

27 Wild J, Bleiberg H, Blighan G, *et al.* Phase II study of epirubicin in advanced adenocarcinoma of pancreas. *Eur J Cancer Clin Oncol* 1985;**21**:191–4.

28 Schein PS, Lavin PT, Moertel CG. Randomised phase II clinical trial of adriamycin in advanced measurable pancreatic carcinoma: a GITSG report. *Cancer* 1978;**42**:19–22.

29 Topham C, Glees J, Rawson NSB, *et al.* Randomised trial of epirubicin alone versus 5-FU, epirubicin and mitomycin C in locally advanced carcinoma of pancreas. *Br J Cancer* 1991;**64**:179–81.

30 Smith DB, Kenny JB, Scarffe JH, *et al.* Phase II evaluation of melphalan in adenocarcinoma of the pancreas. *Cancer Treat Rep* 1985;**69**:917–8.

31 De Forni M, Rougier P, Adenis A, *et al.* Phase 2 study of taxotere in locally advanced and/or metastatic pancreatic cancer [abstract]. *Ann Oncol* 1994;**5**(suppl):202.

32 Brown T, Tangen C, Flemming T, *et al.* A phase 2 trial of taxol and G-CSF in patients with adenocarcinoma of the pancreas [abstract]. *Proc Am Soc Clin Oncol* 1993;**12**:200.

33 Casper ES, Green MR, Brown TD. Phase 2 trial of gemcitabine in the treatment of advanced carcinoma of the pancreas [abstract]. *Proc Am Soc Clin Oncol* 1991;**10**:143.

34 Mallinson CN, Rake MO, Cocking JB, *et al.* Chemotherapy in pancreatic cancer: results of a controlled, prospective, randomised, multicentre trial. *BMJ* 1980;**281**:1589–91.

35 Palmer K, Kerr M, Knowles G, *et al.* Chemotherapy prolongs survival in inoperable pancreatic carcinoma. *Br J Surg* 1994;**81**:882–5.

36 Smith FP, Hoth DF, Levin B. 5-Fluorouracil, adriamycin and mitomycin C (FAM) chemotherapy for advanced adenocarcinoma of the pancreas. *Cancer* 1980;**46**:2014–8.

37 Bitran JD, Desser RK, Kozloff MF. Treatment of metastatic pancreatic and gastric cancer with 5-FU, adriamycin and mitomycin c. *Cancer Treat Rep* 1979;**63**:2049.

38 Rothman H, Cantrell JE, Lokich J, *et al.* Continuous infusion of 5-fluorouracil plus weekly cisplatin for pancreatic carcinoma. A Mid-Atlantic Oncology Program Study. *Cancer* 1991;**68**:264–8.

39 Sindelar WF, Hoekstra HJ, Kinsella TJ. Surgical approaches and techniques in intra-operative radiotherapy for intra-abdominal, retroperitoneal and intrapelvic neoplasms. *Surgery* 1988;**103**:247–56.

40 Abe M, Takahashi M. Intra-operative radiotherapy: the Japanese experience. *Int J Radiat Oncol Biol Phys* 1981;**7**:863.

41 Nishamura A, Nakano M, Otsu H. Intraoperative radiotherapy for advanced carcinoma of the pancreas. *Cancer* 1984;**54**:2375.

42 Roldan GE, Gunderson LL, Nagorney DM, *et al.* External beam versus intraoperative radiotherapy and external beam irradiation for locally advanced pancreatic cancer. *Cancer* 1988;**61**:1110–6.

43 Mohiuddin M, Rosato F, Schuricht A, *et al.* Carcinoma of the pancreas—the Jefferson experience 1975–1988. *Eur J Surg Oncol* 1994;**20**:13–20.

44 The Gastrointestinal Tumour Study Group. Treatment of locally unresectable carcinoma of the pancreas: comparison of combined modality therapy (chemotherapy plus radiotherapy) to chemotherapy alone. *J Natl Cancer Inst* 1988;**80**:751–5.

45 The Gastrointestinal Tumour Study Group. Further evidence of effective adjuvant combined radiation and chemotherapy following curative resection of pancreatic cancer. *Cancer* 1987;**59**:2006.

46 Johnstone PA, Sindelar WF. Patterns of disease recurrence following definitive therapy of adenocarcinoma of the pancreas using surgery and adjuvant radiotherapy: correlations of a clinical trial. *Int J Radiat Oncol Biol Phys* 1993;**27**:831–4.

47 Cannobio L, Boccardo F, Cannata D, *et al.* Treatment of advanced pancreatic carcinoma with the somatostatin analogue BIM 23014. Preliminary results of a pilot study. *Cancer* 1992;**69**:648–50.

48 Bramhall S, Lemoine N. 72 kDa collagenase, stromelysin-1 and tissue inhibitor of metalloproteinase-1 expression in pancreatic cancer. *Digestion* 1994;**55**:286.

49 Davies B, Brown P, East N, *et al.* A synthetic matrix metalloproteinase inhibitor decreases tumour burden and prolongs survival of mice bearing human ovarian cancer xenografts. *Cancer Res* 1993;**53**:2087–91.

50 Teicher BA, Holden SA, Ara G, *et al.* Potentiation of cytotoxic cancer therapies by TNP-1470 alone and with other anti-angiogenic agents. *Int J Cancer* 1994;**57**:920–5.

51 Nicolson M, Webb A, Cunningham D, *et al.* Cisplatin and protracted venous infusion 5-fluorouracil—good symptom relief with low toxicity in advanced pancreatic cancer. *Ann Oncol* 1995;**6**:801–4.

8: Liver and biliary tract

Proximal bile duct cholangiocarcinoma

SHINICHI MIYAGAWA, MASATOSHI MAKUUCHI
and DERRICK F MARTIN

Extrahepatic bile duct carcinoma is an uncommon malignant tumour. It tends to occur in older patients over the age of 70 years. Slightly more males than females are affected. The neoplasm tends to grow slowly and to infiltrate surrounding structures, such as the liver parenchyma, intrahepatic bile ducts, and the hepatoduodenal ligament. Until recently, palliative percutaneous, endoscopic or surgical biliary drainage procedures were considered the most acceptable treatment in terms of operative mortality and long term survival when compared with more aggressive methods. Although rare in the western hemisphere, liver fluke infestation in the Orient may be complicated by bile duct carcinoma. In the East, *Clonorchis sinensis* is prevalent, and *Opisthorchis viverrini* infestation is important in the South East. Bile duct carcinomas are associated with ulcerative colitis, with or without sclerosing cholangitis. It is unclear whether sclerosing cholangitis is a premalignant lesion or whether the usually present inflammatory bowel disease predisposes the patient to the development of both lesions. The role of hepatic calculi is uncertain, although bile duct carcinoma has been found in 5–10% of patients with hepatolithiasis. The congenital fibropolycystic family of conditions, including congenital hepatic fibrosis, cystic dilatation (Caroli's disease), choledochal cyst, and polycystic liver and von Meyenburg complexes, may be complicated by bile duct carcinoma. The most important aspect to be considered both diagnostically and therapeutically is the location of the tumour because this will affect the preoperative management, operative methods, and prognosis of patients. Of all bile duct neoplasms, about 35% arise in the middle or lower third of the main bile duct, and diffuse types account for approximately 10% of cases, whereas about 55% occur in the upper third of the main bile duct.

Clinical presentation

The most common clinical manifestation is obstructive jaundice. This occurs relatively late in the course of the disease because jaundice will not develop until a major duct is completely obstructed. While a distended gall bladder may be palpated with tenderness and pain in patients with middle or lower third bile duct carcinoma, this is not demonstrable in patients with upper third biliary carcinoma. Uncommonly, pruritus may precede clinical jaundice. Fever and pain associated with the jaundice are unusual, unless the bile duct has been interfered with surgically, endoscopically, or percutaneously. The faeces are pale and fatty and occult blood is often present. The serum biochemical findings are those of cholestatic jaundice. The serum bilirubin, alkaline phosphatase, and γ-glutamyl transferase levels may be very high. The serum mitochondrial antibody test is negative and α fetoprotein (AFP) is not increased. Serum carcinoembryonic antigen (CEA) and/or carbohydrate antigenic determinant 19-9 are useful markers for cholangiocarcinoma. Biliary carcinoma presents difficult diagnostic problems because the presenting symptoms may mimic benign biliary disease.

Staging

The most useful and convenient diagnostic device for obstructive jaundice is ultrasonography (US), which can provide information regarding dilatation of the intrahepatic bile duct, obstructed sites in the biliary tree, and some causes of obstruction. When US shows dilatation of the intrahepatic biliary tree, no dilatation of the common bile duct, and a non-distended gall bladder (unless it has been removed or has been the site of previous disease), the common hepatic duct is obstructed. US can also show cancerous infiltration into the hepatic parenchyma and the portal vein. Intraoperative US can reveal extramural infiltration and vascular involvement more precisely. Obstructed sites can also be identified by computed tomography (CT). Bile duct carcinoma is recognised as thickening of the wall of the bile duct by low density tumour, which occupies the ductal lumen. Some of these cancers are enhanced by contrast material. Vascular involvement and lymph node metastasis can also be evaluated by US and CT. The presence of biliary dilatation can be detected easily by US and CT in all patients, but these imaging modalities cannot predict correctly the underlying pathology of the stricture.

Arterial encasement and narrowing and obstruction of the portal vein are features of extramural cancer extension. This information is essential for deciding whether surgery is indicated and for assessment of the necessity of combined vascular resection and reconstruction during surgery. Contrast enhanced CT, supplemented with visceral angiography in selected patients, will provide the images required for judging resectability in the majority of cases. It is generally considered that angiographically demonstrated vascular involvement implies malignancy. Vascular encasement does not, however, always reflect malignant changes because severe inflammation can induce

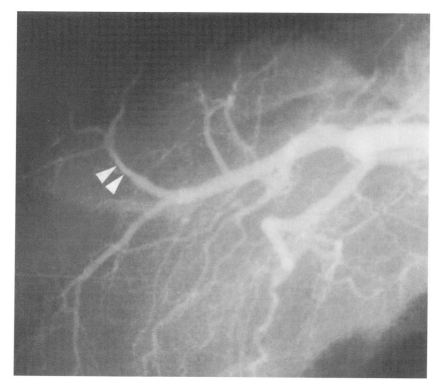

FIGURE 8.1—*Angiography shows a narrowed anterior segmental branch of the hepatic artery (arrow heads). There is no evidence of malignancy in the resected specimen, and only fibrous replacement of the arterial media is apparent.*

morphological changes in vessels (Figure 8.1). Thus it appears that accurate preoperative diagnosis of the nature of hilar bile duct strictures is difficult even when using angiography.[1]

Bismuth and Corlette described patterns of involvement of the proximal biliary system by tumour.[2] In type I (cancer extends to but does not involve the bifurcation) and II (cancer involves the bifurcation but does not extend up either hepatic duct) lesions, the proximal right and left hepatic ducts may be uninvolved by the tumour and resection margins can be established without the need for hepatic parenchymal resection; however, when involvement of a unilateral hepatic duct without extension into secondary radicles (type III) occurs, resection of the involved lobe may be necessary. In some type III and most type IV (cancer involves the secondary biliary radicles) lesions, an extended hemihepatectomy may be necessary to encompass all tumour in the contralateral duct system. Even in types I and II, however, concomitant hepatectomy (resection of segments 4 and 1 or extended hemihepatectomy) with resection of the extrahepatic bile duct is recommended to ensure a microscopically clear resection, leading to an improved long term survival rate, because proximal bile duct carcinoma has the pathological characteristic of extramural extension.

Interventional radiology

Ultrasonography, having determined that jaundice is obstructive, will also provide some indication of the level of tumour obstruction. Tumour extending into sectoral or segmental ducts within the liver may be detected by US (Figure 8.2); these involved ducts will not be dilated but the presence of proximally dilated ducts can give an indication of the extent of the tumour. The next logical radiological investigation is direct cholangiography in order to determine the nature and extent of an obstructing lesion. Percutaneous transhepatic cholangiography and endoscopic retrograde cholangiography can demonstrate the stenotic portion of the bile duct precisely (Figure 8.3), but will give no direct information about its histological nature. Malignant disease may be visualised arising directly within the bile duct system and this is most commonly due to cholangiocarcinoma. Benign biliary strictures of the intrahepatic ducts or major hepatic confluence are also very rare. Typical images of primary sclerosing cholangitis obtained by direct cholangiography show multiple strictures, the appearance of beading, a small lumen calibre, and failure of the biliary tree to dilate proximal to a stricture (Figure 8.4). Atypical primary sclerosing cholangitis can mimic bile duct carcinoma.

Cholangiocarcinoma can affect any part of the biliary system but is most commonly clinically evident when it involves the common bile duct or the confluence of the hepatic ducts (Klatskin tumour). The tumour can be a localised, relatively soft lesion or a focal, polypoid, predominantly intraluminal lesion (Figure 8.5). Some tumours are very tough and fibrotic, often associated with very little by way of tumour mass. Cholangiocarcinoma

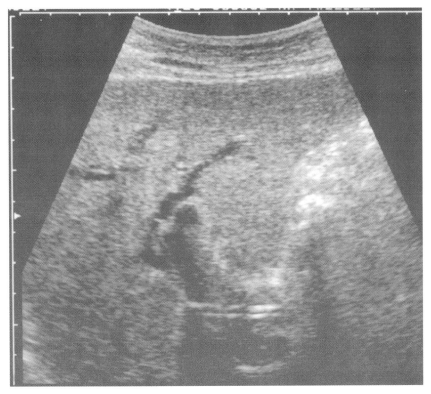

FIGURE 8.2—*A paracentrical ultrasound image through the right lobe of the liver at the level of the porta hepatis. The double hyperechoic lines of the biliary stent within the common duct can be seen. Anterior to this is a low density infiltrative area of cholangiocarcinoma. The tubular structures converging on the tumour are dilated segmental ducts.*

can be multiple but published figures of the incidence of multiple tumours of up to 10% are probably exaggerated. The tumour tends to extend longitudinally from its original focus along the duct system.

Whether the initial approach to direct cholangiography is percutaneous or endoscopic depends on the availability of local expertise. Whichever method of approach is chosen, it is vital that the radiologist or endoscopist should be able to progress immediately to a therapeutic procedure to decompress the duct system. There is no place for the limited diagnostic evaluation of an obstructing biliary lesion that does not progress immediately to therapeutic decompression. Whether the approach is percutaneous or endoscopic, the addition of bile duct decompression does not limit the surgical therapeutic options.

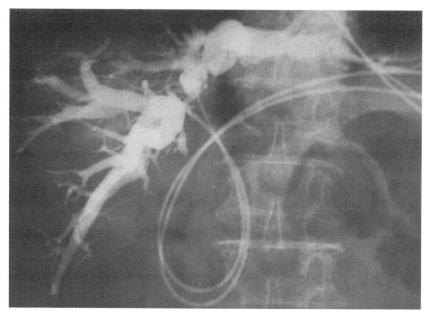

FIGURE 8.3—*The right and left hepatic ducts are obstructed completely at the hepatic hilum. Two biliary drainage tubes are inserted by the retrograde endoscopic route.*

Biopsy

Histological proof of cholangiocarcinoma is difficult to obtain. The sensitivity of diagnostic cholangiography itself, for the diagnosis of cholangiocarcinoma, is very high, probably over 95%. This is mainly because there are very few other conditions that lead to a focal bile duct obstruction. Cytology of aspirated bile has a sensitivity of approximately 30%, while brush cytology of a focal lesion is a little more sensitive but still only around 50–60%. Direct biopsy of a focal lesion can be performed with endoscopic biopsy forceps or a variety of devices that can be passed into the bile duct, through the stricture, often over a guidewire. Percutaneous, image guided fine needle aspiration biopsy, or cutting needle biopsy can all be performed but none of these methods has a sensitivity much over 70%. From the point of view of clinical management, this relatively low sensitivity of histology causes difficulty. A positive biopsy is valuable but a negative biopsy is of very limited clinical value because the result is likely to be incorrect. Although many endoscopists and radiologists feel the need to support a radiological diagnosis of cholangiocarcinoma with histology, the techniques available at present need refinement and many therefore forego biopsy, relying upon cholangiographic features to make the diagnosis.

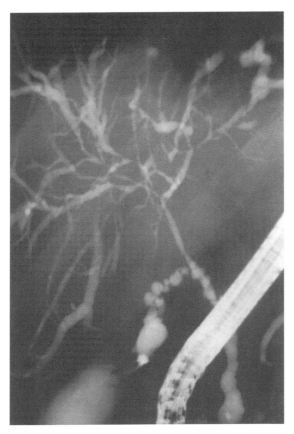

FIGURE 8.4—*Endoscopic cholangiogram demonstrating widespread changes of severe sclerosing cholangitis. There are multiple strictures associated with alternating areas of ectasia involving the common duct, cystic duct, and virtually all of the intrahepatic duct system.*

If a diagnostic tissue sample from the biliary tree is considered necessary for definitive diagnosis, brush cytology and endobiliary biopsy may be available for histological examination, but these methods present technical problems, are difficult to repeat, and frequently do not obtain a sufficient amount of tissue for diagnosis. The sensitivity of bile cytology in patients with malignant biliary stricture is reported to vary between 30 and 73%, that of brush cytology between 50 and 66%, that of endobiliary biopsy between 30 and 100%, and that of fine needle aspiration cytology between 42 and 67%, although the number of patients undergoing these biopsy techniques was small.[3]

249

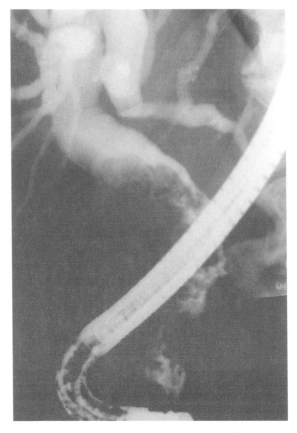

FIGURE 8.5—*An extensive polypoid cholangiocarcinoma involving much of the common duct. These lesions tend to be soft and fleshy.*

It has been suggested that a preoperative histological diagnosis obtained from a small biopsy specimen does not always predict the postoperative histological findings in biliary stricture. Percutaneous transhepatic cholangioscopy is useful for differential diagnosis between benign and malignant biliary stenosis and for estimation of the tumour extent in the superficial or superficially spreading type of hilar cholangiocarcinoma, because mucosal changes can be seen directly and the appropriate site for performing a diagnostic biopsy can be identified. Demerits of this method are the risk of infecting the biliary tree and the possibility of cancer seeding along its route. Once direct cholangiography and drainage have been performed, further imaging using CT, magnetic resonance, or angiography can be undertaken to assess the suitability of the patient for attempted

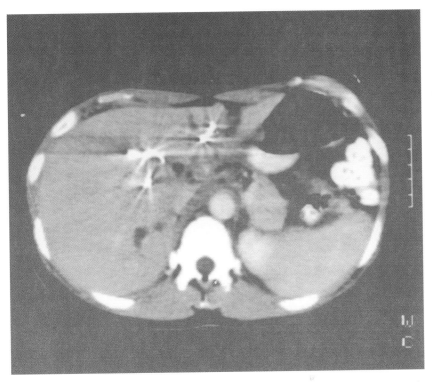

FIGURE 8.6—*A single axial CT image taken just above the level of the porta hepatis. Left and right percutaneous drainage catheters have been placed, which have decompressed the bile duct system. A single segmental (segment 6) posterior duct can be seen, which has not been decompressed. This indicates that there is tumour invasion of this segmental duct stem.*

curative surgery (Figure 8.6). Most patients are not suitable for surgery on the basis of age or the presence of other limiting disease, and therefore further imaging is not necessary; however, as a basic principle it is important to remember that it is easy to adopt a nihilistic approach to bile duct malignancy because palliative stenting is so effective. It is important that patients with surgically treatable lesions should be evaluated further, if at all possible, so that curative surgery can be undertaken at an early stage.

Endoscopic retrograde cholepancreatography (ERCP)

ERCP is the preferred option for direct cholangiography by most gastroenterologists and surgeons. It has the advantage that a thorough inspection of the upper gastrointestinal tract is possible, and a particular

251

advantage under the circumstances currently being considered, that, where a distal bile duct stricture is evident, pancreatography can be performed to differentiate carcinoma of the pancreas from carcinoma of the bile duct. The main indication for ERCP is therefore to provide a diagnosis. While US indicates the presence of bile duct obstruction, cholangiography indicates the nature and precise site of the obstruction.

Once the diagnosis of malignant bile duct obstruction is established with cholangiography, ERCP has subsidiary indications. Firstly, to make an attempt to assess operability, and, secondly, to provide drainage, which can be used as temporary therapy pending surgery or as definitive therapy where the lesion is considered inoperable.

Where there is a tumour involving the common bile duct, ERCP alone does little to define the ability of the surgeon to resect the lesion. Proximal lesions which extend into the sectoral ducts (Figure 8.7), or even segmental

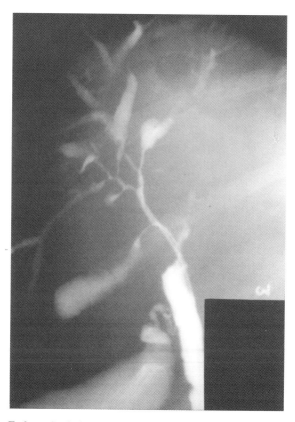

FIGURE 8.7—*Endoscopic cholangiogram showing extensive involvement of the common hepatic duct extending into the left, right, and sectoral ducts.*

ducts on the right, may be resectable by right hepatectomy if the left duct system and its associated vasculature are clear of tumour. Once tumour has extended into the left hepatic duct an extended right hepatectomy is necessary. Less commonly a tumour limited to the left hepatic duct system can be dealt with by left hepatectomy. Careful endoscopic cholangiography with selective cannulation of right and left ducts may allow the detection of patients who are clearly inoperable, or may select those patients who require further imaging and assessment before proceeding to surgery.

For drainage a single 10 or 12 Fr plastic stent is sufficient in the majority of patients with a common duct neoplasm. Similarly for the majority of patients with tumours involving the confluence of the hepatic ducts, a

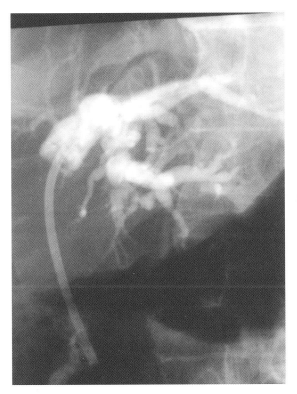

FIGURE 8.8—*An endoscopically placed stent draining the left hepatic duct system. Good drainage of segments 2 and 3 and possibly of segment 4 is achieved. This is the endoscopic equivalent of a segment 3 bypass.*

single stent draining either the left (Figure 8.8) or right lobes is sufficient in the majority. It is not necessary as a routine to drain the left and right hepatic duct systems.

From a clinical standpoint the most important indication for therapy is jaundice, which is relieved in most. Other clinical factors, such as itching, anorexia, and general malaise, can be improved after stenting. In particular, itching resolves rapidly after establishment of drainage.

Techniques

ERCP technique starts with patient preparation.[4] Because many patients are anorexic and may additionally undergo periods of fasting for radiological investigations, negative fluid balance can become a clinical problem. If there is deep jaundice or any risk of sepsis, prerenal failure can intervene unless careful attention is paid to fluid balance, intravenous fluids being administered if necessary.

It is routine to check parameters of coagulation before ERCP but this is in fact superfluous. Patients with obstructive jaundice require ERCP, irrespective of coagulation abnormality, and as sphincterotomy is not needed for the placement of a single stent, no bleeding complication is anticipated. In fact even if sphincterotomy is performed, minor abnormalities of coagulation do not predict risk of bleeding and assessment of coagulation abnormalities can therefore be dispensed with. Where there is clinical evidence of a coagulation problem, evaluation and correction are probably worthwhile.

In patients with bile duct obstruction, intravenous antibiotics should be given before ERCP. Colonisation of bile by bacteria in malignant obstruction is uncommon before instrumentation but is almost invariable after ERCP. The use of broad spectrum antibiotics that penetrate into bile (piperacillin, mezlocillin, cefuroxime) provides effective prophylaxis against sepsis; they should be given about one hour before ERCP. Antibiotic therapy need not be continued unless drainage is inadequate. Naturally, careful explanation of the procedure and the acquisition of informed consent is necessary.

Elderly ill patients undergoing endoscopy tend to become hypoxic during sedation and intubation. Hypoxia can be avoided by preoxygenation. It is wise to give approximately 4 litres of oxygen a minute through a nasal cannula for up to five minutes before sedation. Pulse oximetry should be available throughout ERCP, although when preoxygenation is used and oxygen delivery is maintained throughout, it is uncommon for oxygen saturation to drop below 95% at any time during ERCP.

Adequate sedation is important. ERCP can be uncomfortable and occasionally distressing for the patient. There is a vogue for a minimalist approach to sedation in endoscopy on the grounds of improved safety; however, sphincterotomy or stent insertion in an inadequately sedated and uncomfortable patient can be dangerous, and failure to allow adequate

254

drainage may be much more risky than an increased level of sedation carefully monitored but allowing successful drainage. Many patients with malignant disease return for stent exchange. Adequate sedation during their first procedure will allow them to embark upon further procedures in a relaxed and confident frame of mind. An unpleasant first experience will lead to unnecessary anxiety.

There are two hurdles for the endoscopist during ERCP in a patient with bile duct malignancy. The first is to gain deep access to the duct through the papilla; the second is to negotiate a guidewire and catheter across the stricture before stent insertion. In most patients deep bile duct cannulation is straightforward and can be assisted by the use of sublingual trinitrin or intravenous glucagon (or both simultaneously), which relax the choledochal sphincter. It is wise to gain access to the bile duct using a cannula which can accept a 0·035 inch guidewire so that once access is achieved it need never be lost. A finely tapered catheter may allow easier access but finer guidewires should also be available. When deep bile duct cannulation is not immediately achievable, precut papillotomy (needle knife papillotomy) is an invaluable technique. This procedure, well described in standard endoscopic texts, is considered by some to be risky but in fact it is extremely safe when used judiciously and carefully. It can easily turn potential failure to success.

Contrast injection into the bile duct below the level of the stricture most commonly allows contrast to pass through into the dilated duct above. It is often easy to pass a cannula through such a stricture, particularly if this is introduced carefully together with a standard 0·035 inch, Teflon coated, long, floppy tipped, straight guidewire. Even when contrast does not pass through the stricture careful probing with cannula and guidewire will allow access to the ducts above the stricture. This probing should not be vigorous because a false track can readily be made and can lead to failure. It is worth injecting a little contrast medium through the stricture and following this immediately with an attempt at passing a wire. Wires often pass most readily at this time.

If negotiation of a cannula through the stricture proves difficult, then a polymer coated hydrophilic guidewire is an invaluable device that rarely fails to gain access through the stricture. It may be used together with a standard ERCP cannula but works better when loaded into a stiff cannula. A 7 Fr biliary dilatation catheter is best. Of course, having gained access through the papilla to the distal common duct, exchange of catheters should be made over a guidewire in order to maintain access. Once access to the ducts above the tumour is acquired, the catheter is removed, leaving the guidewire in position, and a guiding catheter is introduced. A 10 or 12 Fr stent can then be introduced over the catheter and wire combination. Important points to remember while inserting a stent are: (a) the scope should be kept as close to the papilla as possible at all times; (b) a careful eye should be kept on the catheter and guidewire combination to ensure that displacement does not occur; and (c) it is best to insert the stent by using the torque power of the endoscope, its forceps elevator, and its angulation controls, rather than brute force in simply pushing the stent over the guidewire. The stent is pushed partially from the scope over the catheter and guidewire combination and then pushed up into the tumour by upward angulation of the scope and upward movement of the forceps elevator. This cycle of movements is repeated until the stent is in position. The stent is held in position with the pusher tube whilst the coaxial catheter and guidewire are removed. If a single stent is to be inserted, sphincterotomy is not necessary. For the insertion of two or more stents, sphincterotomy is helpful. Curved or angled guidewires allow selective access to right or left hepatic ducts, particularly if used in conjunction with a stiff catheter. Axial rotation of the endoscope tends to direct the catheter towards right or left duct, whereupon gentle probing with the guidewire allows deep access to the duct. A polymer coated guidewire is best for this manoeuvre but should be exchanged for a standard, Teflon coated working wire before catheter exchange takes place.

Plastic or metal stents

Over recent years it has been routine to use 10 or 12 Fr plastic stents for drainage but these invariably occlude because of an accumulation of biliary and bacterial debris. The likelihood of stent occlusion is dependent upon diameter and therefore the large (30 Fr; 1 cm) diameter of expandable metal stents makes these devices attractive. For cholangiocarcinoma, where disease progress is slower than with pancreatic carcinoma, it is tempting to use metal stents in order to achieve a prolonged period of drainage. The disadvantage, however, is that when metal stents occlude, management can be difficult, although insertion of a plastic stent through the metal stent is the simplest way to resolve the problem. If plastic stents are used initially the time to reintervention is shorter but stent exchange tends to be easier.[5] As yet there are limited data comparing the two types of stent in cholangiocarcinoma and, while the costs of metal stents are very high compared with plastic, the decision as to which to use is not simply to be made on reintervention rates alone.

Complications

Potential complications fall into a number of categories.

Complications from sedation can be minimised by cautious use of benzodiazepines and analgesics. While the margin of safety with these drugs is fairly wide, their dosages should be modified depending upon the patient's age and physical status. Drugs for the reversal of sedation should be routinely available. Oxygen desaturation is prevented by preoxygenation but the risk of hypercapnia and respiratory acidosis due to hypoventilation should be remembered.

Complications from endoscopy are unusual. It is possible to perforate any part of the upper gastrointestinal tract during ERCP, particularly when there is pre-existing pathology. Unexpected oesophageal strictures, benign or malignant, as well as large hiatus hernia can cause trouble for the endoscopist. Duodenal scarring and active ulceration can make the duodenum more vulnerable to perforation. Other injuries, such as splenic laceration and tearing of the splenic pedicle, have been described and presumably result when the endoscopist uses a long loop of scope in order to gain access. ERCP is best performed using gentle refined endoscopy. It rarely needs a heavy hand.

Complications caused by diagnostic ERCP relate to the injection of contrast medium into the duct systems. A sterile bile duct may be contaminated by bacteria after ERCP and in the presence of obstruction this may lead to cholangitis. Antibiotic prophylaxis and the provision of adequate drainage after ERCP guard against cholangitis. Acute pancreatitis occurs with a documented incidence of approximately 1% after ERCP, although its true incidence in clinical practice is probably higher. While there is continuing debate concerning the role of ionic and non-ionic contrast media and their relative risks of acute pancreatitis, there is no firm evidence that the more expensive non-ionic media offer any advantage. Acute pancreatitis is probably more related to trauma to the papilla, the rate of contrast injection and other factors which elevate intrapancreatic duct pressures. The risk is minimised by gentle manipulation of the papilla, slow contrast injection and the use of very dense (370 mg iodine/ml) contrast medium, which can be seen easily on the fluoroscopic screen and is highly viscous, thereby preventing rapid injection.

Endoscopic sphincterotomy is now extremely safe. Although the reported frequency of complications is in the region of 7–10%, with 1–2% mortality, most expert operators can now offer a complication rate of under 4% with virtually no mortality related to sphincterotomy itself. Some minor venous oozing is quite common (about 20%) after sphincterotomy but invariably stops without intervention. Heavier bleeding that persists can be managed with injection of adrenaline, alcohol, water, or even contrast medium under the cut edge of the sphincterotomy in order to tamponade, constrict, or thrombose bleeding vessels. The need for surgery or gastroduodenal artery embolisation is rare. Retroperitoneal perforation, previously recorded in up to 1%, is now rare. Sphincterotomy for stenting is rarely necessary except where two stents are planned. Even though the risks of sphincterotomy are small, they are better avoided.

Cholangitis is the most common complication after stenting and relates to the adequacy of drainage. A single 10 Fr stent through a common duct lesion is infrequently complicated by cholangitis but a single stent through a lesion isolating the hepatic ducts is occasionally complicated by cholangitis in the undrained lobe of the liver and requires initial therapy with intravenous fluids and antibiotics, with speedy progress to endoscopic or percutaneous drainage if cholangitis does not settle.

Outcome

After a single stent has been placed through an obstructing lesion, jaundice will clear promptly in the majority of patients, although significant improvement in deep jaundice may take up to one week to become evident. Jaundice clears more slowly after prolonged obstruction, with drainage of only part of the intrahepatic duct system or after cholangitis. If jaundice does not clear, this indicates that the stent is not functioning. Jaundice because of intrahepatic metastatic disease is unusual. Stents of 10 or 12 Fr remain patent for an average of about six months and there is no known method of prolonging stent patency at present. When the stent occludes, jaundice and often cholangitis develop. If stent occlusion leads to cholangitis, this can usually be managed conservatively with fluids and antibiotics, to be followed by elective stent exchange. Compared with patients who have no treatment for bile duct obstruction, patients managed by endoscopic stenting survive significantly longer. While a small proportion, perhaps 5%, of patients survive up to two years after initial diagnosis and undergo a number of stent changes, survival beyond one year from diagnosis is not common.

Percutaneous transhepatic procedures

Since ERCP is the dominant diagnostic and therapeutic method of management of bile duct malignancy, percutaneous procedures have assumed a secondary role.[6] Specific indications are:

(1) Where ERCP is not available or is inappropriate (for example after partial gastrectomy).
(2) Where endoscopic access across a stricture is not possible.
(3) When selective intrahepatic duct cholangiography is necessary to assess resectability.

Techniques

As for ERCP, patient preparation is important. The same principles that govern preparation before ERCP apply, and sedation, oxygenation, and monitoring are similarly involved. Percutaneous transhepatic cholangiography is performed with the patient supine. Using ultra-sonographic and fluoroscopic guidance, the needle tip is aimed at about the midpoint of the right 11th rib, the entry site being as far cranially as the pleural reflection will allow and in the anterior axillary line. Using this approach the needle can normally be aligned so that it points caudally and the line of approach to the bile duct allows a smooth obtuse angle and easy access to the common duct. The traditional approach, whereby the needle is inserted low in the right lobe of the liver and points cranially towards the xiphisternum, is better avoided as this forms an acute angle with the common duct, making passage of wires and catheters down the duct more difficult and more uncomfortable for the patient. If access to a suitable duct is provided by this approach and the distal duct stricture is to be negotiated, then a fine 0·018 inch guidewire can be passed through the needle, which is then removed. A dilator is passed over this wire to allow access for a larger 0·035 inch guidewire, which can then be used as a working wire. If a proximal duct lesion is to be stented, then it is perhaps best to enter the bile duct system peripherally in order to allow sufficient room within the ducts above the stricture to place a stent. If the initial duct puncture is too central, then a second needle can be used to puncture a selected peripheral duct while the initial needle is left in situ. Passage of a guidewire through the stricture rarely fails with a percutaneous approach. A 6 Fr polyethylene, angled tip, torque catheter can be used, together with a hydrophilic, polymer coated wire, to find a route through into the duodenum. This guidewire is then replaced with a standard 0·035 inch Teflon coated steel wire.

If a previous ERCP has failed to allow access to the ducts above a stricture, once percutaneous passage of a wire into the duodenum has succeeded there are two possible options. Firstly, a 400 cm endoscopic guidewire can be passed through the transhepatic catheter into the duodenum and grasped with a basket passed through an endoscope. The wire is withdrawn up through the endoscope and used for the standard endoscopic placement of a 10 Fr stent. In the past this combined procedure has been extremely effective in allowing a 10 Fr stent to be placed within the biliary system while needing only a 6 Fr track through the liver. The risk of complications from percutaneous procedures is dependent upon the size of the transhepatic track. Alternatively a transhepatic expanding metal stent (Figure 8.9) can be placed over a transhepatic guidewire. The Wallstent has a 7 Fr delivery system and this keeps the risks of transhepatic placement to a minimum. The Wallstent expands to 1 cm (30 Fr). The choice between percutaneous metal stent insertion and a combined percutaneous and endoscopic procedure depends upon personal and local factors. The costs of the two procedures are roughly similar. If a left duct approach is

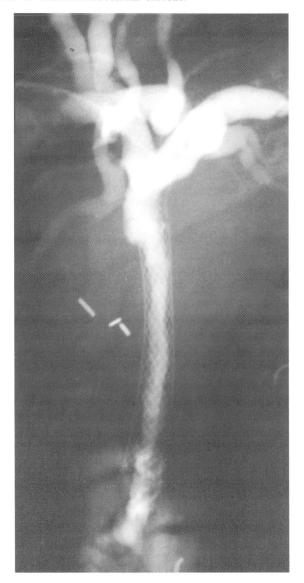

FIGURE 8.9—*A percutaneous transhepatic metal stent has been placed. The fully extended diameter of the stent and the drainage which it allows is clearly seen.*

necessary, it is best to select as peripheral an entry point as possible into the segment 3 duct, using ultrasound to guide the approach. The needle should be inserted subxiphisternally and aimed towards the porta hepatis to provide as little angulation as is possible along the line of approach to the common duct. The principles of access to the duct system and across the stricture are as for a right sided approach. If bilateral insertion of metal stents is anticipated, it is best to place bilateral guidewires through into the duodenum before deploying the stents. Because one expanded stent can occlude access for the second stent, stents are best deployed after passage of an 8 Fr sheath over each guidewire, stents being deployed within the sheaths, which are withdrawn during deployment. The stents should be deployed one immediately after the other.

If good drainage is not established immediately, percutaneous drainage can be provided while the stent expands.

Occasionally ERCP does not give sufficient information regarding involvement of the intrahepatic duct system with tumour: bilateral percutaneous transhepatic cholangiography may be necessary to provide an accurate assessment. This is performed as described above, percutaneous transhepatic drainage catheters being left in position after cholangiography. An assessment of the degree of involvement can be made immediately or later using catheter cholangiography. If the lesion is considered operable, then surgery can be undertaken promptly. If not, then the transhepatic catheters can be used to place bilateral metal stents.

Complications

The risks of percutaneous transhepatic procedures exceed those of endoscopic stenting and, as noted above, relate to the size of the transhepatic track necessary. If this is kept to a minimum, then complications can be expected in about one third of patients, although most are minor and include local pain, minor pleural effusions, transient haemobilia (Figure 8.10), and pyrexia without other evidence of cholangitis. Significant complications of haemorrhage, peritoneal bile leakage and cholangitis occur in 2–3% and can usually be managed conservatively. Bile leakage can be managed by the insertion of a drainage catheter under image guidance. Most bile leaks are self limiting and drainage need only be for a short period. Cholangitis normally indicates inadequate drainage and can be avoided by leaving transhepatic catheters in situ until adequate antegrade drainage is established and confirmed by catheter cholangiography. Normally antibiotic therapy is continued until full internal drainage is established.

Outcome

It is very uncommon for percutaneous transhepatic stent insertion to fail, although it may be necessary to complete the procedure in stages, perhaps 70% of stent insertions being possible at the first sitting. Relief of jaundice is equally as good as for endoscopic stent placement and, if

261

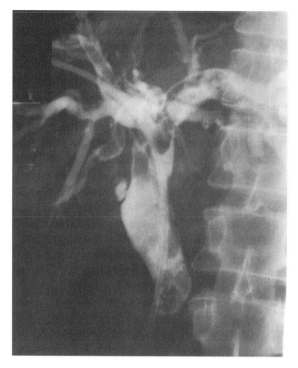

FIGURE 8.10—*A percutaneous transhepatic cholangiogram has allowed placement of an internal external drainage catheter. The cast-like objects within the bile duct system are blood clots. A mild degree of haemobilia is not uncommon after percutaneous procedures but rarely has significant consequences.*

transhepatic metal stents are used, the period of intervention-free drainage may be long enough to allow most patients to need only one procedure.

Surgical therapy

The first resection of a primary cancer originating in the hepatic duct confluence was reported by Brown and Mayers in 1954.[7] Soon the pathological characteristics of this kind of tumour were described in detail, although hilar bile duct cancers were regarded as practically irresectable. In 1965, Klatskin reviewed 13 cases of a distinctive tumour, described as a localised sclerosing adenocarcinoma at the hepatic duct bifurcation resulting in death due to progressive hepatic failure, and recommended aggressive palliative treatment utilising surgical or catheter drainage of the obstructed biliary system.[8] Since then, long term survival has been reported in a small but significant percentage of patients who had undergone excision of hilar cholangiocarcinoma. Resection has rapidly gained ground and is now regarded in many centres as the treatment of choice.

There is general agreement that extrahepatic metastasis, hepatic metastasis not encompassed in planned en bloc hepatic resection, or lymph node involvement outside the hepatoduodenal ligament preclude removal. When tumour invades the hepatic artery and/or portal vein at the hepatic hilum, it is necessary to secure these vessels for the safety of the patient and to reconstruct them, if they are concomitantly removed. Although there is little argument for preservation of portal blood flow, interruption of hepatic arterial flow during tumour resection may have dismal consequences. Because the blood supply to the biliary tree is derived from the hepatic artery and not the portal vein, transection of the choledochus with division of the ascending pericholedochal arteries and interruption of the hepatic artery induces necrosis of the biliary tree. Therefore, if extended surgery including vascular resection has to be performed, reconstruction of the hepatic artery and portal venous branch is important.

Resection cannot be performed in patients in whom vascular encasement extends from the first to the third order branches and tumour invasion beyond the third order biliary tree occurs in both lobes of the liver, or in those in whom multiple liver metastasis or distant metastasis (lymph node, other organs) are proved by preoperative imaging modalities. Such patients may need multiple external biliary drainage catheters for biliary decompression in place, even after discharge from hospital. These catheters can be replaced by indwelling stents (endoprostheses). The former requires daily catheter care and spoils the patient's quality of life, while the latter carries a risk of catheter obstruction followed by cholangitis.

Intrahepatic enterobiliary anastomosis and operative biliary drainage using catheters are alternative palliative measures. Intrahepatic cholangio-enteric anastomosis using ducts discovered by amputation of the tip of the right or left liver lobe has proved only partially satisfactory because of the small calibre and fragility of these ducts, leading rapidly to stenosis of the anastomosis with subsequent cholangitis. Other techniques have included wedge resection of the anterior edge of segment 3, and a transscissural approach through the umbilical cleavage plane, known as the round ligament approach. These result in a wide orifice and secure anastomosis can be performed.

Right side anastomosis can also be performed by wedge resection of segment 5 or 6, and bilateral intrahepatic anastomosis by combined resection of the inferior portions of segments 4 and 5 to expose the segment 4 and 5 biliary ducts; however, persistent and recrudescent jaundice and cholangitis cannot be avoided, even using these three techniques. This is because interruption of the biliary tree cannot be restricted to two areas at the hepatic hilum (right and left hepatic ducts), and the biliary tree is interrupted segmentally, so cholangitis occurs repeatedly with the progression of the hilar cholangiocarcinoma. Other problems include the possibility of undrained portions remaining in the liver at the site of the intrahepatic anastomosis as the result of improper interpretation of a cholangiogram. The mortality rate at 30 days for surgical bypass in patients with hilar carcinoma is between zero and 31%. Quality of life is poor due to repeated high fever, and the mean survival time is 13–16 months, with an occasional long term survivor. Operative mortality rates in patients with surgically placed catheters vary from 10 to 21%, and a median survival of approximately one year is frequently seen. The postprocedure mortality rate at 30 days after percutaneous or endoscopic drainage for various causes of malignant obstruction is comparable at 17–38%. Median survival is approximately six months. In patients with endoscopically placed endoprostheses, repeated cholangitis (0–42%) and no decline in bilirubin (0–28%) are common.[9]

Liver transplantation has been attempted but the results are disappointing.[10] At the present time this procedure is not indicated. There are occasional reports of good results with irradiation and chemotherapy; however, these therapeutic methods bring about an improvement in only a small number of patients with hilar carcinoma.

Pathologically, patients with hilar tumours limited to the mucosa or reaching the fibromuscular layer tend to develop no lymph node metastasis, no invasion of lymphatics or veins, and no perineural infiltration, while patients with more advanced tumours, reaching the submucosal layer or serosa or invading adjacent organs, have a high incidence of lymph node metastasis, lymphatic permeation, venous invasion, and perineural infiltration.

Hilar tumour extends extramurally by lymphatic permeation, venous invasion and perineural infiltration. This extension occurs more commonly in the transverse direction than in the longitudinal direction along the bile duct, and infiltration in the hepatic direction is more frequent than in the duodenal direction. The incidence of cancerous invasion at the surgical margin is less frequent in patients with extrahepatic bile duct resection alone.[11] Based on investigation of the macroscopic form in extrahepatic bile duct cancer, the cancer is limited to the area around the main tumour in the papillary and nodular types. In the superficial or superficially spreading type, the cancer is located in the mucosa without infiltration into the fibromuscular layer or Glisson's fibrous layer. This mucosal change cannnot be revealed by cholangiography but seems granular or papillary on percutaneous transhepatic cholangioscopy. In the nodular infiltrative and infiltrative types, thickening of the fibromuscular or Glisson's fibrous layer is induced by cancer involvement, and this histological finding is reflected by irregular narrowing of the biliary duct from the main tumour on cholangiography. In these types of bile duct cancer, a tumour-free surgical margin can be obtained by dividing the bile duct at a dilated site without such narrowing. Especially in the superficially spreading type of hilar cholangiocarcinoma, cholangiography shows multiple separate irregular narrowings.

Para-aortic lymph node metastasis in hilar carcinoma occurs via lymph nodes around the common hepatic artery and behind the head of the pancreas, but the incidence of para-aortic lymph node metastasis is usually lower than in middle and lower bile duct carcinomas. Bilateral biliary branches of the caudate lobe join to the right hepatic duct, the left hepatic duct, the confluence of these, and/or the right posterior hepatic duct. The biliary branches of the caudate lobe are involved in over 95% of patients with hilar carcinoma.

Resectability rates of hilar cholangiocarcinoma vary from 16 to 92·3% and mortality rates from zero to 33·3%. Morbidity rates are around 50%. The mean survival time is 9·3 months to 3·6 years and the median survival time 7–15 months. Improved resectability and mortality rates parallel the continuous development of resection modalities. Five year survival rates are reported to be 22–38%; however, in our study of 25 patients (no obstructive jaundice in nine and jaundice followed by biliary drainage in 19) with hilar or diffuse bile duct carcinoma who had undergone extended right hemihepatectomy, with or without pancreatoduodenectomy, there were no hospital deaths and the cumulative one and three year survival rates were 95% and 80·4%, respectively. The mean survival time was 21·5 ± 2·4 months (ranging from 3 to 40 months).[12]

There are three surgical methods of removal for hilar cholangiocarcinoma: extrahepatic bile duct resection without hepatectomy, with central hepatectomy, or with major hepatectomy. The first procedure is indicated only in selected patients with cancer limited to the extrahepatic bile duct with a depth of cancer infiltration limited to the mucosa or fibromuscular layer. After laparotomy and examination of the peritoneal cavity, skeletonisation of the vessels in the hepatoduodenal ligament and lymph node dissection around the head of the pancreas are carried out. The distal side of the common bile duct is transected at a tumour free position. The left hepatic duct is dissected in the cranial area of the transverse portion of the portal vein and the transected stump of the common bile duct is pulled up and transected at a tumour free position. The bilateral biliary branches of the caudate lobe are then dissected and transected, with subsequent transection of the right hepatic duct at a tumour free position, if necessary transected around the confluence of the anterior and posterior branches of the right hepatic duct. Hepaticodochojejunostomy is performed in a Roux-en-Y fashion.

The second method is used in patients who have hilar carcinoma not limited to the mucosa or fibromuscular layer but who have poor liver function. After skeletonisation of the hepatoduodenal ligament, with lymph node dissection around the pancreas head and division of the distal common bile duct, the proximal bile duct is dissected free from the hepatic artery and the portal vein to the level of the secondary and tertiary hepatic radicles, excising hepatic parenchyma surrounding the bile duct and leaving two or more intrahepatic ducts exposed for anastomosis. A Roux-en-Y jejunal limb is brought up to the hepatic hilum and the proximal end is oversewn. This procedure does not involve the caudate lobe. As mentioned before, the biliary branches of the caudate lobe are inevitably involved by hilar carcinoma; complete removal of the caudate lobe with resection of the extrahepatic bile duct is therefore recommended. Caudate lobectomy in isolation, using a transhepatic approach, is not easy to perform. In patients with poor liver function, caudate lobectomy with partial or complete resection of segment 4 is an acceptable alternative to allow a wide operative field for resection of hilar carcinoma and bilioenterostomy (Figure 8.11).

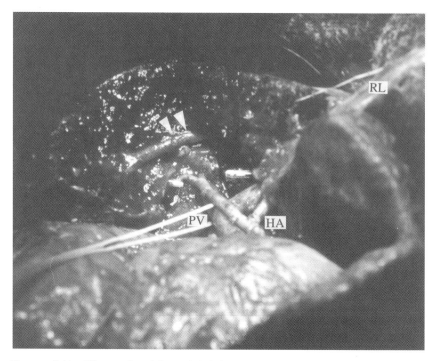

FIGURE 8.11—*The caudate lobe and inferior portion of segment 4 are removed. The skeletonised hepatic artery (HA), portal vein (PV), and a thick tributary of the middle hepatic vein-drained segment 5 (arrow heads) are seen. RL = round ligament.*

During this procedure, mobilisation and isolation of the liver from the retrohepatic inferior vena cava is carried out from both sides by dissecting and dividing the short hepatic veins. After skeletonisation of the hepatoduodenal ligament, with lymph node dissection around the pancreas head and division of the distal common bile duct, the left and right hepatic arteries and portal venous branches are identified and isolated, and the caudate branches of the portal vein are transected. After that, the hepatic parenchyma is divided from the right side of the umbilical portion to the fissure for the Arantius duct, after transection of the hepatic arterial and portal venous branches of segment 4 in the umbilical fossa. The left hepatic duct is transected at the distal end of its transverse portion. Parenchymal transection is begun on the inferior surface to expose the total length of the middle hepatic vein on its left side, then the parenchymal transecting plane is directed to the right side of the inferior vena cava. The right hepatic duct is transected around the bifurcation of its anterior and posterior branches; however, this method carries a risk of cancer persistence in the bile duct stumps.

The third method is indicated in patients with normal liver function. In most cases, the right hepatic artery passes under the common hepatic duct. In contrast, the left hepatic artery runs away from the bile duct and toward the umbilical portion of the left portal vein. Furthermore, the left hepatic duct is longer than the right hepatic duct. As a result of these anatomical features, the left hepatic artery is rarely involved by carcinoma originating from the major hepatic duct confluence, and a cancer-free margin is more easily obtained in the left hepatic duct than in the right. As the bifurcation of the portal vein lies behind the hepatic duct bifurcation and is vulnerable to cancerous invasion, resection of the venous bifurcation is recommended for curative resection. Reconstruction of the left portal venous branch is less likely to result in stricture than that of the right sided branch because of the narrow angle of the main and left portal vein. In patients with the same extent of cancerous invasion into both hepatic ducts, or predominant invasion into the right hepatic duct, extended right hemihepatectomy with complete caudate lobectomy and resection of the extrahepatic bile duct is chosen; however, in patients with obviously predominant invasion into the left hepatic duct, extended left hemihepatectomy with total caudate lobectomy and resection of the extrahepatic bile duct is chosen. In extended left hemihepatectomy, reconstruction of the right hepatic artery is usual and a microsurgeon needs to be on standby. In extended right hemihepatectomy, after lymph node dissection and transection of the common bile duct, the right hepatic artery and portal venous branch are ligated and divided, and the left hepatic artery and portal venous branch are isolated down to the umbilical portion, with severing of their caudate lobe branches. Complete mobilisation of the right lobe and isolation of the liver from the retrohepatic inferior vena cava is then carried out, followed by transection of the left hepatic duct. The left hepatic duct is transected at the right side of the umbilical portion of the portal vein in extended right hemihepatectomy with complete caudate lobectomy; the transection point is at the same level in right trisegmentectomy. Extended right hemihepatectomy with caudate lobectomy is therefore our standard procedure (Figure 8.12).

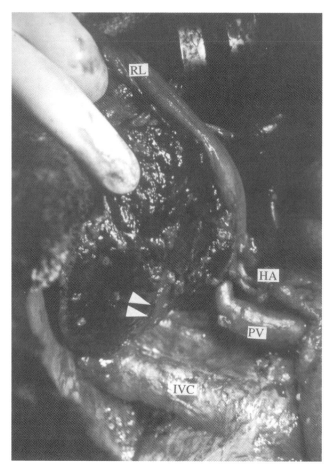

FIGURE 8.12—*Transected plane after extended right hemihepatectomy with removal of the caudate lobe. The middle hepatic vein (arrow heads) can be seen in the plane. The hepatic artery (HA) and portal vein (PV) are skeletonised. RL = round ligament; IVC = inferior vena cava.*

Extended left hemihepatectomy retains a larger hepatic parenchymal volume and is technically easier than extended right hemihepatectomy; however, it carries a risk of residual cancer, as described previously. Left hepatectomy with extrahepatic duct resection is reported to be the most versatile surgical procedure for hilar cholangiocarcinoma, providing a high resectability rate, safety, and a good quality of postoperative life, although better long term survival cannot be expected for the aforementioned reason. Extended left hemihepatectomy may therefore be limited to patients with predominant cancerous invasion into the left hepatic duct or slightly deteriorated liver function.

Suggested plan of surgical management

Although biliary drainage may not always be required before surgical treatment not involving hepatic resection, biliary decompression may be necessary before hepatectomy when major hepatectomy is intended for curative resection of hilar bile duct carcinoma; however, the ideal degree and extent of biliary decompression for hepatic resection has not yet been established because appropriate evaluation of liver function is difficult, nor has it been determined how much liver volume can be removed in the cholestatic state. So far, operative methods have been decided upon following a single measurement of liver function in the jaundiced state, and patients with limited reduction of the serum total bilirubin level have been postulated to have poor liver function. Palliative operation or minor hepatectomy combined with bile duct resection has been thought to be appropriate for these patients. It is unclear whether widely used liver function tests performed in the jaundiced state can justify the selection of a therapeutic modality in patients with malignant biliary obstruction.

In our series of 25 patients we demonstrated that, after the serum bilirubin level had decreased almost into the normal range after biliary drainage, extended right hemihepatectomy with or without pan-creatoduodenectomy could be performed without hospital death. Even in patients with an extremely slow rate of decrease in serum total bilirubin after biliary drainage, such extensive surgery was as safe as in those without previous jaundice. In patients who underwent biliary drainage only in the part of the liver to be preserved, that area of the liver hypertrophied, while the volume of liver to be preserved did not change in patients who underwent whole liver biliary drainage.[12] Biliary decompression is therefore a therapeutic necessity before extended right hemihepatectomy with or without pancreatoduodenectomy and the surgical procedure should not be decided by the rate of decrease in serum total bilirubin after biliary drainage.

Partial biliary drainage in the area of liver to be preserved is suitable for obtaining hypertrophy of the future remnant liver.

Hepatic failure is a fatal postoperative complication particularly related to hepatic resection. Its occurrence is related to the quantity and quality of the remaining liver parenchyma. When the remnant liver is normal, hepatic failure hardly ever occurs, except when extensive resection of normally functioning parenchyma is required for removal of an awkwardly located small lesion, particularly in cases of hilar cholangiocarcinoma or small cancer invading the trunk of the right portal venous branch. Preoperative portal embolisation is useful for preventing the occurrence of postoperative hepatic failure in cases of extensive resection of normally functioning hepatic parenchyma. When the serum total bilirubin level decreases to below 85·5 mmol/l (5·0 mg/dl) in jaundiced patients, right portal venous branch embolisation can be performed in an attempt to induce atrophy of the right lobe and hypertrophy of the left lobe.[13, 14] A balloon catheter is inserted into the portal vein at laparotomy through an ileocolic vein. After portography has defined the intrahepatic portal anatomy, the portal venous branch of the lobe to be resected is embolised under fluoroscopic control (Figure 8.13). The embolisation material consists of a mixture of 0·5–1·0 g Gelfoam Ô (absorbable gelatin sponge) powder, 2500–5000 units thrombin, diatrizoate sodium meglumine (60% Urografin Ô, 10–20 ml) and 40 mg gentamicin. When the serum bilirubin level falls to below 34·2 mmol/l (2·0 mg/dl) in jaundiced patients after right portal venous branch embolisation, hepatectomy is carried out.

A combination of biliary decompression of the liver remnant, with subsequent portal venous branch embolisation of the part of the liver to be resected, is recommended to obtain lower mortality and morbidity in extended right hemihepatectomy or parenchymal resections.

Radiochemotherapy

Radiobiology of liver

Any therapeutic schedule involving ionising radiation must take into account the radiosensitivity of the surrounding normal tissues. Clearly, the radiobiology of the liver is critical in terms of delivery of radiotherapy for hepatobiliary tumours. Radiation hepatitis has been reported with whole liver irradiation doses greater than 2500 cGy, with a big increase in the risk of centrilobular necrosis at doses >3500 cGy. Local application of radiotherapy by intracavitary treatment through the biliary tree or hepatic

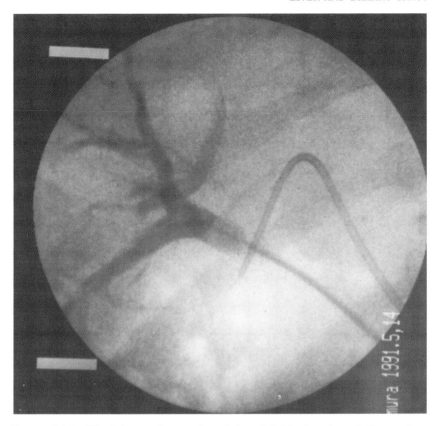

FIGURE 8.13—*The right portal venous branch is occluded by inserting a balloon catheter through an iliac vein and is embolised. A transhepatic biliary drainage tube inserted through a biliary branch of segment 3 can also be seen.*

arterial administration of radionuclides bound to microspheres demonstrates that much higher "doses" of ionising radiation can be administered when there is an element of selective targeting.

Radiotherapy

Ionising radiation has been used for the primary treatment of extrahepatic biliary cancers and has been evaluated as an adjuvant treatment after surgical resection. There is a seeming paradox in the literature. Several series indicate that radiotherapy prolongs survival in patients who have not had a complete resection. Given the relative rarity of the cancer, these trials have been small and tend not to be randomised. There is even less evidence

271

to support the role of adjuvant postoperative irradiation and it is impossible to recommend routinely on the basis of currently available evidence.

Intraluminal brachytherapy has been used in the treatment of cervical, oesophageal, and lung cancer to deliver high regional doses of ionising radiation by the insertion of a radioactive source into the hollow viscus. This technique has been used through the bile ducts, either transcutaneously or by ERCP, for the treatment of extrahepatic biliary tumours. The penetration depth of ionising radiation from the radioactive source is only 0·5 cm, therefore most studies have combined brachytherapy with external beam irradiation. Again, although these developments are logical, the existing database, which predominantly compares phase II trials with historical controls, does not support a clear survival benefit from this type of radiotherapy.

External beam radiotherapy has little to offer the patient with cholangiocarcinoma; however, there has been a vogue in recent years for intraluminal radiotherapy using either iridium wires or more recently microselection afterloading therapy. Although it is tempting to take the opportunity to provide intraluminal radiotherapy before withdrawal of transhepatic catheters, there is as yet no clear evidence that this technique has any benefit for the patient. The extra period of time necessary for the catheters to remain in position while radiotherapy is given often causes discomfort and sometimes distress for the patient. It is unlikely that intraluminal radiotherapy has a useful role in the management of cholangiocarcinoma.

Chemotherapy

Most reports of chemotherapy for cancers of the biliary tract are based on relatively small patient numbers. Tumour response rates are similar for tumours of the gall bladder, bile ducts or intrahepatic cholangiocarcinomas; this section therefore groups these indistinguishably together. A wide range of antineoplastic agents, such as 5-fluorouracil (5FU), streptozoticin, methyl-CCNU, mitomycin C, doxorubicin, and etoposide, have been assessed in the treatment of cholangiocarcinoma, with little evidence of worth. Similarly, combinations of these agents provide no additional benefit but worse toxicity. Given the advances that have been made by combining 5FU and folinic acid in the treatment of advanced colorectal cancer (Chapter 10), one would predict that it would be worthwhile testing this strategy in the treatment of cholangiocarcinoma, but initial small trials have proved disappointing.

Metastatic liver tumours

KENICHI SUGIHARA, NICHOLAS D JAMES and
DAVID KERR

Most patients with metastatic tumours who are referred for liver resection are those with colorectal secondaries.[15-17] Of 351 patients with metastatic liver tumours who underwent liver resection at the National Cancer Center Hospital during the last 14 years, 284 (80·9%) had colorectal secondaries, 28 had gastric secondaries, and 11 had sarcomatous tumours from the digestive tract. Most clinical studies on liver resection for metastases have therefore focused on colorectal secondaries.

Staging

Synchronous liver metastases are found in 12–14% of patients with colorectal cancer at diagnosis or primary surgery, and metachronous metastases develop in 8–11% of patients undergoing potentially curative surgery.[18, 19] The resection rate (the number of patients who undergo liver resection/the number of patients with liver metastases), which will depend on the criteria for liver resection used by each surgeon, is roughly 12% in the USA,[20] 24% in Germany,[19] and 45% in the National Cancer Center Hospital, Tokyo.

All patients with colorectal cancer should be recommended to have US for detection of liver metastases before colorectal surgery. After surgery, regular follow up with CEA assay and US every three months may allow detection of liver tumours at an earlier stage. Elevated CEA levels and/or suspicious appearances on US require further examination by contrast enhanced dynamic CT to confirm the presence, number, and localisation of metastases. Improved delineation may be obtained by CT angiography

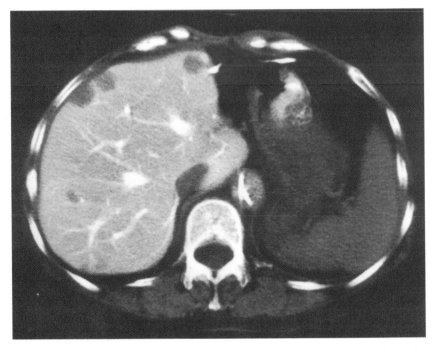

FIGURE 8.14—*The CT arterial portography demonstrates three tumours of the medial and anterior segment, which have been detected by US, and additional tumour 6 mm in diameter of the posterior segment which was not detected by US and dynamic CT.*

and CT arterial portography (Figure 8.14).[21, 22] US performed by experienced examiners, however, can achieve almost the same accuracy as CT using contrast media. A combination of US and CT helps to decide the feasibility of liver resection, based on the number and localisation of tumours and their structural relation to the intrahepatic vascular and biliary systems. The volume of the normal liver parenchyma that will be removed should be calculated from CT when extended right lobectomy, trisegmentectomy, or right lobectomy combined with limited resection of the left lobe is proposed (Figure 8.15). Preoperative[9] portal embolisation, as described earlier in this chapter when considering resection for proximal bile duct cancer, may increase the safety of liver resection where more than 60% of the normal liver is to be removed. Patients who are determined to have resectable liver tumours should undergo examinations to exclude extrahepatic metastases, including chest radiography or pulmonary CT for lung tumours, abdominal US or CT for retroperitoneal lymph node swelling, pelvic CT for local recurrence of rectal cancer, and colonoscopy for anastomotic recurrence and metachronous colorectal cancer.

Interventional radiology

For patients with colorectal liver metastases the five year survival rate is more favourable than for patients with metastases from a variety of other primary malignancies, particularly the gastrointestinal tract, lung, and breast, in which the prognosis is poor.[23] For the majority of patients, clinical presentation with right upper quadrant pain, abdominal mass, weight loss, and anorexia usually indicates the presence of disease that is largely untreatable.

When metastases are present, standard radiological investigation with US, contrast enhanced CT, hepatic scintigraphy, or magnetic resonance imaging (MRI) will confirm disease in over 80%, a combination of techniques improving accuracy still further. Of course, the main factor that governs the sensitivity of imaging is the bulk of metastatic disease, and sensitivity is reduced when disease is clinically occult—for example, when there are only one or two small liver lesions or when micrometastases are present. There is therefore a need for improvements in imaging techniques to detect these early metastatic lesions which may be suitable for resection.

Imaging techniques

Intraoperative and laparoscopic US can detect metastatic lesions within the liver with greater sensitivity than routine abdominal US. This is because the direct contact between the transducer and the liver allows the use of high frequency (7–10 MHz) probes, which have better spatial resolution, enabling the detection of smaller lesions. Abdominal US has difficulty in detecting subcapsular lesions that are in the near field of the image. While these too may be detectable by intraoperative or laparoscopic US, they are also likely to be palpable at operation or visible laparoscopically, thus improving the sensitivity of these techniques still further. For the routine evaluation of patients after colorectal cancer surgery, these two techniques are, however, too invasive.

Abdominal US, contrast enhanced CT, and MRI are at the moment the mainstays of the investigation of possible metastatic disease in colorectal cancer but, as noted above, all have a significant false negative rate. MRI is likely to improve technically still further, particularly with the development of better receiver coils, better image sequences, and the use of paramagnetic

---

FIGURE 8.15—Opposite top: *the dynamic CT shows multiple tumours of the lateral, medial and posterior segment.* Opposite bottom: *right portal vein embolisation using Gelfoam two weeks before liver resection increases the safety of extended right lobectomy combined with partial resection of the lateral segment.*

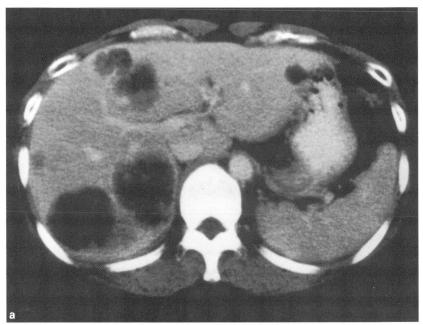

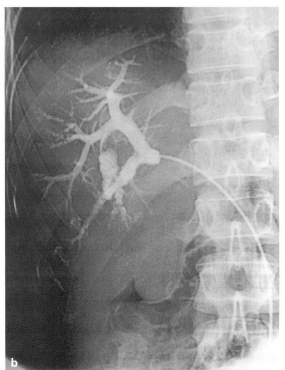

contrast agents. Also, the development of ultrasound contrast agents may improve detection of smaller lesions in the future. Standard, contrast enhanced CT can already be manipulated in a variety of techniques. Dynamic contrast enhancement in which imaging takes place during the injection of 80–120 ml of iodinated contrast medium is already routinely performed and is more sensitive than non-enhanced CT. Delayed scanning after contrast injection has its proponents because metastatic lesions may undergo differential enhancement compared with adjacent liver, allowing clearer definition, but this technique has so far been disappointing for the demonstration of lesions not visible during dynamic contrast enhanced CT. Normally, approximately 70% of liver blood flow is via the portal vein but metastatic lesions tend to derive their blood supply from the hepatic artery and therefore enhance earlier than the adjacent normal liver. CT performed during the direct intra-arterial injection of contrast into the hepatic artery via a femoral catheter may clarify the presence of metastases as early enhancing areas. CT portography, in which contrast is injected directly into the superior mesenteric artery and CT of the liver performed during the portal phase in order to detect poorly enhancing areas of liver, may also detect lesions. Both of these techniques are invasive and not suited to routine use.

There are two non-invasive techniques that take advantage of the altered hepatic artery and portal vein supply to the liver in metastatic disease and which may, with technical improvements, become acceptable routine investigations for the detection of occult disease. During the immediate postintravenous injection blood pool phase of hepatic scintigraphy, there is an initial peak of hepatic activity due to arterial flow, followed by a later peak due to portal flow. The normal ratio of these flows has been defined and an alteration of the ratio, with increased hepatic arterial component, has been shown to correlate with the later development of metastatic liver disease. This was the first radiological investigation that allowed the prediction of metastatic disease before lesions could be individually detected. More recently, the arterial and venous flows and their ratio have been defined using Doppler assessment of flow in the artery and vein and similarly an alteration in the ratio has been shown to correlate with the development of metastatic disease. It can be expected that with the use of ultrasound contrast agents the sensitivity of the hepatic artery to portal vein blood flow ratio will improve further. Of course, the ability to predict the development of metastatic disease does not as yet necessarily impart an advantage to the patient. The main thrust of therapeutic management of colorectal liver metastases has been to remove the affected segment or lobe of liver at surgery. While this is straightforward when metastases are visible, it is not possible when the liver appears normal and an abnormal flow ratio is the only abnormality. None the less, it may be that in some patients the demonstration of an abnormal flow ratio may prompt more invasive investigation with CT portography or laparoscopic US, thereby directing the surgical approach more specifically.

Image guided therapy

Although surgical liver resection is the ideal for the management of patients with colorectal metastases, it is estimated that this is only appropriate therapy in 5–10% of such patients. Approximately 50% of patients with colorectal carcinoma will develop liver metastases. Other methods of treatment are therefore required for the majority of patients who are not suitable for surgery. Ultrasound guided injection of alcohol is a popular and effective treatment for hepatocellular carcinoma and has also been used for patients with colorectal metastatic disease. Unfortunately, the results available have been disappointing as it seems that necrosis is patchy and therefore relatively ineffective. Treatment can be painful. Other techniques, such as freezing or heating metastases, show greater promise and in particular the ultrasound guided insertion of fine optical fibres for interstitial laser photocoagulation seems effective. Laser photocoagulation seems to result in better local necrosis of tumour and fewer side effects when compared with alcohol injection.[24] These modalities have the advantage of being repeatable, allowing management of recurrence or new lesions that become evident during follow up. Theoretically, image guided therapy could be used to reduce the total number of metastases within the liver together with surgery to deal with larger localised tumours.

Hepatic arteriography is now rarely indicated for the diagnosis of liver metastases. In the past, embolisation of the hepatic artery was in vogue for the management of metastatic disease, particularly when this was bulky and painful, but this has been a disappointing method of treatment. Low volume metastatic disease responds poorly to hepatic arterial embolisation and, where disease is extensive, side effects due to necrosis of tumour result in there being no benefit to the patient from this method of treatment. Surgically implanted arterial catheters are used for regional chemotherapy. The one circumstance in which arterial embolisation may be of benefit is in the management of metastatic endocrine tumours which cause symptoms not only because of bulk but more particularly because of hormonal activity. This may be reduced by embolisation; however, this method of therapy is likely to be surpassed by the use of somatostatin and its synthetic analogues.

Outcome of liver resection

Despite many studies on liver resection for colorectal metastases, selection criteria that can accurately identify patients who will benefit from resection are not yet established. It is apparent that all liver tumour must be removed for there to be a chance of long term survival. The next step is to discover determinants that predict accurately an unfavourable outcome after apparently complete removal of all tumour tissue. The generally agreed indications for liver resection have been extended from a solitary lesion to up to three metastases in the same lobe, after analysis of early experience;[25 26] however, a small group of patients with more than three tumours, can survive more than five years after histologically complete resection.[18 27 28] It is difficult to place a firm limit on the number of tumours that should be resected because complete removal depends on many factors, particularly their number, size, and distribution, and the structural relation of each tumour to the vascular and biliary system. Rather than the number of tumours that are resected, curative removal, that is with a negative histological margin, is the most important predictor of possible long term survival.[18 27]

At present no modality other than resection can provide prospects for long term survival or improved prognosis. The author believes that technically feasible liver resection is indicated when all tumours, even if more than three in number, can be removed, provided that adequate normal parenchyma can be preserved, no extrahepatic metastases are detectable, and the patient is considered fit for operation. In addition, liver resection may sometimes be considered in patients with synchronous extrahepatic tumours which are resectable. Contraindications to surgery include the presence of metastases in the hepatic or coeliac lymph nodes and tumours invading the inferior vena cava or the hepatic hilus. These criteria for liver resection are supported by recently reported large series that revealed 5 year survival rates between 30 and 47·9% with a low mortality rate (Table 8.1).[18 27 29] The surgical

TABLE 8.1—*Outcome of curative liver resection for colorectal metastases*

Author	Term of patient accrual	No. of patients	Five year survival rate (%)	Mortality (%)	Morbidity (%)	Hepatic recurrence (%)
Scheele[27]	1960–1988	219	39	5·5	22	
Steele[28]	1984–1988	69	37·1	2·7	13	41·4
Doci[29]	1980–1989	100	30	5	11	41
Sugihara[17]	1978–1989	109	47·9	1·3	22·4	31·8

strategy employed in the majority of large series reported to date has been anatomical major resection.[25–29] Ultrasound guided, limited liver resection is the method of choice in the author's unit. Intraoperative US is essential to detect deposits not seen before operation, to confirm relationships between tumours and the intrahepatic vascular system, and to retain an adequate surgical margin. The caudate lobe should be carefully examined:

the paracaval portion by US, the Spigelian portion and the caudate process by US and palpation. In limited liver resection it is difficult to get a resection margin of more than 10 mm, which has been regarded as an important determinant of long term survival.[26 30] Our experience, however, suggests that complete tumour removal with a negative histological margin, even when this is less than 10 mm, provides an equivalent chance of prolonged survival.[17] Scheele also stressed the importance of a negative histological margin in his leading article on hepatectomy for liver metastases.[31] A histopathological study of colorectal liver metastases, which found no microscopic deposits in the liver parenchyma around tumours and no evidence of intrahepatic metastases from metastatic liver tumours, provides support for non-anatomically limited resection as the procedure of choice for colorectal liver metastases.[32] This contrasts with the inadequacy of this approach in hepatocellular carcinoma (see later).

In synchronous liver metastasis, liver resection can be performed simultaneously with colorectal surgery, but where possible it is better delayed, providing the initial tumour size is less than 2 cm, for up to three or four months. During the observation time, additional deposits that were not detected at the time of colorectal surgery may develop and can be removed with the initial deposits if they do not preclude surgery.

After potentially curative liver resection, the predominant site of recurrence is the liver remnant (Table 8.1), followed by the lung.[17 18 26 28 29] Most recurrences develop within 18 months.[18] An aggressive approach to recurrent metastatic tumour, including repeat liver resection or pulmonary resection, may provide long term survival if the deposits can be removed curatively.[33] Repeat liver resection does not increase the mortality rate nor the morbidity rate.[33 34] The indications for repeat liver resection should be the same as for the first resection.

Cryosurgery with ultrasonic guidance may yield a small success rate in patients with unresectable and/or multiple bilobar metastases.[35] Complete destruction of whole tumour deposits by cryofreezing may be difficult, especially when the tumour is large. A combination of lobar resection and cryosurgery for small deposits in the contralateral lobe may expand our indications for surgery to some patients with tumours currently considered to be unresectable.

Radiochemotherapy

In contrast to the stark and discouraging results of systemic chemotherapy, regional hepatic arterial infusion therapy (HAIT) offers a more targeted opportunity, particularly for patients with unresectable liver tumours. The simple premise underlying the use of HAIT is that most cytotoxic drugs have very steep dose–response curves, so that a small increment in drug dose will result in a large increase in cell kill. Clearly this limits the systemic use of antineoplastic agents because toxicity to normal host cell compartments (bone marrow, crypt cells of the gastrointestinal tract, hair follicle cells, etc) soon intervenes. There are, however, certain anticancer drugs that enjoy a significant pharmacokinetic advantage in that they are extracted in large quantities by the liver on first arterial pass, meaning that much higher drug concentrations (up to 300–400 times for 5FU) can be generated in the body compartment harbouring the bulk of the tumour.

In technical terms, the drug can be administered by a Seldinger approach with a hepatic arterial catheter being manipulated through the femoral artery, allowing intermittent delivery of chemotherapy every 3–4 weeks. Alternatively, the surgeon can implant an indwelling hepatic arterial catheter, inserted through the gastroduodenal artery, at laparotomy, which is connected externally to a subcutaneous injection port, allowing repeated access for chemotherapy treatment.

In the West, there is most experience with regional chemotherapy for hepatic metastatic colorectal cancer, and pharmacokinetic studies have shown that there is a regional advantage for delivery of 5FU, doxorubicin, mitomycin C and cisplatin.

Intra-arterial chemotherapy has the advantage of bringing a high dose of cytotoxic agents to the target organs with minimum toxicity to other organs.[36] Although HAIT was started in the 1960s,[37] the introduction of an implantable vascular access device and pump has provided a new stimulus for the development of this therapy. These advances permit the continuous infusion of chemotherapy with less impairment of the quality of life than was possible in the past.

A widely utilized schedule of HAIT with 5-fluoro-2'deoxyuridine (FUDR) for unresectable colorectal liver metastases is continuous infusion given by an implantable pump at a dose of 0·2–0·3 mg/kg/day for 14 days every 28 days. This consistently yields a response rate of 40–60% (Table 8.2). Several randomised trials using FUDR for HAIT, and FUDR or 5FU for systemic infusion have shown significantly higher response rates for HAIT than for systemic chemotherapy in the treatment of colorectal liver metastases.[38–42] A survival benefit was observed only in the study by Rougier and colleagues;[42] however, their control group included patients who did not receive any treatment. Reasons why the good objective response rate of liver metastases is not always reflected in survival benefits may include the forced termination of HAIT by biliary toxicity, and the high incidence of extrahepatic tumour progression during treatment.

Biliary sclerosis, the most serious complication of HAIT using FUDR, occurred in 3–25% of cases (Table 8.2).[38–42] Its incidence increased with increases in the dose[40] and duration of infusion.[42] Shortening of infusion duration, lower dosage, and coinfusion of dexamethasone with FUDR[43]

TABLE 8.2—*Outcome of hepatic arterial infusion therapy for unresectable colorectal liver metastases*

Author	Drug	No. of patients	Response (%)	Median survival (months)	Sclerosing cholangitis (%)
Kemeny[38]	FUDR	31	50	17	8
Chang[39]	FUDR	32	62	17	21
Hohn[40]	FUDR	50	42	17	52*
Martin[41]	FUDR	33	48	12·6	3
Rougier[42]	FUDR	81	43	15	25
Stagg[44]	FUDR+5FU	64	50	22·4	0
Sugihara[45]	5FU	53	51	11	0

* Termination of treatment due to biliary toxicity.

have been attempted to reduce this toxicity. Other trials of HAIT, which aimed to yield a high response rate with low toxicity, have studied alternating low dose intra-arterial FUDR plus 5FU[44] and 5FU alone by continuous infusion[45] (Table 8.2).

Systemic metastases ultimately develop in 35–55% of patients receiving HAIT.[38 39 42 45] As HAIT has little or no effect on extrahepatic metastases, HAIT combined with systemic chemotherapy may resolve this problem.[46] In five previous randomised studies of HAIT versus systemic chemotherapy,[38–42] FUDR or 5FU was used for systemic infusion. The recent reports of improved response rate for systemic chemotherapy with 5FU plus leucovorin[47 48] may necessitate a new randomised trial of HAIT versus systemic chemotherapy.

The initial enthusiasm for HAIT has been tempered by a number of factors, including liver toxicity resulting from the infusion of FUDR, the development of systemic disease in patients receiving HAIT, the improved results of systemic chemotherapy with 5FU and leucovorin, the cost of arterial cannulation and pump placement, and the uncertainty of survival benefit; however, HAIT may still play an important part as a palliative modality in the treatment of unresectable colorectal liver metastases, given that most patients with systemic disease ultimately die of tumour progression in the liver and that HAIT can reduce tumour burden by more than 50% in nearly 50% of patients with liver metastases.

Hepatocellular carcinoma

TADATOSHI TAKAYAMA, MASATOCHI MAKUUCHI,
NICHOLAS D JAMES and DAVID KERR

Hepatocellular carcinoma (HCC), one of the most common malignancies, with an estimated one million new cases a year worldwide, has an incidence which varies from more than 20/100 000/year in high risk regions such as South East Asia and sub-Saharan Africa to less than 5/100 000/year in low risk regions such as northern Europe and North America.[49] Without regard to geography, HCC is more common in men than in women: men have a 3–8 times greater risk. Epidemiological studies have identified several risk factors associated with the development of HCC.[50] In high risk regions, a strong link between infection with hepatitis B or C and the development of HCC has been suggested, and there is underlying chronic liver disease, notably cirrhosis, in 80–90% of patients with HCC in most countries. Dietary ingestion of large amounts of aflatoxin B_1 appears to be a special environmental cocarcinogen to carriers of hepatitis B virus among rural Africans. In the West, alcohol induced liver injury is a leading cause of cirrhosis and thus an important risk factor for HCC. In addition, the long term use of anabolic steroids or oral contraceptives, and the association of metabolic disorders such as haemochromatosis, α_1 antitrypsin deficiency, and tyrosinaemia, may increase the risk.

Clinical presentation

HCC is usually asymptomatic in its early stages, and no specific clinical symptoms can indicate the presence of a small tumour. Commonly presenting symptoms include upper abdominal discomfort or pain, weight loss, ascites, a palpable tumour, or other sequelae of portal hypertension. Most of the patients with apparent symptoms, however, may present too late to receive effective treatment because of extensive intrahepatic extension, portal or hepatic vein involvement, or extrahepatic metastases.[51]

283

The early diagnosis of HCC is therefore a clinical priority. Identification of small HCC is theoretically possible because (a) it is well known that patients with chronic hepatitis B or C virus infection are at high risk of HCC; (b) elevated serum AFP may give a lead to imaging detection of small HCC; and (c) ultrasonographic imaging can now detect small HCC around 2 cm or less in diameter. Thus combined AFP and ultrasonographic monitoring of such high risk patients should be effective in detecting HCC at earlier stages.

Prospectively, Colombo et al examined the value of a combination of AFP and US as screening tests in the early detection of HCC in 447 Italian patients with cirrhosis.[52] They reported a yearly HCC incidence rate of 3%, and their screening programme failed to achieve the goal of early detection of surgically treatable tumours. Oka et al, however, demonstrated a risk of HCC of 8% a year in 140 clinic based Japanese patients.[53] During a six year follow up period, they detected a small HCC of 2 cm or less in 26 (65%) of 40 patients who were found to have HCC, and this early detection seemed to be helpful in prolonging survival after subsequent optimal treatment. Although the recommendations may be different in different countries, it is desirable to monitor high risk patients every 3–6 months by AFP and/or US, at least in high risk regions.[54] It remains to be clarified by large scale trials in various countries how these patients may best be screened and, more importantly, whether screening can really improve the survival of such patients.

Staging

Ultrasonography, CT, and angiography are used commonly to diagnose HCC, with sensitivities around 90% for tumours less than 3 cm.[55] Newer imaging modalities including angio-CT, lipoidol-CT, and intraoperative US are more sensitive.[55 56] US is the examination of first choice, and any ultrasonographic mass in patients with chronic liver disease must be considered a possible malignancy. The ultrasonographic findings typical for HCC include a smooth, round boundary, internal echoes with a mosaic pattern, a marginal hypoechoic zone, posterior echo enhancement, and lateral shadows.[56]

As a complement to US, dynamic CT with bolus contrast injection is the next investigation to arrive at a qualitative diagnosis of the tumour, as it is a non-invasive method that can evaluate the tumour vascularity. Typically, HCC appears hyperdense in the arterial dominant phase and then becomes hypodense in the portal dominant phase. Once HCC lesions have been confirmed, angiography will be performed for the purposes of preoperative work up or interventional radiology. In Japan, it is commonly combined with CT to detect small intrahepatic metastases that would be undetectable by other imaging methods.[55]

For angio-CT, contrast medium is injected into the superior mesenteric artery during sequential scanning of the liver, and the tumour is visualised as a portal perfusion defect. In lipoidol-CT, injection of 2–5 ml of lipoidol into the hepatic artery is followed by its prolonged retention within HCC, as seen on CT obtained 2–3 weeks later.[57] The lesion appears as a high density area or deposit compared with the non-tumorous liver parenchyma. It is possible by these two methods to identify more and smaller HCC and satellite nodules of 1 cm or less. Such progress in imaging diagnosis has made it possible to identify early and precancerous lesions for HCC, which we demonstrated to undergo malignant transformation.[58] Occasionally, despite extensive radiological examinations, the imaging diagnosis of HCC may be equivocal. For such cases clinical judgment, assisted by fine needle biopsy or by follow up with reimaging, should be of value to avoid possible misdiagnosis.[59]

The current staging system for HCC according to the clinical tumour, node, and metastasis (TNM) classification of the International Union against Cancer (UICC) is shown in Table 8.3.[60] The level for each of three items is determined and the highest values are selected. The T factor is crucial and depends on tumour size (less or more than 2 cm) and number (single or multiple), and the presence of vascular invasion. The stage indicates the degree of extension of the HCC and should reflect the prognosis of the patients.

Despite numerous options for treatment of HCC, patients with clinical stage I or II tumours can be candidates for surgery unless their hepatic function is extremely poor. Ultimately, the limiting factor is a determination of the hepatic functional reserve of each patient. We have defined criteria for operability using the presence or absence of ascites, the level of serum total bilirubin, and the indocyanine green (ICG) clearance at 15 minutes.[61] In brief, patients with no ascites and with a normal bilirubin level (<1·0 mg/dl) are considered good candidates, and are then classified according to their ICG clearance value; lobectomy is considered possible when the patient has an ICG value <10%, segmentectomy at <20%, subsegmentectomy at <30%, and limited resection at >30%. Our policy originated from the need to resect HCC radically and safely because the majority of the patients are functionally impaired but asymptomatic. Recently, Fan et al proposed the use of perioperative nutritional support to reduce complications after hepatectomy in patients with HCC associated with cirrhosis.[62]

TABLE 8.3—*Stage of hepatocellular carcinoma*[60]

Definition of TNM
Primary tumour (T)
TX   Cannot be assessed
T0   No evidence of primary tumour
T1   Solitary tumour ≤ 2 cm, no vascular invasion
T2   Solitary tumour ≤ 2 cm, with vascular invasion; or
       Multiple tumours, one lobe, ≤ 2 cm, no vascular invasion; or
       Solitary tumour >2 cm, no vascular invasion
T3   Solitary tumour >2 cm, with vascular invasion; or
       Multiple tumours, one lobe, ≤ 2 cm, with vascular invasion; or
       Multiple tumours, one lobe, >2 cm, with/without vascular invasion
T4   Multiple tumours, both lobes; or
       Any tumour(s) involving major branch of portal or hepatic veins

Regional lymph nodes (N)
NX   Cannot be assessed
N0   No regional lymph node metastases
N1   Regional lymph node metastases

Distant metastases (M)
MX   Cannot be assessed
M0   No distant metastases
M1   Distant metastases

Stage grouping
  I   T1N0M0
  II   T2N0M0
  III   T1N1M0
        T2N1M0
        T3N0M0
        T3N1M0
  IVA T4, any N, M0
  IVB Any T, any N, M1

Surgical therapy

Resection

Standard procedures

Among various therapeutic options, surgery is the leading form of treatment because it may offer a chance of long term cure in patients with HCC.[63] In the 1970s, Western surgeons established major hepatectomy procedures for patients with large tumours,[64] while surgeons in the East, where HCC arises frequently in a cirrhotic liver, have been in a dilemma as to how to balance treatment of the tumour with preservation of remnant hepatic function. In cirrhotic patients the major cause of mortality and morbidity after hepatectomy is liver failure, and the risk rises with the volume of functional parenchyma resected. One striking Eastern experience reported postoperative liver failure in 64% of cirrhotic patients undergoing right hepatic lobectomy and in 28% of those having left lobectomy.[65] This indicates that major lobectomy should not be the procedure of choice in patients with cirrhosis.

Our clinicopathological study of resected HCC showed that the frequency of tumour thrombus in the regional portal venous branch was 15% macroscopically and 73% microscopically.[66] This finding led to speculation that HCC infiltrates the nearby portal vein and then forms intrahepatic metastases in the regional area. For this reason, limited or local resection seemed inadequate for removing all possible HCC lesions in these patients. In 1981, the concept of the subsegment, which represents the minimum surgical unit of the liver, became available clinically through the use of intraoperative ultrasonography.[67] Makuuchi's systematic subsegmentectomy[66 67] made it possible to remove the HCC-related portal domain on an anatomical basis, and to spare as much HCC-free functional parenchyma as possible (Figure 8.16). This requires intraoperative ultrasonography,

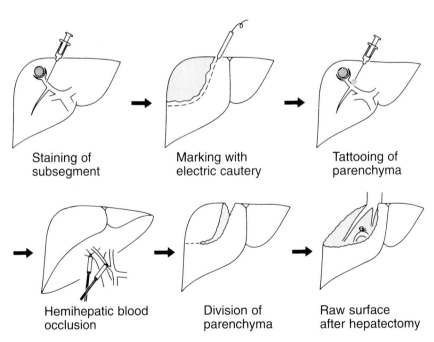

Staining of subsegment	Marking with electric cautery	Tattooing of parenchyma
Hemihepatic blood occlusion	Division of parenchyma	Raw surface after hepatectomy

FIGURE 8.16—*Operative procedure for systematic subsegmentectomy (from reference 66 with permission of* Surg Gynecol Obstet*). Under ultrasound guidance, the portal venous branch is punctured and blue dye is injected to identify the subsegment harbouring the HCC. With hemihepatic vascular occlusion, liver transection is carried out along the marked line. After subsegmentectomy, major hepatic veins that run between the subsegments can be exposed on the raw surface of the liver. (Reproduced with permission from Makuuchi et al.[66])*

which allows precise identification of the site and number of the lesions and the relationship between tumour and intrahepatic vascular systems. Because of its superior outcome to more limited resection,[68] sub-segmentectomy is our procedure of choice for patients with a small HCC and cirrhosis.

Modified procedures

The criteria for excluding patients from surgery include serious hepatic impairment, bilobar tumour dissemination, extrahepatic metastases, and tumour involvement of the great vessels. The last criterion has become a relative contraindication: recently many surgeons have been seeking new means by which HCC and involved portions of these vessels can be removed while preserving remnant liver function, even in patients with cirrhosis. In cirrhotic patients, radical resection of HCC that involves the root of the right hepatic vein is less practicable because right hepatic lobectomy may cause postoperative liver failure. As an alternative, Makuuchi *et al*[69] proposed resection of segments 7 and 8 including the right hepatic vein, while preserving segment 6, which could be drained by the inferior right hepatic vein.[70] Besides this, three new procedures based on the same policy were introduced. As the most extensive procedure, subtotal hepatectomy that would leave only segment 6 was reported by Baer *et al.*[71] In cases without this accessory vein, Nakamura *et al* recommended reconstruction of the right hepatic vein with an autograft to save segment 6.[72] They confirmed experimentally the need for venous drainage to preserve the function of the segment in the remnant liver. Patients in both series had an uneventful postoperative course.

The inferior vena cava may be involved most frequently by HCC that originates in the caudate lobe. Surgery is seldom indicated in this situation. Takayama *et al* demonstrated the successful resection of caudate tumours that involved the vena cava using combined left and caudate lobectomies with or without resection of the vena cava.[73 74] Recently, Sauvanet *et al* reported ex situ resection of a caudate tumour with prosthetic caval replacement and reimplantation of the three hepatic veins.[75] In those cases, evidence of lack of cirrhosis allowed an associated hepatic lobectomy, which greatly facilitated the radical resection. For cirrhotics, however, the authors have reported various procedures smaller than segmentectomies that allow safe resection of caudate tumours, while preserving sufficient functional parenchyma.[76–78]

The presence of tumour thrombus of HCC in the portal vein trunk seems a contraindication to operation, especially in patients with cirrhosis; however, Kumada *et al* reported a series of aggressive procedures by which more than one segment having primary HCC tumour and concomitant thrombi in the portal trunk were removed, and about half of the patients had a cirrhotic liver.[79]

Using or adopting transplantation techniques, Pichlmayr *et al* described a new technique of ex vivo hepatic operation, which was applied to the patients with tumours otherwise deemed unresectable by conventional procedures.[80] Extracorporeal tumour resection on a side table was undertaken using hypothermic preservation and followed by autotransplantation of the remnant part of the liver. The authors suggest that hepatic tumours not compromising global hepatic function or causing cholestasis would be suitable conditions. The assessment of its final therapeutic value requires further experience.

Cryosurgery has been advocated as an alternative to resection for HCC.[81] With this technique, liquid nitrogen is circulated through a metal probe placed on/in the tumour, and each freezing time takes about 15 minutes. This has generally been reserved for patients with unresectable HCC, although it can be used in combination with resection or other techniques. The actual five year survival rates are around 10%. Cryosurgery may be a useful adjunct to resection or palliation, but its role as the first choice of treatment is difficult to interpret because of the multiple combinations of the treatment applied.

Follow up results

The survival rates after hepatic resection for HCC (Table 8.4)[82–95] and for small HCC of less than 5 cm (Table 8.5)[61 68 82 96–100] are summarised. Most recent series after the mid-1980s have reported a one year survival rate of between 56 and 87% and a five year survival rate of between 25 and 44%. A nation based Japanese study demonstrated one, three, and five year survivals of 67, 40, and 29% in 2174 consecutive resected cases,[88] which may represent an average outcome in Japan. Cirrhosis was the background in half or more of these patients.

Perioperative mortality limited to 10% or less was achieved by all teams. Although the results vary among authors, it is obvious that the survival rate is much better for small HCC: one year survival exceeds 80% in all of five Eastern reports, and five year survival is over 40% in most reports, and 60% in two reports from China. These excellent outcomes for small HCC emphasise the importance of detecting small lesions, and of precise and safe resection. How to achieve a still better prognosis for cirrhotic patients with small HCC is a matter for discussion. As to the optimal procedure, Table 8.5 demonstrates two series in which survival rates achieved by different operative procedures were compared. Kanematsu *et al* failed to find any difference between standard and limited resection,[96] while our series showed a superior outcome after subsegmentectomy compared with outcome after limited resection.[68] The prognostic factors after hepatic resection for HCC, such as tumour size, capsular infiltration,

TABLE 8.4—*Overall survival rate after resection of HCC*

Author	Country	Year	Cases resected	With cirrhosis (%)	Operative mortality (%)	Survival rate (%)		
						1 year	3 years	5 years
Wu[82]	China	1986	283	78	4	60	40	26
Lee[83]	Taiwan	1986	109	64	3	84	52	28
Nagao[84]	Japan	1987	94	75	11	73	42	25
Sesto[85]	USA	1987	22		8		50	33
Iwatsuki[86]	USA	1988	67	46	7	76	49	25
Chen[87]	Taiwan	1989	120	74	4	56		26
LCSGJ*[88]	Japan	1990	2174	80	4	67	40	29
Yamanaka[89]	Japan	1990	295	67		76	44	31
Tsuzuki[90]	Japan	1990	119	63	9		47	39
Kosuge[91]	Japan	1993	480		2	87	63	44
Tang[92]	China	1993	314			86	68	61
Nagasue[93]	Japan	1993	229	77	7	80	51	26
Gozzetti[94]	Italy	1993	168	69	8		57	36
Bismuth[95]	France	1993	60	100	10	90	52	

* Liver Cancer Study Group of Japan.

Table 8.5—*Survival rate after resection of HCC smaller than 5 cm*

Author	Country	Year	Cases resected	With cirrhosis (%)	Operative mortality (%)	Survival rate (%)		
						1 year	3 years	5 years
Kanematsu[96]	Japan	1984						
Standard*			13		15	79		23
Limited			37		11	80		33
Wu[82]	China	1986	65	78	4	83	74	64
Li[97]	China	1986	23	79	9	90	71	41
Tang[98]	China	1989	132	90	2	92	76	63
Franco[99]	France	1990	50			67	42	
Makuuchi[68]	Japan	1991						
Subseg*			87		0·8	86	61	45
Limited			168		0·8	89	58	30
Paquet[100]	Germany	1991	23	100	13	77	66	49
Makuuchi[61]	Japan	1993	349	74	2	90	66	44

* Hepatectomy procedures: standard resection, limited resection, and subsegmentectomy.

portal vein invasion, and intrahepatic metastasis, are accepted as significant.[61] Others, including tumour number, surgical procedure, and surgical margin, remain controversial.

Transplantation

Orthotopic liver transplantation appears to be a rational form of therapy for patients with HCC. Indeed, patients who have undergone liver transplantation for severe cirrhosis, and in whom incidental HCC is found in the removed liver, have an excellent prognosis,[10] and Bismuth *et al*[95] have proposed the so called 3-3 rule, which means that transplantation may offer good outcomes in patients with HCC no more than 3 cm in diameter and with less than three nodules. In this context, patients with small HCC and severe cirrhosis may be suitable candidates for transplantation; however, patients with diseases accepted as good indications take priority for transplants, ahead of patients with HCC. Severe hepatic dysfunction and multifocal or bilobar HCC are strong factors favouring transplantation over hepatic resection;[101] however, long term results in such indications are disappointing, with recurrence rates as high as 65% and overall survival rate at 3 years of 30%.[101] At present, whether patients with small HCC should be listed as candidates for transplantation depends on organ availability in each clinical situation.

Recommendations for surgical management

Among the many available treatment options, surgery has played the greatest role in treating patients with HCC. Improved techniques have led to increasing resectability, decreasing operative mortality, and improving long term survival. In the 1980s, Eastern surgeons sought a reasonable strategy for resection of HCC in patients with cirrhosis. The proposed criteria for surgery select suitable patients and procedures, thereby minimising fatal liver failure after hepatectomy. Our evidence of superior efficacy of ultrasonically guided subsegmentectomy compared with limited resection has underlined the importance of anatomical resection of the relevant portal domain in the treatment of small HCC. Other efforts to render resectable initially unresectable tumours are being evaluated, but may aid only a lucky minority. Western surgeons have demonstrated that liver transplantation is a rational treatment form in some of these patients, but its role remains limited. The authors recommend early diagnosis by screening and anatomical resection of small HCC as the most reasonable treatment option for patients with cirrhosis until controlled studies provide objective information. The frequent recurrence of HCC seen after otherwise curative surgical treatment remains a crucial unresolved issue.[102]

Radiochemotherapy

There is no convincing evidence that external beam radiotherapy has any role to play in the primary or adjuvant therapy of HCC other than for occasional palliative use to reduce hepatic capsular pain in patients with advanced disease. An interesting development is of glass microspheres, 40 μm in diameter, with yttrium-90 attached irreversibly to their surface. It is possible to deliver these microspheres via the hepatic artery, either through an indwelling catheter or via a Seldinger technique, and manipulate tumour blood flow, with vasoactive drugs like angiotensin 2, to increase cancer delivery selectively. The results of trials with these new agents are awaited with interest.[103]

5-Fluorouracil, doxorubicin, mitomycin C, and cisplatin have been shown to have significant effects on tumour shrinkage when administered to HCC patients by the IHA route, but do not have convincing survival benefits. In Japan there has been considerable interest in a macromolecular polymer (SMANCS) combining the anticancer drug neocarzinostatin with the block copolymer of stearic and maleic acids. This polymer is solubilised in the contrast medium lipoidol and has an additional targeting effect in that tumours tend to have a disorganised and leaky vasculature and deficient lymphatic drainage, which leads to accumulation of certain macromolecules within the tumour interstitium. Maeda and coworkers have developed a rational dosing regimen for SMANCS based on tumour uptake as assessed by lipoidol trapping, as demonstrated on a hepatic CT scan performed 7–10 days after drug injection.[104] A multi-institutional phase II study of IHA SMANCS in the treatment of HCC was performed in Japan, accruing more than 200 patients. It was found that patients with no active cirrhosis, and tumour involving no more than two segments of the liver, had a 50% chance of survival for five years after a median of four injections of SMANCS. The survival trends after SMANCS therapy in this large phase II trial require further validation in randomised phase III studies and SMANCS should be tested in Western patients.

Most conventional cytotoxic drugs have undergone phase II trial evaluation, alone or in combination. None of these, including 5FU, cisplatin, mitomycin C, etoposide, and mitoxantrone, have shown significant worth (i.e. consistent tumour response rate of more than 20% and/or survival benefit), and although there is a lingering myth that doxorubicin as single agent has useful activity, following from an initially promising African trial, this has not been confirmed by subsequent studies.

There is little justification for the use of systemic chemotherapy in the treatment of this condition unless the patient has been entered in a clinical trial.

Novel therapeutic strategies

Modulation of drug resistance

P glycoprotein (P-gp) is a membrane glycoprotein which, when expressed by cancer cells, can confer resistance to a wide range of cytotoxic drugs.

P-gp functions as a multidrug transporter with a relatively broad spectrum of activity. HCC cells have been shown to express high levels of P-gp using molecular and immunocytochemical methods and it is possible that elevated P-gp expression at least partially explains the relative resistance of HCC to conventional antineoplastic agents. A number of inhibitors of P-gp have been described and drugs such as verapamil, quinidine, and cyclosporin A can bind to P-gp and reverse the multidrug resistant phenotype in vitro. Early clinical trials combining standard chemotherapy with P-gp modulators have shown promising results in the treatment of myeloma and leukaemia.[105]

It is conceptually attractive to consider combining hepatic arterial infusion of doxorubicin and a P-gp blocker like verapamil as this could sensitise the HCC cells to the chemotherapeutic agent, and verapamil would have the added advantage of increasing the ratio of tumour:normal blood flow by virtue of its vasodilatory properties and therefore increasing tumour drug delivery.

Gene therapy

Given the extraordinary increase in the availability of molecular technologies, the prospect of gene therapy, whereby a structural gene is introduced into the genome of the cancer cell with therapeutic intent, has reached the realm of the clinical trial—for example, it is possible to insert genes that code for bacterial enzymes such as cytosine deaminase into an adenovirus or retrovirus. Cytosine deaminase is not produced by mammalian cells but if it can be introduced into cancer cells via the virus and then expressed, the enzyme is capable of converting an inactive prodrug (5-flucytosine) to the active, cytotoxic species (5FU) within the microenvironment of the tumour. The key to virally directed enzyme prodrug therapy (VDEPT) is to build in an element of tumour cell selectivity in terms of enzyme expression. Of HCCs, 70–80% express the oncofetal antigen AFP and viral constructs have been made that linked the promoter sequence for AFP to the gene for cytosine deaminase.[106] Subsequent experiments have shown that the bacterial enzyme is only expressed in

AFP positive cells after viral infections. One could envisage a clinical trial combining hepatic arterial infusion of viral particles followed after an interval by the inactive prodrug 5-flucytosine. The hypothesis to be tested would be that selective expression of cytosine deaminase in HCC would generate very high local concentrations of 5FU, which could lead to useful antitumour activity with acceptable toxicity.

References

1 Verbeek PCM, Leeuwen J, Wit LT, *et al.* Benign fibrosing disease at hepatic confluence mimicking Klatskin tumors. *Surgery* 1992;**112**:866–71.

2 Bismuth H, Corlette MB. Intrahepatic cholangioenteric anastomosis in carcinoma of the hilus of the liver. *Surg Gynecol Obstet* 1975;**140**:170–8.

3 Kurzawinski T, Deery A, Davidson BR. Diagnostic value of cytology for biliary stricture. *Br J Surg* 1993;**80**:414–21.

4 Siegel JH. *Endoscopic retrograde cholangio-pancreatography: technique, diagnosis and therapy.* New York: Raven Press, 1992.

5 Davids PHP, Groen AK, Rauws EAJ, *et al.* Randomised trial of self-expanding metal stents versus polyethylene stents for distal malignant biliary obstruction. *Lancet* 1992;**ii**: 1488–92.

6 Martin DF. Combined percutaneous and endoscopic procedures for bile duct obstruction. *Gut* 1994;**35**:1011–2.

7 Brown G, Mayers N. The hepatic duct. A surgical approach for resection of tumor. *Aust N Z J Surg* 1954;**23**:308–12.

8 Klatskin G. Adenocarcinoma of the hepatic duct and its bifurcation within the porta hepatis: an unusual tumor with distinctive clinical and pathological features. *Am J Med* 1965;**38**:241–56.

9 Boerma EJ. Research into the results of resection of hilar bile duct cancer. *Surgery* 1990; **108**:572–80.

10 Iwatsuki S, Gordon RD, Shaw BW, *et al.* Role of liver transplantation in cancer therapy. *Ann Surg* 1985;**202**:401–7.

11 Ogura Y, Mizumoto R, Tabata M, Matsuda S, Kusada T. Surgical treatment of carcinoma of the hepatic duct confluence: analysis of 55 resected carcinomas. *World J Surg* 1993; **17**:85–93.

12 Miyagawa S, Makuuchi M, Kawasaki S. Outcome of extended right hepatectomy after biliary drainage in hilar bile duct cancer. *Arch Surg* 1995;**130**:759–63.

13 Makuuchi M, Thai BL, Takayasu K, *et al.* Preoperative portal embolization to increase safety of major hepatectomy for hilar bile duct carcinoma: preliminary report. *Surgery* 1990;**107**:521–7.

14 Kawasaki S, Makuuchi M, Miyagawa S, *et al.* Radical operation after portal embolization for tumor of hilar bile duct. *J Am Coll Surg* 1994;**178**:480–6.

15 Iwatsuki S, Shaw BW Jr, Starzl E. Experience with 150 liver resections. *Ann Surg* 1983; **197**:247–53.

16 Kortz WJ, Meyers WC, Hanks JB, *et al.* Hepatic resection for metastatic cancer. *Ann Surg* 1984;**199**:182–6.

17 Gazzaniga GM, Cogolo LA, Ciferri E, *et al.* Liver surgery for metastases: clinical results. *J Surg Oncol* 1991;**2**(suppl):59–62.

18 Sugihara K, Hojo K, Moriya Y, *et al.* Pattern of recurrence after hepatic resection for colorectal metastases. *Br J Surg* 1993;**80**:1032–5.

19 Scheele J, Stangl R, Altendorf-Hofmann A. Hepatic metastases from colorectal carcinoma: impact of surgical resection on the natural history. *Br J Surg* 1990;**77**:1241–6.

20 Cady B, Stone MD. The role of surgical resection of liver metastases in colorectal carcinoma. *Semin Oncol* 1991;**18**:399–406.

21 Brown G, Mayers N. The hepatic duct. A surgical approach for resection of tumor. *Aust NZ J Surg* 1954;**23**:308–12.
22 Klatskin G. Adenocarcinoma of the hepatic duct and its bifurcation within the porta hepatis: an unusual tumor with distinctive clinical and pathological features. *Am J Med* 1965;**38**:241–56.
23 Benomark S, Haestrom L. The natural history of primary and secondary malignant tumour of the liver. *Cancer* 1969;**23**:198–202.
24 Amin Z, Bown SG, Lees WR. Local treatment of colorectal liver metastases: a comparison of interstitial laser photocoagulation (ILP) and percutaneous alcohol insertion (PAI). *Clin Radiol* 1993;**48**:166–71.
25 Iwatsuki S, Esquivel CO, Gordon RD, *et al.* Liver resection for metastatic colorectal cancer. *Surgery* 1986;**100**:804–10.
26 Ekberg H, Tranberg K, Andersson R, *et al.* Pattern of recurrence in liver resection for colorectal metastases. *World J Surg* 1987;**1**:541–7.
27 Scheele J, Stangl R, Altendorf-Hofmann A, *et al.* Indicators of prognosis after hepatic resection for colorectal secondaries. *Surgery* 1991;**110**:13–29.
28 Steele G Jr, Bleday R, Mayer RJ, *et al.* A prospective evaluation of hepatic resection for colorectal carcinoma metastases to the liver: gastrointestinal study group protocol 6584. *J Clin Oncol* 1991; **9**:1105–12.
29 Doci R, Gennari L, Bignami P, *et al.* One hundred patients with hepatic metastases from colorectal cancer treated by resection: analysis of prognostic determinants. *Br J Surg* 1991;**78**:797–801.
30 Hughes K, Scheele J, Sugarbaker PH. Surgery for colorectal cancer metastatic to the liver. *Surg Clin North Am* 1989;**69**:339–59.
31 Scheele J. Hepatectomy for liver metastases. *Br J Surg* 1993;**80**:274–6.
32 Yamamoto J, Sugihara K, Kosuge T, *et al.* Pathological support for limited hepatectomy in the treatment of liver metastases from colorectal cancer. *Ann Surg* (in press).
33 Elis D, Lasser PH, Hoang JM, *et al.* Repeat hepatectomy for cancer. *Br J Surg* 1993;**80**: 1557–62.
34 Kakazu T, Makuuchi M, Kawasaki S, *et al.* Repeat hepatic resection for recurrent hepatocellular carcinoma. *Hepatogastroenterology* 1993;**40**:337–41.
35 Ravikumar TS, Kane R, Cady B, *et al.* A 5-year study of cryosurgery in the treatment of liver tumors. *Arch Surg* 1991;**126**:1520–3.
36 Collins JM. Pharmacologic rationale for regional drug delivery. *J Clin Oncol* 1984;**2**: 498–504.
37 Sullivan RD, Zurek WZ. Chemotherapy for liver cancer by protracted ambulatory infusion. *JAMA* 1965;**194**:481–6.
38 Kemeny N, Daily J, Reichman B, *et al.* Intrahepatic or systemic infusion of fluorodeoxyuridine in patients with liver metastases from colorectal carcinoma. *Ann Intern Med* 1987;**107**:459–65.
39 Chang AE, Schneider PD, Sugarbaker PH, *et al.* A prospective randomized trial of regional versus systemic continuous 5-fluorodeoxyuridine chemotherapy in the treatment of colorectal liver metastases. *Ann Surg* 1987;**206**:685–93.
40 Hohn D, Stagg R, Friedman M, *et al.* A randomized trial of continuous intravenous versus hepatic arterial floxuridine in patients with colorectal cancer metastatic to the liver. *J Clin Oncol* 1989;7:1646–54.
41 Martin JK Jr, O'Connell MJ, Wieland HS, *et al.* Intra-arterial floxuridine vs systemic fluorouracil for hepatic metastases from colorectal cancer. *Arch Surg* 1990;**125**:1022–6.
42 Rougier P, Laplanche A, Huguier M, *et al.* Hepatic arterial infusion of floxuridine in patients with liver metastases from colorectal carcinoma: long term results of a prospective randomized trial. *J Clin Oncol* 1992;**10**:1112–8.
43 Kemeny N, Seiter K, Niedzwiecki D, *et al.* A randomized trial of intrahepatic infusion of fluorodeoxyuridine with dexamethasone versus fluorodeoxyuridine alone in the treatment of metastatic colorectal cancer. *Cancer* 1992;**69**:327–34.
44 Stagg RJ, Venook AP, Chase JL, *et al.* Alternating hepatic intra-arterial floxuridine and fluorouracil: a less toxic regimen for treatment of liver metastases from colorectal cancer. *J Natl Cancer Inst* 1991;**83**:423–8.

45 Sugihara K. Continuous hepatic arterial infusion of 5-fluorouracil for unresectable colorectal liver metastases: phase II study. *Surgery* (in press).

46 Kemeny N, Conti JA, Sigurdson E, *et al.* A pilot study of hepatic artery floxuridine combined with systemic 5-fluorouracil and leucovorin. *Cancer* 1993;**71**:1964–71.

47 Poon MA, O'Connell MJ, Moertel CG, *et al.* Biochemical modulation of fluorouracil: evidence of significant improvement of survival and quality of life in patients with advanced colorectal carcinoma. *J Clin Oncol* 1989;**7**:1407–17.

48 Petrelli N, Douglass HO Jr, Herrera L, *et al.* The modulation of fluorouracil with leucovorin in metastatic colorectal carcinoma: a prospective randomized phase III trial. *J Clin Oncol* 1989;**7**:1419–26.

49 Munoz N, Bosch X. Epidemiology of hepatocellular carcinoma. In: Okuda K, Ishak KG, eds. *Neoplasms of the liver.* Tokyo: Springer, 1987:3–19.

50 Okuda K. Hepatocellular carcinoma: recent progress. *Hepatology* 1992;**15**:948–63.

51 Maraj R, Kew MC, Hyslop RJ. Resectability rate of hepatocellular carcinoma in rural southern Africans. *Br J Surg* 1988;**75**:335–8.

52 Colombo M, de Franchis R, del Ninno E, *et al.* Hepatocellular carcinoma in Italian patients with cirrhosis. *N Engl J Med* 1991;**325**:675–80.

53 Oka H, Kurioka N, Kim K, *et al.* Prospective study of early detection of hepatocellular carcinoma in patients with cirrhosis. *Hepatology* 1990;**12**:680–7.

54 McMahon BJ, London T. Workshop on screening for hepatocellular carcinoma. *J Natl Cancer Inst* 1991;**83**:916–9.

55 Takayasu K, Moriyama N, Muramatsu Y, *et al.* The diagnosis of small hepatocellular carcinomas: efficacy of various imaging procedures in 100 patients. *Am J Roentgenol* 1990;**155**:49–54.

56 Makuuchi M. Intraoperative ultrasonography for hepatic surgery. In: Makuuchi M, ed. *Abdominal intraoperative ultrasonography.* Tokyo: Igaku-shoin, 1987:89–123.

57 Nakakuma K, Tashiro S, Hiraoka T, *et al.* Hepatocellular carcinoma and metastatic cancer detected by iodized oil. *Radiology* 1985;**154**:15–7.

58 Takayama T, Makuuchi M, Hirohashi S, *et al.* Malignant transformation of adenomatous hyperplasia to hepatocellular carcinoma. *Lancet* 1990;**336**:1150–3.

59 Shimizu S, Takayama T, Kosuge T, *et al.* Benign tumors of the liver resected because of a diagnosis of malignancy. *Surg Gynecol Obstet* 1992;**174**:403–7.

60 UICC International Union against Cancer. Digestive system tumours, liver. In: Hermanek P, Sobin LH, eds. *TNM classification of malignant tumours.* 4th ed. Berlin: Springer, 1987:53–5.

61 Makuuchi M, Kosuge T, Takayama T, *et al.* Surgery for small liver cancers. *Semin Surg Oncol* 1993;**9**:298–304.

62 Fan ST, Lo CM, Lai ECS, *et al.* Perioperative nutritional support in patients undergoing hepatectomy for hepatocellular carcinoma. *N Engl J Med* 1994;**331**:1547–52.

63 Okuda K, Obata H, Nakajima Y, *et al.* Prognosis of primary hepatocellular carcinoma. *Hepatology* 1984;**4**(suppl):3–6.

64 Fortner JG, Maclean BJ, Kim DK, *et al.* The seventies evolution in liver surgery for cancer. *Cancer* 1981;**47**:2162–6.

65 Lin TY. Resectional therapy for primary malignant hepatic tumors. In: Murphy GP, ed. *International advances in surgical oncology.* New York: Alan R Liss, 1979:25–54.

66 Makuuchi M, Hasegawa H, Yamazaki S. Ultrasonically guided subsegmentectomy. *Surg Gynecol Obstet* 1985;**161**:346–50.

67 Makuuchi M, Hasegawa H, Yamazaki S. Intraoperative ultrasonic examination for hepatectomy. *Jpn J Clin Oncol* 1981;**11**:367–90.

68 Makuuchi M, Takayama T, Kosuge T, *et al.* The value of ultrasonography for hepatic surgery. *Hepatogastroenterology* 1991;**38**:64–70.

69 Makuuchi M, Hasegawa H, Yamazaki S, *et al.* Four new hepatectomy procedures for resection of the right hepatic vein and preservation of the inferior right hepatic vein. *Surg Gynecol Obstet* 1987;**164**:68–72.

70 Makuuchi M, Hasegawa H, Yamazaki S, *et al.* The inferior right hepatic vein: ultrasonic demonstration. *Radiology* 1983;**148**:213–7.

297

71 Baer HU, Dennison AR, Maddern GJ, *et al.* Subtotal hepatectomy: a new procedure based on the inferior right hepatic vein. *Br J Surg* 1991;**78**:1221–2.

72 Nakamura S, Sakaguchi S, Hachiya T, *et al.* Significance of hepatic vein reconstruction in hepatectomy. *Surgery* 1993;**114**:59–64.

73 Takayama T, Makuuchi M, Takayasu K, *et al.* Resection after intraarterial chemotherapy of a hepatoblastoma originating in the caudate lobe. *Surgery* 1990;**107**:231–5.

74 Takayama T, Makuuchi M, Kosuge T, *et al.* A hepatoblastoma originating in the caudate lobe radically resected with the inferior vena cava. *Surgery* 1991;**109**:208–13.

75 Sauvanet A, Dousset B, Belghiti J. A simplified technique of ex situ hepatic surgical treatment. *J Am Coll Surg* 1994;**178**:79–81.

76 Makuuchi M, Kawasaki S, Takayama T, *et al.* Caudate lobectomy. In: Lygidakis NJ, Makuuchi M, eds. *Pitfalls and complications in the diagnosis and management of hepatobiliary and pancreatic diseases.* Stuttgart: Thieme, 1993:124–32.

77 Takayama T, Tanaka T, Higaki T, *et al.* High dorsal resection of the liver. *J Am Coll Surg* 1994;**179**:72–5.

78 Yamamato J, Takayama T, Kosuge T, *et al.* An isolated caudate lobectomy by the transhepatic approach for hepatocellular carcinoma in cirrhotic liver. *Surgery* 1992;**111**:699–702.

79 Kumada K, Ozawa K, Okamoto R, *et al.* Hepatic resection for advanced hepatocellular carcinoma with removal of portal vein tumor thrombi. *Surgery* 1990;**108**:821–7.

80 Pichlmayr R, Grosse H, Hauss J, *et al.* Technique and preliminary results of extracorporeal liver surgery (bench procedure) and of surgery on the in situ perfused liver. *Br J Surg* 1990;**77**:21–6.

81 Zhou XD, Tang ZU, Yu YQ, *et al.* Clinical evaluation of cryosurgery in the treatment of primary liver cancer: report of 60 cases. *Cancer* 1988;**61**:1889–92.

82 Wu MC, Zhang XH, Chen H. Hepatic resection for primary liver cancer. *Chin Med J* 1986;**99**:175–80.

83 Lee CS, Sung JL, Hwang LU, *et al.* Surgical treatment of 109 patients with symptomatic and asymptomatic hepatocellular carcinoma. *Surgery* 1986;**99**:481–90.

84 Nagao T, Inoue S, Goto S, *et al.* Hepatic resection for hepatocellular carcinoma: clinical features and long term prognosis. *Ann Surg* 1987;**205**:33–40.

85 Sesto ME, Vogt DP, Hermann RE. Hepatic resection in 128 patients: a 24 year experience. *Surgery* 1987;**102**:846–51.

86 Iwatsuki S, Starzl TE. Personal experience with 411 hepatic resections. *Ann Surg* 1988;**208**:421–34.

87 Chen MF, Hwang TL, Jeng LBB, *et al.* Hepatic resection in 120 patients with hepatocellular carcinoma. *Arch Surg* 1989;**124**:1025–8.

88 The Liver Cancer Study Group of Japan. Primary liver cancer in Japan: clinicopathologic features and results of surgical treatment. *Ann Surg* 1990;**211**:277–87.

89 Yamanaka N, Okamoto E, Toyosaka A, *et al.* Prognostic factors after hepatectomy for hepatocellular carcinomas: a univariate and multivariate analysis. *Cancer* 1990;**65**:1104–10.

90 Tsuzuki T, Sugioka A, Ueda M, *et al.* Hepatic resection for hepatocellular carcinoma. *Surgery* 1990;**107**:511–20.

91 Kosuge T, Makuuchi M, Takayama T, *et al.* Long-term results after resection of hepatocellular carcinoma: experience of 480 cases. *Hepatogastroenterology* 1993;**40**:328–32.

92 Tang ZY, Yu YQ, Zhou XD, *et al.* Subclinical hepatocellular carcinoma: an analysis of 391 patients. *J Surg Oncol* 1993;**3**(suppl):55–8.

93 Nagasue N, Kohno H, Chang YC, *et al.* Liver resection for hepatocellular carcinoma: results of 229 consecutive patients during 11 years. *Ann Surg* 1993;**217**:375–84.

94 Gozzetti G, Mazziotti A, Luca Grazi G, *et al.* Surgical experience with 168 primary liver cell carcinomas treated with hepatic resection. *J Surg Oncol* 1993;**3**(suppl):59–61.

95 Bismuth H, Chiche L, Adam R, *et al.* Liver resection versus transplantation for hepatocellular carcinoma in cirrhotic patients. *Ann Surg* 1993;**218**:145–51.

96 Kanematsu T, Takenaka K, Matsumata T, *et al.* Limited hepatic resection effective for selected cirrhotic patients with primary liver cancer. *Ann Surg* 1984;**199**:51–6.

 97 Li GH, Li JQ, Zhou YQ. Surgical treatment of small primary liver carcinoma. *Chin Med J* 1986;**99**:827–8.

 98 Tang ZY, Yu YQ, Zhou XD, *et al*. Surgery of small hepatocellular carcinoma: analysis of 144 cases. *Cancer* 1989;**64**:536–41.

 99 Franco D, Capussotti L, Smadja C, *et al*. Resection of hepatocellular carcinomas: results in 72 European patients with cirrhosis. *Gastroenterology* 1990;**98**:733–8.

100 Paquet KJ, Koussouris P, Mercado MA, *et al*. Limited hepatic resection for selected cirrhotic patients with hepatocellular or cholangiocellular carcinoma: a prospective study. *Br J Surg* 1991;**78**:459–62.

101 Farmer DG, Rosove MH, Shaked A, *et al*. Current treatment modalities for hepatocellular carcinoma. *Ann Surg* 1994;**219**:236–47.

102 Belghiti J, Panis Y, Farges O, *et al*. Intrahepatic recurrence after resection of hepatocellular carcinoma complicating cirrhosis. *Ann Surg* 1991;**214**:114–7.

103 Anderson JH, Goldberg JA, Bessent RG, *et al*. Glass yttrium 90 microspheres for patients with colorectal liver metastases. *Radiother Oncol* 1992;**25**:137–9.

104 Maeda H. SMANCS and polymer conjugated macromolecular drugs: advantages in cancer chemotherapy. *Adv Drug Deliv Rev* 1991;**6**:181–202.

105 Ferry D, Kerr DJ. Multidrug resistance in cancer. *BMJ* 1994;**308**:148–9.

106 Huber BE, Richards CA, Krenitsky TA. Retroviral mediated gene therapy for the treatment of hepatocellular cancer: an innovative approach for cancer therapy. *Proc Natl Acad Sci USA* 1991;**88**:8039–43.

9: Endocrine tumours

DONAL O'SHEA, STEPHEN R BLOOM, and
ROBIN C N WILLIAMSON

Gastrointestinal neuroendocrine tumours originate from a common cell type. They present widely variable and sometimes dramatic clinical syndromes. They run an unpredictable course, and only curative resection has been shown to alter the outcome of the disease. Palliative treatment, which may include chemotherapy, hepatic arterial embolisation, or somatostatin analogue therapy, can provide prolonged symptom free survival.[1][2]

In this chapter, the epidemiology and clinical features of the different tumours and the general principles that guide management decisions will be reviewed.

Epidemiology

Gut neuroendocrine tumours (gastroenteropancreatic tumours, gut hormone tumours) are rare. The annual incidence is about 1 in 500 000 for pancreatic islet cell tumours (gastrinomas, insulinomas, vipomas, glucagonomas, somatostatinomas, other hormone secreting neoplasms, and non-functioning tumours) and 1 in 500 000 for tumours associated with the carcinoid syndrome.

Pancreatic endocrine tumours

These tumours were originally described as apudomas because it was thought that they had a common origin from neural crest cells with the ability to perform amine precursor uptake and decarboxylation. This theory has since been disproved, and it has been proposed that the neuroendocrine and mucosal endocrine cells of the gastroenteropancreatic axis are derived from a common bipotential stem cell.

The genetic basis for the development of sporadic pancreatic endocrine tumours remains largely unknown. Gastrinomas and insulinomas are the most common manifestations of multiple endocrine neoplasia type I (MEN I), in which allelic deletion in the q13 region of chromosome 11 is found;

loss of heterozygosity for this region has been demonstrated in some patients with sporadic gastrinoma and insulinoma. Twenty five per cent of pancreatic islet cell tumours are associated with the MEN I syndrome, and 45% of these are malignant.[3] The remaining 75% are sporadic, and 70% of these are malignant.

Islet cells are pluripotential with respect to peptide production. Some 70% of tumours are associated with elevated pancreatic polypeptide levels. In a small proportion of cases other hormones, particularly gastrin, may become elevated and cause secondary syndromes during the course of the disease. Altered processing of peptide precursor molecules may result in a variety of molecular weight forms of the same peptide being secreted. This fact can have clinical implications: for example, large molecular forms of glucagon (enteroglucagon) can cause villous hypertrophy and prolonged intestinal transit times. Large forms of somatostatin have been reported to cause hypoglycaemia, rather than the hyperglycaemia usually associated with the somatostatinoma syndrome. Not all the immunoreactive peptide is bioactive.

Carcinoid tumours

The annual incidence of the carcinoid syndrome is about 1 in 500 000. The term carcinoid was first used by Obendorfer in 1907 to describe a carcinoma-like lesion without malignant qualities. It is now used to describe tumours containing or producing serotonin (5-hydroxytryptamine, 5HT). Several different cell types either synthesise or take up 5HT. The term carcinoid is applied to a variety of malignant tumours, with different biological behaviour, grouped by their similar histology.

Primary gastrointestinal carcinoid tumours are derived from the embryonic foregut (thyroid, bronchus, stomach, common bile duct, and pancreas), midgut, or hindgut. The most common sites for carcinoid tumours are the appendix, ileum, and rectum, but these tumours are often found incidentally on histological examination of gastrointestinal biopsy specimens. These tumours are almost always benign. Rectal tumours are often multicentric and even when they metastasise are rarely associated with the carcinoid syndrome. The carcinoid syndrome occurs in about 10% of patients with carcinoid tumours. It does not develop when the tumour drains through a normal liver, and so midgut tumours have almost always metastasised, usually to the liver, before symptoms develop. The carcinoid syndrome is most commonly due to a metastatic midgut tumour, about 50% of which metastasise to the liver. Primary carcinoid tumours are bronchial in origin in about 10% of cases, and rarely occur in the ovary and testis. Tumours in these sites may be associated with the syndrome in the absence of metastases because they drain directly to the systemic circulation and not through the portal venous system.

Clinical presentation and diagnosis

The clinical presentation is dependent on the type and amount of hormone being produced. The diagnosis of specific syndromes is based on the demonstration of elevated levels of the relevant hormone. Different antisera, which may identify alternative hormone forms, are used by various laboratories. Results cannot therefore be standardised, although there is consistency in the order of magnitude of hormone levels.

Confirmation of the diagnosis can be provided by immunohistochemical analysis of a resection specimen or liver biopsy. The histological appearance is characteristic. The tumour cells are usually cuboidal, with a normal chromatic nucleus and well developed eosinophilic cytoplasm, and cells are arranged in nests, trabeculae, or glandular structures. Features suggesting malignancy such as cytologic atypia, perineural infiltration, or invasion of blood vessels, are rarely found, and permeation of lymphatics or blood vessels by these tumours does not correlate with malignant potential.

Clinical syndromes

Pancreatic islet cell tumours

Non-functioning tumours

These tumours by definition are not associated with a recognised hormonal syndrome but they account for up to half of all pancreatic endocrine tumours. They usually present late with symptoms attributable to tumour bulk, such as anorexia and weight loss, or to effects on local structures, such as obstructive jaundice or intestinal obstruction or haemorrhage. They are often mistakenly diagnosed as adenocarcinomas, but the presence of elevated circulating gut hormones, such as pancreatic polypeptide or neurotensin, and the use of immunocytochemical analysis can point to the correct diagnosis. Other clues to the fact that a pancreatic mass may be a neuroendocrine tumour rather than the more common ductal carcinoma are substantial size, slow growth, calcification, and marked vascularity on imaging (contrast enhanced computed tomography (CT) or angiography). Non-functioning tumours usually respond poorly to chemotherapy. Debulking surgery or hepatic embolisation may be beneficial. They have a relatively poor prognosis as a result of their late presentation and lack of response to therapy, although prolonged survival is possible in the presence of metastases, unlike survival in pancreatic adenocarcinoma.

Gastrinoma

Gastrinomas have an incidence of 1 in 500 000. Although many are extremely slow growing, they are usually malignant. At time of diagnosis,

50% of patients have metastases and up to 30% of patients have the MEN I syndrome. The majority of tumours are pancreatic, but between 20 and 40% are duodenal and these are usually microadenomas, as little as 1 mm in diameter. Sporadic duodenal microgastrinomas are solitary. In those patients with MEN I they are usually multiple and associated with pancreatic microadenomas. Primary lymph node gastrinomas have been described but these probably represent metastases from duodenal microgastrinomas.

The gastrinoma syndrome was first described in 1955 by Zollinger and Ellison, who reported the triad of fulminating ulcer diathesis, recurrent ulceration with a poor response to therapy, and pancreatic non-β cell islet tumours. The syndrome is the result of excess gastrin stimulated gastric acid secretion. This hyperacidity causes severe, multiple peptic ulcers, which are usually duodenal, but may occur in the oesophagus and jejunum. They are often associated with complications such as haemorrhage, perforation, and stricture formation. Diarrhoea and steatorrhoea due to acid inactivation of small bowel enzymes and mucosal damage may be prominent features, preceding ulcer disease by 12 months or more in up to 10% of cases.

The diagnosis of the gastrinoma syndrome requires the demonstration of a raised fasting gastrin concentration while the patient is off H_2 receptor antagonists (cimetidine/ranitidine) or proton pump inhibitors (omeprazole) and in the presence of increased basal gastric acid secretion. The peak acid response to exogenous pentagastrin is modest because the parietal cell mass is already under constant stimulation. Hypergastrinaemia and raised acid output may result from retained antrum after partial gastrectomy or the very rare condition of G cell hyperplasia. The intravenous secretin test may distinguish between these conditions and can sometimes aid diagnosis when other investigations are equivocal. In the presence of a gastrinoma, gastrin levels should be increased by at least 50% after secretin, while there is no such increase in association with G cell hyperplasia or retained antrum. Gastrin levels are increased in response to a test meal in the last two conditions but not in association with a gastrinoma. Endoscopy may be valuable in demonstrating oesophageal and duodenal ulceration and hypertrophy of the gastric mucosa, while immunocytochemical analysis of antral biopsies may demonstrate G cell hyperplasia.

Insulinoma

Insulinomas and gastrinomas are the most common functioning pancreatic endocrine tumours. The incidence of insulinomas is 1 in 1 000 000. They are less common in MEN I than gastrinomas. Ninety per cent are sporadic, 80% are benign, and they are invariably pancreatic in origin. Patients often present with a longstanding history that includes bizarre behaviour, episodes of violence, blackouts, and in most individuals weight gain. The weight gain is seen because patients learn that eating will avert their incipient hypoglycaemia. The diagnosis is confirmed by finding a blood sugar less than 2·2 mmol/l with a raised or inappropriately normal insulin level. With these samples an assay for C peptide must be performed. This is the endogenous flanking peptide of insulin and is not present in those who are self administering exogenous insulin as part of a personality disorder. The last element of the diagnosis is a negative sulphonylurea screen to exclude self administration of these agents. These individuals will have a raised insulin and C peptide and performing the sulphonylurea screen coincident with the hypoglycaemia may be the only way to prevent a futile search for an occult tumour. In subjects with a history consistent with recurrent hypoglycaemia the investigation of choice is a supervised prolonged fast with normal exercise levels. If after 72 hours the blood glucose has not fallen to less than 2·2 mmol/l, the possibility of an insulinoma being present is remote. Twenty four hours into a fast 70% of patients with an insulinoma will have experienced hypoglycaemia; by 72 hours this is over 97%.

Vipoma

In adults 90% of vasoactive intestinal polypeptide (VIP) producing tumours (vipomas) arise in the pancreas. The remaining tumours are mainly gangliomas or ganglioneuroblastomas, originating in the sympathetic chain or adrenal medulla, and these are especially common in children. Most extrapancreatic tumours are benign. At the time of diagnosis 50% of pancreatic vipomas have metastasised, usually to local lymph nodes and the liver.

The features of the vipoma (Verner–Morrison, pancreatic cholera) syndrome reflect the known biological actions of VIP. The cardinal symptom is the large volume diarrhoea, without steatorrhoea. Patients excrete more than three litres daily, with volumes of over 20 litres described. In severe crises the volume loss, coupled with the vasodilator effects of VIP and the associated hypokalaemia, may precipitate cardiovascular collapse, as in infective cholera.

Hypokalaemia results from stool loss and activation of the renin-angiotensin system. The loss of bicarbonate in the stool leads to the associated acidosis. The achlorhydria or hypochlorhydria, which occurs in over 50% of patients, distinguishes this diarrhoeal syndrome from that associated with the gastrinoma syndrome. Its absence in a proportion of patients makes the eponym WDHA (watery diarrhoea, hypokalaemia, and achlorhydria) syndrome inappropriate. In up to 50% of cases there is glucose intolerance as a result of the glucagon-like actions of VIP. Hypercalcaemia occurs, probably due to parathyroid hormone related peptide (PTHrP) secretion, and is exacerbated by the dehydration. Hypomagnesaemia arises as a result of magnesium loss in the stool. Flushing of the head and neck, which can occur on tumour palpation, may be associated with a marked fall in systemic blood pressure. In advanced cases there is extreme weight loss. Vipomas are usually associated with markedly raised plasma VIP concentrations, but the half life of VIP in the circulation is only two minutes. The diagnosis can be confirmed by the finding of elevated circulating peptide histidine methionine (PHM), which is produced from the preproVIP molecule, is more stable in plasma, and is cosecreted by vipomas. Pancreatic polypeptide levels are elevated in 75% of cases and neurotensin in 10%. Ganglioneuroblastomas may secrete noradrenaline and adrenaline and so be associated with elevated urinary catecholamines and catecholamine metabolites.

Glucagonoma

Glucagonomas are α cell tumours of the pancreas that secrete various forms of glucagon and other peptides derived from the preproglucagon molecule. They have an estimated annual incidence of 1 in 20 million, with a marginal female preponderance, and invariably present in adulthood. Over 70% of patients have metastases at the time of diagnosis.

The characteristic feature of the glucagonoma syndrome is the necrolytic migratory erythematous rash, which occurs in almost all patients, although it often remains undiagnosed for many years (Figure 9.1a). The rash usually starts in the groins and perineum and migrates to the distal extremities. The initial lesions are erythematous patches, which become raised and may be associated with bullae. These lesions break down and gradually heal, often leaving an area of hyperpigmentation, only to recur in another site. All mucous membranes may be involved, commonly leading to angular stomatitis, cheilitis, and glossitis (Figure 9.1b). The cause of the rash is unknown. A direct effect of glucagon on the skin, glucagon induced prostaglandin release, amino acid or free fatty acid deficiency, or zinc deficiency due to the similarity with acrodermatitis enteropathica, have all been proposed as the underlying mechanism. The rash has been reported in a few patients without glucagonomas, who either had coeliac disease or cirrhosis, both of which may have led to elevation in glucagon and glucagon-like peptides. Impaired glucose tolerance and occasionally mild diabetes requires insulin therapy. There is marked progressive weight loss, which is occasionally severe enough to be fatal. Venous thrombosis is enhanced and may be life threatening. Normochromic normocytic anaemia probably results from direct bone marrow suppression by glucagon. Disturbance of bowel function and nail dystrophy are also common features of the syndrome. Mental slowness, depression, and other paraneoplastic neurological syndromes may also occur.

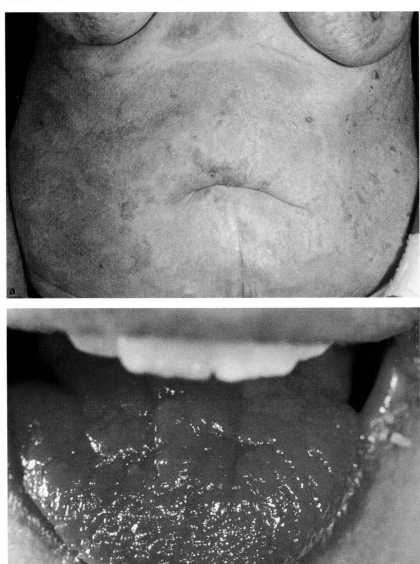

FIGURE 9.1—(a) *Necrolytic migratory erythema. Extensive truncal involvement is seen here. The raised areas have overlying scales where the skin is necrolysing. (b) The glossitis associated with a glucagonoma is extremely painful and may account for the prominent weight loss seen in this syndrome prior to presentation.*

The diagnosis of glucagonoma is confirmed by demonstrating raised fasting plasma glucagon concentrations by radioimmunoassay, and the elevation is usually clear cut.

Somatostatinoma

Somatostatinomas are extremely rare, with an estimated annual incidence of about 1 in 40 million. The tumours are usually pancreatic, although some arise in the duodenum. Approximately 50% of duodenal somatostatinomas occur in association with neurofibromatosis type I (NF I, von Recklinghausen's disease), where the tumours are usually periampullary and may be associated with phaeochromocytoma. Pancreatic tumours usually present late with hepatic metastases. Duodenal tumours are frequently identified early, as a result of local effects.

The somatostatinoma syndrome is characterised by the triad of cholelithiasis, diabetes, and steatorrhoea, which occurs in almost all patients with pancreatic tumours. These features result from the inhibitory actions of somatostatin on gall bladder contraction and secretion, insulin secretion, and pancreatic exocrine secretions. Hypoglycaemia has occasionally been described, possibly due to larger molecular forms of somatostatin having a greater inhibitory effect on counterregulatory hormones than on insulin. Other features of the syndrome include hypochlorhydria, anaemia, postprandial fullness, and weight loss. The syndrome is rarely seen in association with duodenal somatostatinomas, gall bladder disease being the only common manifestation. Duodenal tumours usually present as a result of effects on local structures, causing jaundice, pancreatitis, intestinal obstruction, or haemorrhage.

Circulating levels of somatostatin are usually elevated more than 10-fold in association with pancreatic tumours. Duodenal tumours are associated with much lower somatostatin levels, probably because they are usually about one tenth the size of the pancreatic lesions. Multiple molecular weight forms of somatostatin may be demonstrated by columning of plasma or tumour extracts, and these may explain unusual clinical features.

Carcinoid syndrome

The cardinal feature of carcinoid syndrome is the flush. This predominantly involves the head and upper thorax, and may be associated with tachycardia, hypotension, and increased skin temperature. Patients often complain of a sensation of intense heat, and wheezing may occur. Rarely flushing extends to the trunk and limbs, and may be associated with lacrimation and facial oedema. Attacks are paroxysmal and often unprovoked. Recognised precipitating factors for a flushing attack include alcohol or food ingestion, stress, emotion, and exertion. Flushing initially lasts for only a few minutes but as the disease progresses may become almost continuous. Such patients often develop a chronically reddened and cyanotic facial hue with widespread telangiectasia and leonine facies. This fixed flush is more commonly seen with bronchial carcinoids, in whom flushing can last for hours or days, occasionally with profound hypotension and even anuria. Gastric carcinoids are often associated with raised, localised wheal-like areas of flushing, which are usually pruritic and may migrate.

The other characteristic feature of the syndrome is secretory diarrhoea, which may be profuse, with passage of several litres a day, occasionally accompanied by electrolyte disturbance. There may be associated cramping abdominal pain, nausea, and vomiting. Rarely these symptoms may result from small bowel obstruction from a large ileal carcinoid tumour, but the majority of primary tumours are small. Hepatic metastases may cause right hypochondrial pain, particularly if the liver capsule is involved or stretched, and acute exacerbations may occur if metastases become ischaemic and infarct. Weight loss and, in the later stages, cachexia are common as a result of anorexia, malabsorption, and increased conversion of 5-hydroxytryptophan into 5-hydroxytryptamine causing nicotinamide deficiency.

Cardiac valve abnormalities affect about 50% of patients. They occur as a result of endocardial fibrosis, with plaques of smooth muscle in a collagenous stroma deposited on the valves. Lesions are almost always right sided. Left sided valve damage only occurs in association with bronchial carcinoids, which drain into the left atrium, or atrioseptal defects with right to left shunting. The most common lesions are tricuspid incompetence and pulmonary stenosis, which may result in right ventricular failure. The other causes of breathlessness in association with the carcinoid syndrome are bronchospasm, which affects a small number of patients, often occurring with flushing attacks, and metastatic involvement of the lung and pleura. Arthritis occurs in a small number of patients, and sclerotic bone metastases are seen, often in association with foregut tumours.

Carcinoid tumours, in common with other gastroenteropancreatic tumours, have the potential to produce a variety of peptide products and may be associated with other syndromes, with or without the carcinoid syndrome. The most common of these associated syndromes is Cushing's syndrome due to an ectopic adrenocorticotrophic hormone (ACTH)-secreting bronchial or pancreatic carcinoid. Carcinoid tumours may also be a feature of MEN I.

The diagnosis of carcinoid syndrome is made on the basis of elevated levels of 5-hydroxyindole acetic acid (5HIAA) in a 24 hour urine collection. Urinary 5HIAA acts as a marker of disease progression. Various foods, including avocados, bananas, aubergines, pineapples, plums, and walnuts should be avoided while collecting specimens, to prevent false positive results. A number of drugs and other substances interfere with the spectrophotometric assay. Paracetamol, fluorouracil, methysergide, and caffeine give false positive results. ACTH, phenothiazines, methyldopa, monoamine oxidase inhibitors, and tricyclic antidepressants give false negatives. The other products of carcinoid tumours are not routinely assayed. Circulating markers of neuroendocrine tumours, such as pancreatic polypeptide and chromogranin, may corroborate the diagnosis. Other gut hormones are occasionally elevated in association with carcinoid tumours, most frequently gastrin.

Staging

Staging of gastrointestinal endocrine tumours is not complicated. The slow growing nature of these tumours means that they have often been present for many years before they come to clinical attention. They have often metastasised by presentation. Practically, endocrine tumours of the gut are resectable or irresectable, lone or metastatic. Resection represents the only possibility of cure. If the tumour is not resectable, management is palliative and life expectancy often prolonged but unpredictable, with no therapeutic intervention yet showing a survival benefit. Thus this part of the text will concentrate on localisation of these tumours, which facilitates curative resection of the tumour.

Localisation of tumour

Because of the activity of their hormonal product, gastrinomas and insulinomas tend to present early and can be extremely difficult to localise. Other pancreatic neuroendocrine tumours are large, have metastasised (Figure 9.2), and are easily detected by computed tomography (CT) or abdominal ultrasonography.[4] The small tumour represents the best opportunity for cure. Preoperative localisation improves surgical outcome. It may be achieved non-invasively by transabdominal or endoscopic ultrasonography or by contrast enhanced CT. Highly selective visceral angiography remains the gold standard; it relies on the fact that even small tumours can exhibit an irregular vascular blush as a result of increased vascularity. Angiography is more sensitive for insulinoma than gastrinoma. Recently, success in detecting tiny tumours has been achieved by selective arterial injection with a secretogogue (calcium for insulin or secretin for gastrin), combined with venous sampling to detect which artery is supplying the tumour. Radiolabelled somatostatin scans (Figure 9.3a and b) are unrivalled for defining the extent of the disease but are not as sensitive as had been hoped at detecting the small primary.[5,6]

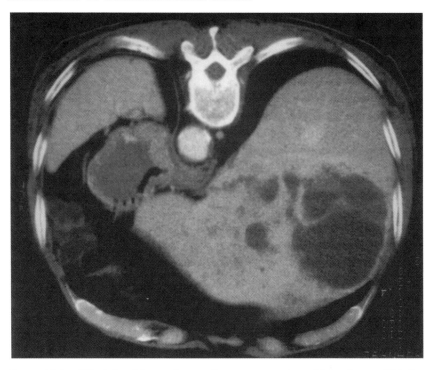

FIGURE 9.2—*CT of the abdomen in a patient at presentation with a vipoma. This is a typical finding in patients with gastrointestinal endocrine tumours where large and extensive intrahepatic metastases are often present.*

Where preoperative efforts have failed, mobilisation of the pancreas and duodenum with thorough examination by an experienced surgeon will usually locate the tumour(s). Intraoperative ultrasonography is helpful at localising the occult endocrine primary. Duodenotomy, transillumination, and careful palpation are helpful in the case of gastrinomas. Preliminary work with intraoperative injection of radiolabelled somatostatin and use of a handheld gamma detecting probe has been associated with wider margins of resection than occurs with intraoperative clinical assessment alone.

Carcinoid

Localisation of carcinoid tumours is rarely a problem. At diagnosis, most have gross hepatic metastases, visible on CT (Figure 9.2) or abdominal ultrasonography. In those rare cases in which the syndrome occurs in the absence of obvious metastases, tumour localisation may offer the prospect

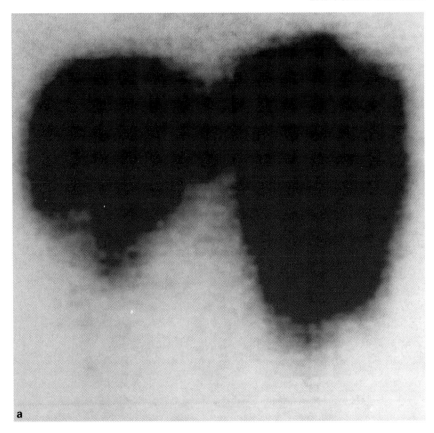

FIGURE 9.3—*Radiolabelled somatostatin scan demonstrating (a) dense uniform uptake in the entire upper abdomen.*

of cure or good palliation for the patient. Symptomatic tumours are unlikely to be confined to the gastrointestinal tract and so chest radiography and CT of the chest and pelvis should be performed. Radiolabelled somatostatin analogues have proven valuable in localising occult carcinoid tumours. The resolution remains only about 1 cm and bronchial carcinoids are frequently atypical and may not express somatostatin receptors. An alternative method of isotopic localisation is using [123]metaiodobenzylguanidine (MIBG) scanning, which is reported to be as effective as labelled somatostatin scans. These scanning techniques can also be useful in patients with metastatic disease as they demonstrate the extent of spread.

311

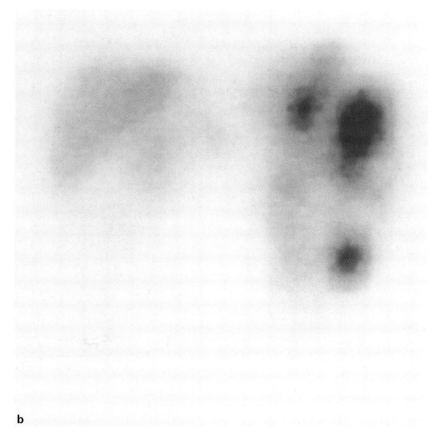

b

FIGURE 9.3—*Radiolabelled somatostatin scan demonstrating (b) patchy uptake in distinct areas in the upper abdomen.*

Surgery

Local disease

Surgical excision is the treatment of choice for all patients with benign disease, which accounts for 80% of insulinomas, 50% of vipomas, and 40% of gastrinomas. Operation is indicated for all patients with apparently benign sporadic lesions that have been localised radiologically. Tumour enucleation can be curative for small pancreatic tumours. Local resection with primary anastomosis is the operation of choice for carcinoid tumours of the ileum. If there are enlarged lymph nodes a wider excision of the mesentery is recommended. More extensive resections may be necessary, particularly for large lesions in the pancreatic head or if multiple tumours are found at operation. Where possible, pancreatic resection should be conservative, with preservation of the spleen during distal pancreatectomy and preservation of the pylorus during proximal pancreatoduodenectomy. A careful search should be made for adjacent lymph node metastases, particularly in gastrinoma patients, as these can often be removed en bloc.

Failure to localise tumours is not uncommon because up to 40% of gastrinomas and insulinomas are microadenomas (less than 1 cm in diameter) and up to 30% of gastrinomas are duodenal. Highly selective angiography increases the localisation rate with conventional radiology to 90%. Management of the remaining 10% of patients should be medical, with repeat of the localisation procedures every 1–2 years. Operation should be performed on detection of a lesion. Dynamic stimulation tests, with calcium for insulinomas and secretin for gastrinomas, combined with selective angiography localises over 90% of tumours. Only in the very rare patient, usually with an insulinoma, who fails to respond to medical therapy, should blind laparotomy be necessary.

Patients with MEN I associated islet cell tumours present a dilemma when considering operative treatment. There are often multiple adenomas, usually less than 1 cm in diameter, which may be widely scattered throughout the pancreas and duodenum. Curative surgery may necessitate a pancreatoduodenectomy, but this can only be justified in patients from families in which the pattern of pancreatic disease has been extremely malignant, or in patients in whom medical therapy is unsuccessful.

Metastatic disease

Surgical resection of metastatic disease is one method of reducing tumour bulk. Options include multiple local excisions of hepatic deposits, formal resection of one or more segments of the liver, or possibly injection of alcohol into the tumour. Occasional cures have been reported after enucleation of tumour deposits. Indeed, several reviews indicate that the metastatic non-functioning tumour group may well benefit from operation over other debulking procedures, with prolonged survival benefit; however, there is an appreciable morbidity rate associated with surgical debulking as these patients are often elderly and a poor operative risk. Other methods of debulking include chemotherapy and hepatic arterial embolisation.

Since the mid-1980s liver transplantation has become a realistic option. It offers a potential long term palliation to patients with metastatic disease confined to the liver and a resectable or previously resected primary tumour. It is recommended that this option be considered in all patients under the age of 50, although few prove suitable candidates, either due to the debilitating consequences of their disease or because of psychological factors. Imaging of the thorax and abdomen, together with radiolabelled somatostatin analogue scans, is performed to determine the extent of the metastatic disease, and angiography is performed to ensure that the portal vein is patent. Eligible patients are then further evaluated before a final decision is made.

Non-surgical therapies

The non-surgical therapies available for neuroendocrine tumours include chemotherapy, hepatic arterial embolisation, and the somatostatin analogues.[7-9] Symptomatic management has greatly improved with the use of somatostatin analogues, but no survival benefit to the tumour group has been demonstrated. Many treatments for specific features of hormone syndromes have been replaced by the somatostatin analogues; however, specific treatments are still the mainstay for some of the major tumours. The use of the proton pump inhibitor omeprazole to switch off gastric acid secretion in the Zollinger–Ellison syndrome, the use of diazoxide to treat the hypoglycaemia of insulinomas, and the use of zinc for the necrolytic migratory erythema of glucagonoma are the most prominent examples.

Chemotherapy

A variety of chemotherapeutic regimens has been advocated for patients with metastatic gut neuroendocrine tumours. The most widely used combines streptozotocin and 5-fluorouracil. Streptozotocin is a nitrosourea antibiotic that was found selectively to destroy the pancreatic β cell and cause diabetes in animals, although not in humans. It is taken up selectively into the pancreatic islets and has proved an effective therapy for pancreatic islet cell tumours when used alone. 5-Fluorouracil is active when metabolised, fluorouridine being incorporated into RNA and another metabolite inhibiting thymidylate synthetase and hence DNA synthesis. It is synergistic with a number of other cytotoxic agents and was found to enhance the response rate of islet cell tumours to streptozotocin. Moertel et al reported a 63% response rate with a median duration of 17 months, including a 33% complete response rate with a median duration of 24 months, in 42 patients treated with streptozotocin and 5-fluorouracil.[7] Other studies have confirmed this response rate.

A widely used regimen is streptozotocin $500\,mg/m^2$ and 5-fluorouracil $400\,mg/m^2$ given by intravenous infusion on alternative days for 10 days. The most common side effects of the regimen are nausea, vomiting, anorexia, and general malaise, which have been reported to occur in over 80% of patients. These symptoms can be reduced by giving lorazepam 2 mg intravenously, dexamethasone 4 mg intravenously, and metoclopramide 1 mg/kg intravenously within the half hour before starting treatment. Four courses of chemotherapy at three month intervals are given before assessing the response. Selection of patients for chemotherapy is determined by the likely responsiveness of the tumour and the efficacy of other therapies. Vipomas respond in over 90% of cases. The response of streptozotocin alone in the case of vipomas may be dramatic, patients often being symptom free for years after just one course of treatment. Glucagonomas respond in 70% of cases, with remissions frequently lasting more than one year. Malignant insulinomas respond in about 40% of cases, and in these patients octreotide is not an option because it exacerbates hypoglycaemia by inhibiting counterregulatory hormones. Thus in patients with vipomas, glucagonomas, and possibly malignant insulinomas, chemotherapy would be considered at an early stage. Gastrinomas respond in only about 40% of cases and the associated syndrome is well controlled by omeprazole. Thus debulking is often not indicated in such patients until non-endocrine manifestations of tumour load become apparent, and hepatic embolisation may be more effective at this point. Tumours associated with the carcinoid syndrome rarely respond to chemotherapy. The response rate for other functioning tumours and non-functioning tumours is about 30%. The choice between hepatic embolisation and chemotherapy will be based on the tumour distribution and the presence of contraindications to either therapy.

Hepatic artery embolisation

Hepatic arterial embolisation, with foreign substances, was first used in the early 1950s. It was reported as effective in patients with metastatic gut neuroendocrine tumours in 1977. Ligation of the hepatic artery is an ineffective procedure because of the rapid development of local anastomotic vessels. The indications for hepatic artery embolisation are palliation of the clinical consequences of hormone production from hepatic metastases and, more controversially, the reduction of tumour load to ameliorate non-endocrine systemic symptoms.[8]

Hepatic metastases are supplied by the hepatic artery alone, but the surrounding liver parenchyma is supplied by both the artery and the portal vein. Thus the metastases can be devascularised by embolisation of their hepatic arterial supply, while blood supply to the normal liver is adequate if the portal vein is patent. Portal vein occlusion is thus an absolute contraindication to the procedure. Other contraindications include a markedly prolonged prothrombin time, replacement of over 50% of the liver parenchyma with tumour in association with marked deterioration in liver function, intercurrent infection, and end stage disease.

Patency of the portal vein should be established by abdominal CT and should be confirmed by angiography immediately before embolisation. The patient should be given prophylactic broad spectrum antibiotics before catheterisation to guard against infection in the necrotic tissue and hepatic abscess formation. Octreotide 500 µg subcutaneously is given if the tumour is functioning, to block the effects of massive peptide release. Once patency of the portal vein has been confirmed catheterisation of the hepatic artery is performed and the arterial supply to the tumour is embolised. It is preferable to occlude collaterals so that the main arterial trunks remain patent for future embolisation. If there is extensive disease in both lobes, it is prudent to embolise each lobe on separate occasions to reduce morbidity. During the procedure the patient should be monitored for hypotension, which may result from release of potent vasodilating peptides, compounded by the contrast load. Antibiotics and octreotide are recommended after embolisation.

Common side effects of the procedure are malaise, mild hypotension, fever, deranged liver function due to tumour necrosis, nausea, vomiting, and abdominal pain. Paralytic ileus may occur. Serious complications are rare and death has only been reported in patients in whom there were relative contraindications to embolisation. Since the introduction of octreotide, life threatening hypovolaemia with renal impairment due to severe peptide mediated vasodilatation and volume depletion is rare. Careful attention must still be paid to fluid balance before, during, and after the procedure. Inadvertent embolisation of other organs, including the pancreas and gall bladder, may occur, and that of the latter may be a common occurrence, although usually asymptomatic. If abdominal symptoms persist, this possibility should be excluded by performing an ultrasound examination.

A partial response to embolisation is seen in 60–80% of patients. Revascularisation, with recurrence of symptoms, can occur (usually after a delay of several months) and embolisation can be successfully repeated at this juncture. Embolisation is most commonly used for patients with carcinoid syndrome in whom chemotherapy is of little benefit, although the initial treatment for these patients is usually octreotide. The procedure should be considered in all patients with gut neuroendocrine tumours with extensive hepatic tumour load in the absence of contraindications.

Octreotide and other somatostatin analogues

Somatostatin is a cyclic tetradecapeptide that was isolated from mammalian hypothalami in 1972. It is the major physiological inhibitor of growth hormone release from the pituitary. It is also a potent inhibitor of release of other pituitary and pancreatic hormones. Ongoing treatment with analogues of somatostatin is now established for the control of excess hormone production and control of symptoms resulting from this hypersecretion. In both carcinoid and pancreatic tumours, somatostatin has been associated with some shrinkage of the tumour mass.[9] Therapeutic use of somatostatin was precluded by its plasma half life of three minutes, but the synthetic analogue octreotide has a plasma half life of nearly two hours when given intravenously and is considerably more potent at inhibiting hormone secretion.

Octreotide therapy is of particular value in treating the glucagonoma, vipoma, and carcinoid syndromes. In patients with the glucagonoma syndrome it reduces circulating glucagon levels in about 75% of patients. It ameliorates the rash in almost all cases, usually for periods in excess of six months, but rarely affects the weight loss or diabetes. It has not been shown to influence the tendency to venous thrombosis. Over 90% of patients with the vipoma syndrome respond to octreotide therapy, commonly within 24 hours. Over 70% of patients with the carcinoid syndrome respond to octreotide, and it is most effective in treating the diarrhoea and flushing.

Octreotide may be effective in treating hypoglycaemia in malignant insulinomas, but great caution is needed because inhibition of the release and action of counterregulatory hormones, such as glucagon, may occur. Recent advances with the cloning and characterisation of the action of the somatostatin receptors in humans may contribute in this area. There are five receptors, labelled SSTR 1 to 5, in order of their discovery. Release of glucagon is modulated by SSTR 2, while that of insulin by SSTR 4. The role of somatostatin analogues in insulinomas has been limited by the concomitant suppression of glucagon release that may potentially occur and thereby accentuate hypoglycaemia. Use of a SSTR 4 selective agonist may reduce this risk. The potential for a range of other somatostatin receptor specific analogues will become clear over the next few years.

Octreotide is administered subcutaneously, starting with a dose of 50 µg twice or three times a day and increasing to a maximum of 500 µg three times a day. It may be given by subcutaneous infusion and higher maximum doses may be achieved this way. It is first line therapy in patients with troublesome symptoms from hormone syndromes, particularly those with the carcinoid syndrome. In patients with other syndromes it is often combined with chemotherapy or hepatic embolisation. The main problem with octreotide is that resistance develops, at least in part due to increased tumour bulk. This resistance can develop after a few months or after many years and can initially be overcome by using increasing doses. After a further 12–24 months most patients will have become unresponsive to octreotide or other therapeutic interventions. This resistance may be delayed by combining octreotide therapy with tumour debulking. We and others have been studying several very slow release preparations of somatostatin analogues. They appear to provide equivalent or better symptom control and require injection from once a week to once a month. This development will undoubtedly further improve the quality of life of these patients.

The side effects of octreotide are minimal. Pain at the injection site due to the acidic medium is usually short lived. Gall stone formation due to cholestasis probably occurs in about half the patients, but rarely results in symptoms. Pancreatic exocrine insufficiency occurs infrequently, and resolves with pancreatic enzyme supplements; glucose intolerance is rarely important.

Omeprazole

Omeprazole is the treatment of choice for patients with the gastrinoma syndrome who are not undergoing curative resection or whose symptoms need controlling before operation. The clinical manifestations of the syndrome result from excess secretion of gastric acid as a result of the stimulatory effect of gastrin. Omeprazole is a substituted benzimidazole, which competitively inhibits gastric hydrogen potassium ATPase, blocking release of gastric acid. Omeprazole produces effectively a medical gastrectomy in doses of 80–240 mg daily, reducing basal acid output to less than 5 mmol/h after two days of treatment, healing 100% of ulcers within one month of therapy, and abolishing diarrhoea. Symptoms do not recur if treatment is maintained. Omeprazole is susceptible to degradation in an acid environment and so it should be combined initially with an H_2 blocker for a few days until acid output is successfully diminished. The dose of omeprazole can be titrated against symptoms until the appropriate dose is achieved. Repeat acid studies are only rarely needed to confirm hypochlorhydria in patients who still complain of symptoms despite very high doses. Side effects of omeprazole are rare but include diarrhoea, headache, skin reactions, and peripheral oedema.

Diazoxide

Hypoglycaemia in patients with insulinomas who are awaiting operation or who are not surgical candidates is a difficult problem. It may be prevented by appropriately spaced carbohydrate meals and guar gum to even carbohydrate absorption, but most patients will require diazoxide. This drug directly inhibits insulin release and enhances glycogenolysis. It is given at a dose of 5–15 mg/kg body weight. Hirsutism is a common side effect. Fluid retention occurs in almost all patients, and a diuretic is therefore also prescribed. Hypertension is rare at these doses.

318

Glucagonoma

Here the specific options available are topical zinc and high protein diet for the rash, insulin for the diabetes, and the range of general debulking therapies.

Evaluation of therapy outcome

In neuroendocrine tumours of the gastrointestinal tract, the criteria by which outcome of therapy is assessed are symptomatic response, biochemical response, and change in tumour size. In general one can consider:

- mechanical or mass effect—pain/obstructive jaundice
- metabolic tumour load effect—fatigue/weight loss
- endocrine hormone effects—specific to the individual tumour.

Surgery

In most cases, curative resection is the surgical objective. Postoperatively, one will expect a return of elevated hormones to within the normal range, full symptomatic resolution, and negative imaging for recurrence. In particular a negative radiolabelled somatostatin analogue scan will be helpful in defining the presence of residual disease. CT and MRI are accurate, if the same imaging modality is used both before and after surgery and images at corresponding levels are taken.

Where surgical treatment is palliative, the degree of reduction of tumour bulk is reflected by a comparable fall in hormone levels and reduction in symptoms.

Chemotherapy and embolisation

The main criteria of response are the reduction in the symptoms that promoted the intervention. If the biochemical and radiological parameters improve but the symptoms persist, then the treatment has failed.

With these palliative options the response of the elevated hormone is a guide to the extent of tumour response to the therapy. The size of the tumour after treatment is an indicator of the response. Again, CT and MRI are accurate if the same imaging modality is used before and after therapy and images at corresponding levels are taken. The recommended interval between assessments is six months.

References

1 Chesyln-Curtis S, Sitaram V, Williamson RC. Management of non-functioning neuroendocrine tumours of the pancreas. *Br J Surg* 1993;**80**:625–7.
2 Oberg K, ed. Neuroendocrine gut and pancreatic tumours. *Acta Oncol* 1989;**28**:301–449.
3 Sheppard BC, Norton JA, Doppman JL, *et al*. Management of islet cell tumours in patients with multiple endocrine neoplasia: a prospective study. *Surgery* 1989;**106**:1108–17.
4 Hammond PJ, Jackson JE, Bloom SR. Localisation of pancreatic endocrine tumours. *Clin Endocrinol* 1994;**40**:3–14.
5 Schrimer WJ, O'Dorisio TM, Schrimer TP, *et al*. Intraoperative localisation of neuroendocrine tumours with 125I-TYR(3)-octreotide and a hand held gamma detecting probe. *Surgery* 1993;**114**:745–52.
6 O'Shea DB, Bloom SR. Somatostatin in the diagnosis and treatment of neuroendocrine tumours. *Current Opin Diabetes Endocrinol* 1995;**2**:177–81.
7 Moertel CG, Hanley JA, Johnson LA. Streptozotocin alone compared with streptozotocin plus fluorouracil in the treatment of advanced islet cell carcinoma. *N Engl J Med* 1980; **303**:1189–94.
8 Allison DJ, Modlin IM, Jenkins WJ. Treatment of carcinoid liver metastases by hepatic arterial embolisation. *Lancet* 1977;**2**:1323–5.
9 Wynick D, Bloom SR. The use of the long acting somatostatin analogue octreotide in the treatment of gut neuroendocrine tumours. *J Clin Endocrinol Metab* 1991;**73**:1–3.

10: Colon and rectum

Tumour biology, investigation, and surgical management

ALISON WAGHORN and WITOLD KMIOT

Colorectal cancer is a common disease of Western society: the annual incidence is 17 000–20 000 in England and Wales and 60 000 in the USA. Despite recent advances in adjuvant therapies, the worldwide mortality has not altered significantly in 50 years.

Epidemiology

Colorectal carcinogenesis is a complex process in which host, environmental, and genetic factors interact.

The incidence of colorectal carcinoma increases with age. The most common age at which patients present with carcinoma is 60–69 years. Incidence also varies enormously between communities and racial groups (see Chapter 1). The sex distribution of colorectal carcinomas overall in England and Wales is approximately equal; however, in most Western countries carcinoma of the colon is slightly more prevalent in women than men, while the reverse is true for carcinoma of the rectum. Parity in women may be protective. Low physical activity has also been implicated, one explanation being that decreased intestinal transit time allows potential carcinogens to have longer contact with the gut mucosa. Physical activity affects prostaglandins and a number of antioxidant enzymes but it is not known whether these play a major role in the development of colorectal carcinoma. Recent authors have also described certain personality types as being associated with higher risks. Diet may play a role in the aetiology of colorectal carcinoma (see Chapter 1). There is an association between obesity, high energy intake, and high fat diets that makes it difficult to decide which of these factors is most directly associated with colorectal cancer risk.

Secondary bile acids and potentially mutagenic or carcinogenic compounds created by cooking meat have both been identified as potential carcinogens (see Chapter 1). Burkitt observed a low rate of colorectal carcinoma in countries where a high fibre diet was consumed. Multivariate analysis has shown a 35% reduction in the relative risk of colonic carcinoma with a high fibre diet. This may be the result of dilution of carcinogens, enhancement of bacteria fermentation (causing a decrease in pH, which in turn leads to a decrease in free bile acid solubility), and the antineoplastic properties of some of the dietary metabolites. There is a large overlap between vegetables and dietary fibre so it is difficult to distinguish between the two when analysing studies, but vegetables and fruit both contain antioxidants and other potentially anticarcinogenic substances.

The potential of a high calcium diet to reduce the risk of colorectal carcinoma remains controversial (see Chapter 1). Calcium may bind to free bile and fatty acids in the bowel lumen or may have a direct protective effect on gut epithelium. Oral calcium supplements decrease colonic mucosal proliferation. Non-steroidal anti-inflammatory drugs may have a beneficial effect. Sulindac has been shown to be protective against colorectal neoplasia and seems to produce regression in colorectal polyps in patients with familial adenomatous polyposis. Some evidence suggests that regular aspirin ingestion is associated with a decreased incidence of colorectal carcinoma. Conflicting data, largely from animal experiments, make this a controversial area. There has been no conclusive evidence that either alcohol or smoking has any major role to play in the aetiology of colorectal carcinoma. No study to date has shown either occupation or industrial chemical exposure as potential causative agents of colorectal carcinoma.

Two other known factors are worthy of mention: having had one colorectal carcinoma markedly increases the risk of a future carcinoma; and pelvic irradiation for gynaecological carcinomas or for benign diseases (for example, ankylosing spondylitis) increases the risk of developing rectosigmoidal cancer by a factor of between 2 and 8—there is a lead time of 10 years or more after the completion of therapy.

Genetic factors

In colorectal cancer there is a recognised pathway of development, from adenoma to carcinoma. Several groups of patients have a genetic predisposition to colorectal carcinoma (see Chapter 1).

Familial adenomatous polyposis

Patients with familial adenomatous polyposis (FAP), an autosomal dominant inherited condition, have a high incidence of colorectal carcinoma, 50% developing cancer by the age of 30 and 100% by the age of 50.[1]

Gardner's syndrome

This syndrome is a variant of FAP in which desmoid tumours, osteomas, and other neoplasms occur together with adenomas of the colon and rectum. Other extra colonic manifestations of this disease include hepatoblastomas, brain, thyroid, duodenal, bile duct, desmoid, small bowel, adrenal, osteogenic and sarcomatous tumours, adenomas of the small bowel, duodenum, and adrenal gland, gastric polyps, retinal pigmentation, and epidermal cysts.

Hereditary non-polyposis colorectal cancer (HNPCC) syndromes

Lynch type 1

This cancer family syndrome was first noted by Warthin in 1925.[2] Lynch and Krush[3] were to go on and show one of these families to have 6500 neoplasms within the family. A dominant pattern of inheritance for susceptibility to adenomatous polyps and colorectal carcinoma exists. The diagnostic criteria include increased incidence of primary adenocarcinomas in the colon and endometrium, increased incidence of multiple primary malignant neoplasms, and early age of onset with autosomal dominant inheritance.

Site specific colon cancer syndrome

There is a tendency for tumours that occur at a younger age to be multiple and to be more frequently situated in the right colon. A patient fitting this description can be assumed to be a member of a family with one of these specific types of HNPCC if three first degree relatives have colorectal carcinomas.

Family history

If the patient does not fit into the above diagnostic grouping, a rough risk estimation can be made according to the number of relatives with adenocarcinomas (see box).

323

Risk estimation for HNPCC[4]

- One first degree relative   1/17
- One first and one second degree relative   1/12
- One first degree relative over 45 years old   1/10
- Two parents   1/8·5
- Two first degree relatives   1/6
- Three first degree relatives   1/2

Molecular genetics
(See also Chapter 4)

The accumulation rather than the sequence of genetic mutations appears to be important in colorectal tumorigenesis. Patients with FAP and Gardner's syndrome have a mutated APC gene on the long arm of chromosome 5. Mutation of this gene appears to be an early event in colorectal carcinogenesis, and carcinoma of the colon in FAP is more commonly left sided, similar to sporadic large bowel carcinoma.

Hypomethylation

Hypomethylation of DNA has been implicated as an early change in the genetic structure of the cell in the adenoma to carcinoma sequence.

Growth promoting oncogenes

A combination of overexpression of these genes and deletion of growth suppressor genes contributes to loss of control of cell replication. The growth promoting oncogene, K-ras, has been found in the stools of patients with carcinomas; this may have potential as a new screening test if confirmed in future studies.

Tumour suppressor genes

Two tumour suppressor genes that have been implicated in colorectal cancer are the DCC gene on the long arm of chromosome 18 and p53 on the short arm of chromosome 17. Inactivation of p53 appears to be a late step in colorectal tumorigenesis. In vitro evidence that replacing a defective tumour suppressor gene may result in cancer cell death has given rise to hopes of developing new cancer therapies using this principle.

Metastases suppressor genes

Increased expression and/or amplification of some oncogenes is associated with human tumour metastatic aggressiveness. Recent evidence implicating variants of the nm23 gene in colorectal cancer metastasis requires further confirmation.

Chromosome 2

Chromosome 2 markers have been closely linked to cancer predisposition in two HNPCC families. In HNPCC and right sided sporadic tumours there is frequent loss of heterogeneity for these markers, despite a similar incidence of mutations in K-ras, p53, and APC in these syndromes. New bands of "satellite" markers have been described, and it is suggested that this phenomenon results from instability in the replication of short repeated DNA sequences. Most HNPCC families show widespread alterations in these sequences, suggesting that numerous errors have occurred during tumour development.[5] A possible further locus on chromosome 3p has recently come to light.

Kinzler and Vogelstein have proposed this model hypothesis to explain the events in colorectal tumorigenesis (see box).

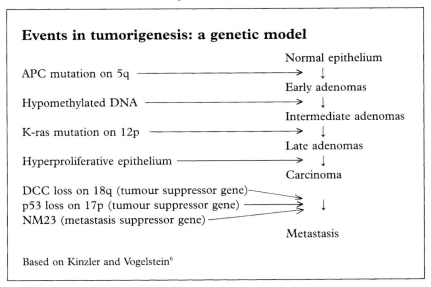

Events in tumorigenesis: a genetic model

		Normal epithelium
APC mutation on 5q →	↓	
		Early adenomas
Hypomethylated DNA →	↓	
		Intermediate adenomas
K-ras mutation on 12p →	↓	
		Late adenomas
Hyperproliferative epithelium →	↓	
		Carcinoma
DCC loss on 18q (tumour suppressor gene)		
p53 loss on 17p (tumour suppressor gene) →	↓	
NM23 (metastasis suppressor gene)		
		Metastasis

Based on Kinzler and Vogelstein[6]

Clinical presentation and diagnosis

Many patients with polyps and Dukes's A carcinomas are asymptomatic; clinical assessment alone is therefore inadequate for population screening.

The World Health Organisation guidelines for screening include the following criteria: improvement of mortality and function, simple and inexpensive test(s), and adequate compliance rates. The long term benefits should outweigh the long term detriments, with a proven benefit to the screened community.

The following procedures have been proposed as screening tests.

- Faecal occult blood studies
- Digital examination of the rectum
- Rigid sigmoidoscopy
- Flexible sigmoidoscopy
- Colonoscopy
- Barium enema
- Tumour markers.

Age incidence and the natural history (the adenoma–carcinoma sequence) should be considered when designing a programme for the prevention of invasive colorectal carcinoma. The incidence of colorectal cancer increases appreciably after the fifth decade.

It is predicted that for an adenoma to develop de novo into a 1 cm lesion requires 2–3 years, and probably a further 7–10 years to develop into a carcinoma. This malignancy therefore has a long silent preclinical phase in which therapeutic intervention is possible.

Faecal occult blood studies

History

In 1864 Van Deen detected the presence of blood in faeces using gum guaiac indicator, but it was not until 1967 that the guaiac slide test was described. Initially, hydrogen peroxide was used as the development agent, but chemical alteration of haemoglobin as it passes through the gastrointesinal tract can diminish its peroxidase-like activity. It is therefore more likely to detect colonic bleeding than upper gastrointestinal tract bleeding.

In 1978 an immunochemical technique specific for human haemoglobin was designed. The slide remains stable for 30 days, but there is a 24–48 hour delay in interpreting the test, and greater technical complexity and cost compared with the other available tests.

Further developments in 1984 enabled the electrostatic binding of haemoglobin to a filter. This method is six times more sensitive than guaiac slide testing, but requires an incubation period and is labour intensive.

Faecal occult blood (FOB) tests are to date the simplest and cheapest method of screening for colorectal carcinoma. Ideally an FOB loss of less than 2 ml/day should be detectable; guaiac testing, however, requires a blood loss of 20 ml/day. Compliance rates for FOB tests vary from 15 to 75% because of differing understanding of the value of such tests and a distaste for the home test.

False positives

The commonly used guaiac test has a high incidence of false positives caused by red meat, uncooked fruit or vegetables, iron-containing drugs, and non-steroidal anti-inflammatory drugs. The newer immunologically based tests may decrease this.

False negatives

The false negative rate is 40% if FOB testing is used alone because tumour bleeding may be intermittent or absent.

At present three long term randomised controlled trials are evaluating FOB as a screening method: the Funen study in Denmark, the Nottingham study in the United Kingdom, and the Minnesota study in the USA.[7] The Sloan Kettering programme is also evaluating FOB tests but is comparing sigmoidoscopy and FOB testing with sigmoidoscopy alone. These studies have yet to be completed. The data so far show the following.

1 FOB testing is a feasible screening method, with a compliance rate varying between 15 and 75%.
2 The positive predictive value is between 22 and 58%, with some studies showing a five times greater incidence of cancer in the study group than in the control population.
3 Cancers detected in the screened population are more likely to be Dukes's A and Dukes's B.
4 Polyps are more likely to be detected in the screened group than in the control population, with some studies showing a threefold increase.
5 The Minneapolis study,[7] which is analysing 45 000 subjects over 50 years, has shown a 33% survival benefit in the screened group. Thirty-eight per cent of those screened annually and 28% of those screened biennially had at least one colonoscopy. Whether a similar result can be obtained without rehydration of the guaiac slides is as yet unknown (rehydration leads to a fourfold increase in positivity). Cost–benefit analysis will be required to determine whether mass screening is more cost effective than other approaches.

Digital examination of the rectum

This method can only detect those 10–15% of colorectal cancers within reach of the examining finger. Most studies do not use digital examination of the rectum alone but combine it with rigid sigmoidoscopy. With the advent of flexible sigmoidoscopy there have not been any further screening studies using this method.

Rigid sigmoidoscopy

The Sloan Kettering group is at present assessing 21 756 patients enrolled between 1975 and 1979 (when they were aged 40 and over) in a randomised controlled trial comparing rigid sigmoidoscopy annually and rigid sigmoidoscopy and FOB annually.[8] Early results show a significantly greater survival probability in the group who underwent sigmoidoscopy and FOB testing than in the sigmoidoscopy alone group (70 versus 48%). The colorectal cancer mortality difference was of no significance (p<0·53).

Flexible sigmoidoscopy

This method is capable of reaching 50–70% of all colorectal neoplasms but no randomised trials have yet been completed to determine whether it can reduce mortality from colorectal cancer. Preliminary data suggest that screening every 10 years with the sigmoidoscope might decrease mortality. Cost effectiveness remains to be considered as flexible sigmoidoscopy requires trained staff, causes discomfort, is time consuming, invasive, has a perforation rate, and needs bowel preparation. A proposed once only programme of population screening for patients over 55 years of age is gaining support.

Colonoscopy

Colonoscopy enables the visualisation of the entire colorectal mucosa and the excision of small polypoid lesions; however, it is expensive, can fail to visualise the proximal colon in 10% of patients, and is associated with a 0·1–0·3% complication rate. It has never been considered justified for screening the asymptomatic average risk population but it does have a role in screening those people with hereditary cancer syndromes and relatives of patients with colorectal cancer, all of whom have an increased risk of colorectal cancer.

Barium enema

Double contrast barium enema provides results comparable to colonoscopy when screening for colorectal carcinomas but has not been advocated as a screening procedure because the compliance rate is low and polyps and Dukes's A carcinomas can be difficult to find on barium enema. The expense, discomfort, and increase in radiology workload associated with the procedure make it inappropriate as a screening investigation. Combined with flexible sigmoidoscopy it may have a role in surveillance.

Tumour markers

Most of the work with tumour markers for screening has been performed with carcinogen embryonic antigen (CEA). There are many problems with this tumour marker as the antigen is not specific to colonic carcinoma and increased levels have been found in patients with tumours of the lung, stomach, and larynx. CEA levels can be increased in benign inflammatory disorders—for example, ulcerative colitis, Crohn's disease, and diverticular disease. This lack of specificity suggests that it is inappropriate for use as a screening marker. CEA is rarely elevated in patients with adenomas and Dukes's A lesions. Other biomarkers (for example, CA 19-9, CA 50, CA 195, and CA 125) have an even worse sensitivity than CEA, but may have a role in improving the prediction of tumour prognosis. K-ras genes are being detected in stools of individuals with colonic carcinoma and may be applicable as a screening method in the future.

Screening in cancer families

The incidence of FAP varies from 1 in 7000 to 1 in 24 000 live births. Polyps tend to develop in the late teens and therefore screening should start at 10 years. If annual colonoscopy is negative for polyps the interval may be extended, but the individuals should be over 50 years old and have no polyps before screening is abandoned.

Linkage analysis is applicable to the screening of FAP families but many of the families carrying the gene do not fulfil the requirements for this analysis. DNA from at least two affected and one unaffected family member should be available. Using a Southern blotting technique with flanking probes for the gene, risk estimates can be produced. Mutation analysis can be performed on individuals in isolation but mutations cannot be detected in 30% of patients.

Management of the premalignant colon

Colonoscopic management of polyps/focal and early carcinoma

Careful evaluation of polyps is necessary before colonoscopic polypectomy, particularly in assessing specific morphology—that is, pedunculated, sessile, flat or elevated, with or without areas of depression. Flat or sessile polyps with or without an area of depression should be considered to be early carcinoma. Colonoscopic polypectomy is adequate for pedunculated adenomas with focal carcinoma not invading the stalk, but a standard bowel resection should be recommended in patients with early carcinoma, poorly differentiated adenocarcinoma, and invasion of lymphatics. Rectal adenomas can also be assessed endosonographically to rule out an occult invasive cancer and assess the need to use more complex techniques for excision.

Surveillance colonoscopy should be carried out once a year for three years after the removal of focal and early carcinomas. After polyps have been detected, annual colonoscopies are advised until there are two sequential years without polyps; a three yearly surveillance programme can then be initiated.

Ulcerative colitis

The patients at greatest risk are those who have had ulcerative colitis for more than eight years. For these people colonoscopy should be performed every 1–2 years and multiple biopsies obtained from every 10–12 cm of normal looking mucosa.[9] Targeted biopsies should be obtained from areas where the surface appears raised as a broad based polyp, regular plaque, villiform elevation, an unusual ulcer (particularly one raised at the edges), or a stricture. Typical inflammatory polyps need not be sampled. Colectomy is recommended in the presence of multiple areas of high grade dysplasia. The identification of a mass lesion with any degree of overlying dysplasia is also an indication for colectomy. Persistent low grade dysplasia without a mass remains more controversial.

Surgery for familial adenosis polyposis syndrome

Eighty per cent of these families have a family history and 20% can be classified as having spontaneous genetic mutations. Eighty per cent of patients will have macroscopic adenomas by the age of 20. Subtotal or complete prophylactic colectomy is not a guaranteed cure of FAP because of its generalised nature: there is a significant mortality from desmoid tumours and periampullary carcinomas.

Recommended treatments

Panproctocolectomy and ileostomy This option is only recommended if there is already a rectal cancer present in the lower third of the rectum.

Colectomy and ileorectal anastomosis This is the most commonly used prophylactic procedure but there is a need for regular follow up as there is a 4% risk of cancer 25 years later.

Colectomy and ileoanal reservoir The colon and rectum are totally removed with preservation of the anal sphincter. This approach is attractive because it removes the large bowel mucosa but avoids the necessity of a permanent ileostomy. Numerous modifications over the years have decreased the complication rate and improved the functional results. At present there is a 10% pelvic sepsis rate and there are some problems with the temporary ileostomy.

Diagnosis and staging

Diagnosis

Colonic malignancy is found in approximately 10% of patients over the age of 40 who present with recent onset of rectal bleeding. Digital examination will find 15–20% of all colorectal cancers.

Clinical symptoms

The typical presentation of the patient with a right sided tumour is non-specific, with a feeling of being generally unwell, anaemia, weight loss, and sometimes an abdominal mass. By contrast, the patient with a left sided colonic carcinoma more often presents with a history of rectal bleeding or change in bowel habit.

Investigations

Haematological and biochemical tests These enable the detection of anaemia and perhaps liver metastases but there usually have to be quite extensive metastases in the liver for a patient to develop abnormal liver function tests.

Colonoscopy Colonoscopy is comparable with barium enema in the detection of lesions of greater than 1 cm and permits simultaneous diagnostic biopsies and therapeutic procedures. There is, however, a minimum reported perforation rate of 0·2%, and a failure to reach the caecum of 10%. Although colonoscopy is three times more expensive than barium enema and has a 10 times higher perforation rate, colonoscopic false negatives are much less common and it has a pivotal role in confirming equivocal lesions seen on barium enema.

Barium enema Barium enema is better than colonoscopy at detecting caecal lesions but it is not as accurate as colonoscopy for assessing the sigmoid colon and the rectum (Table 10.1). Most studies show that there is more discomfort with a double contrast barium enema than with a colonoscopy, especially in the frail and elderly. Residual stool and barium pooling can lead to misdiagnosis. Severe sigmoid diverticulosis and marked luminal narrowing due to muscular hypertrophy may obscure a coexistent carcinoma.

When combining double contrast barium enema and sigmoidoscopy, detection of approximately 95% of tumours greater than 1 cm can be achieved.

TABLE 10.1—*Comparison of the sensitivities of double contrast barium enema (DCBE), sigmoidoscopy, and colonoscopy in the diagnosis of colorectal carcinoma*

	DCBE (%)	Sigmoidoscopy (%)	Colonoscopy (%)
Dukes's A	32	84	88
Dukes's B	79	90	96
Dukes's C	81	81	100

Computed tomography, ultrasonography, and magnetic resonance imaging
Computed tomography (CT) has difficulty in demonstrating the colonic wall when it is less than 5 mm thick. A discrete thickening of the wall may suggest a carcinoma. CT is of limited value in primary diagnosis but is useful if complications have occurred—for example, abscess formation.

Colonic carcinoma can be detected by ultrasonography. Bowel wall thickening due to colorectal carcinoma may result in a "target" or "pseudo kidney" configuration in which the central echogenic mucosa is surrounded by an abnormally thick (>5 mm) hyperechoic rim.

CT and ultrasonographic appearances are not specific for carcinoma and further investigation is required.

Staging

Preoperative staging of tumour and metastases

Before surgical intervention an evaluation should be made of the following.

1 Tumour wall invasion—especially in rectal tumours where there is the possible option of transanal surgery, and palliative surgery might have to be considered.

2 Metastases
   a Lymph node metastases
   b Distant metastases (for example, hepatic, pulmonary).

The following imaging modalities may provide further information:[10]

- Endoluminal ultrasonography
- Computed tomography
- Magnetic resonance imaging (MRI)
- Ultrasonography
- Plain radiography
- Intravenous urography (IVU)
- Immunoscintigraphy

Endoluminal ultrasonography This modality has a role in the assessment of rectal tumours. Five sonographic layers can be determined: mucosa, muscularis mucosa, submucosa, muscularis propria, and perirectal fat. Tumour invasion is characterised by a hypoechoic mass that disrupts surrounding layers. Endoluminal ultrasonography has an accuracy of assessment of tumour depth of 90%, of detection of perirectal spread of 83–94%, and of lymph node involvement of 78%; however, after radiation therapy this decreases to 60% for perirectal invasion and 40% for lymph node involvement. Endosonography is therefore more sensitive than CT for detecting perirectal spread of the tumour. It is also helpful in assessing tumours that are potentially suitable for local excision or endocavity radiation, or sphincter saving procedures.

Computed tomography CT is useful in defining local rectal tumour spread, although mesenteric and mesorectal lymph nodes are poorly visualised. In assessing rectal tumours the specificity of CT in determining local extension of the tumour into or beyond the pericolic fat is 61–77%. For lymph node metastases CT has a substantially lower specificity than endoluminal ultrasonography, at 22–34%. CT with intravenous contrast can provide good evaluation of the ureters and bladder. It can identify liver metastases larger than 2 cm but smaller metastases are often missed. Spiral CT and contrast enhancement techniques have increased the number of liver metastases detected but small metastases still elude detection by these techniques.

Magnetic resonance imaging MRI has not been shown to be superior to contrast enhanced CT but novel techniques utilising endoluminal snake coils may improve resolution.

Ultrasonography This is useful in the assessment of liver metastases. There are rarely any false positives; false negatives do more readily occur. Intraoperative ultrasonography has proven more accurate when assessing numbers of metastases. Some contrast enhancing forms of CT are more accurate (for example, spiral CT, CT combined with portography). Ultrasonography can also look grossly at ureteric involvement (calyceal dilatation).

Plain radiography Radiographs of the chest offer a gross assessment of pulmonary metastases but CT provides a far more accurate assessment.

Intravenous urography Routine preoperative IVU has not been shown to be of any benefit, but if specific features demand assessment of the ureter then it can be valuable. If available, pelvic CT has been shown to demonstrate similar information.

Immunoscintigraphy CEA was the first tumour antibody to be used as a target to detect colorectal cancer. There are, however, problems with the heterogeneity of tumour expression and its cross reactivity with normal tissues. At present we do not have an ideal tumour antibody; most of the work performed so far is with CEA, despite its problems.[11] Many different radioisotopes have been used to label tumour antibodies; the most common of these is indium-111 because of its favourable physical properties. The advantage of radiolabelled antibodies over other modalities is that they can detect metastases simultaneously at multiple sites. In large multicentre studies immunoscintigraphy appeared to be useful in 16–26% of cases when performed preoperatively, by detecting previously occult lesions, identifying localised disease without spread (massive rectal tumours), and the confirmation of adenocarcinoma when other tests were equivocal. It is therefore a relatively ineffective routine preoperative investigation. Immunoscintigraphy has, however, been shown to exhibit a high positivity rate in cases of local recurrence (90%). It is in this role that its future appears to lie. CT and MRI have difficulties differentiating tumour from postoperative and postradiation changes, and the sensitivity of immunoscintigraphy is therefore high compared with other modalities. Its specificity can be as high as 80% (similar to ultrasonography) and its accuracy is as good as MRI, at approximately 86%. Its positive predictive value is comparable with the other modalities and its negative predictive value is lower than that of MRI.

For immunoscintigraphy to have widespread use in colorectal cancer, it needs to be able to detect occult metastases, especially in the liver. At present only 50% of liver metastases are detected by this modality and pulmonary metastases are also poorly detected. This method may, however, allow identification of some smaller tumour deposits and recurrent cancers that elude detection by current methods.

Biomarkers

CEA may give a preoperative baseline that can be compared with postoperative values as an indicator of possible recurrence. Other biomarkers that have been used to aid recurrence detection are CA 19-9, sialic acid, tissue polypeptide antigen, and tumour cell DNA ploidy as determined by flow cytometry. All suffer from lack of specificity and are therefore unhelpful in staging at the present time.

Future advances

New advances include the assessment of tumour proliferation rates using flow cytometry, Ki-67 monoclonal antibodies, or bromodeoxyuridine incorporation. Determination of genetic alterations and deletions on biopsy material may influence treatment strategies as we come to understand their prognostic significance.

A multicentre imaging trial is at present under way to try and determine the relative sensitivity, specificity, and accuracy of CT and MRI in the preoperative detection of hepatic metastases, in the staging of colorectal carcinoma, and in the assessment of locoregional and distant intra-abdominal lymph node metastases. Endoluminal ultrasonography is also being evaluated for its role in the staging of rectal carcinoma.

Intraoperative assessment

Surgeon　It is difficult for a surgeon to assess accurately whether adhesions to the tumour are inflammatory or neoplastic. Hepatic metastases can be seen and felt, and frozen section biopsies can be performed if there is doubt.

Intraoperative ultrasonography　This modality can detect more liver metastases than preoperative imaging.

Frozen section　This can be a useful tool if margins of resection are uncertain—for example, lateral margins on excision of the rectum. It can also be used to assess the appropriate extent of the procedure that needs to be performed—for example, to confirm inoperable tumour or liver metastases.

Pathological staging

It is currently necessary to establish an international terminology that will make it possible to derive all staging systems according to the needs

335

of clinicians and the exchange of information between hospitals. The three main systems used in Europe are:

- Dukes
- tumour, node, metastases (TNM)
- Jass.

Dukes   Dukes's original classification is as follows.

- Dukes's A—tumour does not penetrate into the bowel wall
- Dukes's B—tumour penetrates into the wall with no lymph node involvement
- Dukes's C—tumour has lymph node metastases.

There have been many variations on this classification, including subdivision of Dukes's B and C tumours into subsets. A Dukes's stage D is also now widely accepted as meaning the presence of systemic disease. Five year survival figures of approximately 80% for Dukes's A, 48–62% for Dukes's B, and 22–33% for Dukes's C are reported. The large variation in survival figures suggests that Dukes's staging is clinically unreliable, but it is simple and universally understood.

TNM   The TNM system was originally set up to try and classify all tumours using the same system. It is merely a method of encoding pathological and clinical data; however, it has problems as regards uniformity—for example, T usually represents tumour size, but in colorectal cancer the different numbers are used to define the degrees of direct spread into the bowel wall. The TNM system is complicated, cumbersome, and lacks clinical meaning.

Jass   Jass designed a staging system that identified a small number of important variables that independently influence clinical end points. The four variables listed below were selected as a result of a multivariate analysis of those factors thought to affect prognosis.

1 Number of lymph nodes with metastatic tumour
2 Character of invasive margin
3 Lymphocytic infiltration
4 Local tumour spread.

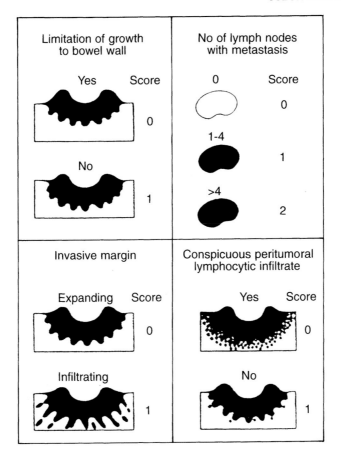

FIGURE 10.1—*Jass* scoring system

A scoring system was devised as seen in Figure 10.1. The groups were then classified as shown in Table 10.2.[12]

The Jass system is the most accurate for pathological staging at present, but is slightly more complex for the pathologist than Dukes's.

TABLE 10.2—*Jass's classification*[12]

Group	Total score	Five year survival (%)
1	0–1	96
2	2	85
3	3	67
4	4–5	27

Surgery

Preoperative evaluation

Colonic tumours

1 History and examination
2 Haematological and biochemical profiles, including liver function tests
3 Colonoscopy ideally, but if inadequate or difficult to perform, barium enema
4 Biopsy—histological assessment and confirmation of tumour
5 Ultrasonography of liver
6 Chest radiograph
7 CT or MRI if a complication is suspected—for example, abscess formation or invasion into nearby structures.

Rectal tumours

As above, with the following additional investigations.

8 Rectal examination—to assess whether the tumour is mobile or fixed and to assess the position of the tumour
9 Proctoscopy—series have shown 18% direct effect on diagnostic and treatment
10 Colonoscopy—to ensure a complete evaluation of the colon
11 Endoluminal ultrasonography and/or CT or RI—for assessment of tumour resectability and lymph node involvement
12 Anorectal manometry—may be required to ensure a sphincter saving procedure is functionally feasible.

Principles of curative surgery

It is of utmost importance to prevent the dissemination of tumour cells during resection and to ensure complete tumour resection wherever possible. When performing colorectal excision an understanding of the modes of spread is therefore essential. There is a sequential invasion of the tumour from mucosa to peritoneum and then into mesorectum or mesocolon and into adherent structures. Other modes of spread include lymphatic, haematological, and transperitoneal spread. Lymphatic spread usually follows the arterial supply to the tumour, but orderly progression is not inevitable and lymph nodes can be skipped. Haematological spread is less common but cancer cells have been isolated from veins draining the tumour. A relationship exists between the degree of differentiation and the presence of tumour cells in the venous drainage. Blood vessel invasion is more common in adenocarcinomas than colloid carcinomas and the most common in the poorly differentiated tumours. Transperitoneal spread is more common than haematological spread, and usually renders the lesion surgically incurable.

Complete tumour excision

En bloc resection Rectal malignancies are found to extend into adjacent structures in up to 20% of primary rectal cancer resections. Palliative diversion or incomplete resection has a reported median 10 month survival. Excision of part or all of any viscus adherent to the tumour should be performed, as although only 20% of adhesions are malignant, it is difficult to differentiate them clinically. However, at autopsies of women with primary rectal carcinoma it was shown that 13% had ovarian involvement and as a result some surgeons have advocated prophylactic oophorectomy.

Lateral margins If the lateral margins are not free of tumour histologically then there is an 85% likelihood of recurrence.

Distal margin In large studies, intramural retrograde spread was shown to be present in 12% of "curative" resections. The extent ranged from 1 to 7 cm. At present there is no consensus on the optimal distal margin. Current recommendations are between 1 and 3 cm, although there is no evidence that a distal margin of 2 cm adversely affects survival.

Complete lymphovascular resection

Colonic resection A complete colonic carcinoma resection means a segmental resection of the colon with its lymphovascular mesocolon.

Mural clearance can be easy to achieve with tumours of the right colon (caecum, ascending colon, hepatic flexure, and proximal half of the transverse colon). They are all supplied by the superior mesenteric artery and resection involves ligation of the colonic branches flush to the parent vessel.

The left colon (distal half of transverse colon, splenic flexure, descending colon, and sigmoid colon) takes its blood supply from the inferior mesenteric artery. This vessel can be taken close to its origin. The rectum is then reliant on its blood supply from the pudendal and middle rectal branches of the internal iliac artery.

Total mesorectal excision Worldwide recurrence rates for rectal cancer range between 20 and 45%. Total mesorectal excision has been advocated to decrease these rates. This involves precise sharp dissection around the integral mesentery of the hindgut, which envelops the entire mesorectum. Recurrence rates as low as 4% have been reported for Dukes's B2 and C tumours, with halving of overall recurrence rates when compared with conventional surgery and adjuvant therapy. The incidence of urinary, sexual, and defecation dysfunction is, however, substantially increased. Further evaluation is needed to confirm the initial results.

High versus low ligation   Early studies showed that 10% of patients undergoing left-sided colonic resection had nodes involved at the inferior mesenteric artery origin. It was therefore felt that a high ligation was mandatory, but recent studies show no survival difference between taking the inferior mesenteric artery at its origin or just distal to its first bifurcation.

Lateral pelvic lymph node dissection   Wide variations in local recurrence rates after anterior resections are probably caused by inadequate lateral margins. No randomised controlled trials have been undertaken but some of the subset analysis of node positive patients demonstrated a trend towards improved results in patients who had extended lateral resection. Similarly, local recurrence rates were lower for patients receiving this extended surgery.

Avoidance of surgical dissemination of the tumour

No touch technique   In 1955 Fisher *et al showed that tumour cells could be demonstrated in the perfusate of mesenteric vessels in resected specimens in up to 60% of patients.*[13] As a result of this, an isolation technique was devised to minimise intravascular and local spread of tumour cells.

This technique involved early wound covering and protection, early exposure and occlusion of the inferior mesenteric and marginal vessels, early bowel occlusion, minimal handling of the cancer, and retroperitoneal node dissection. Early studies showed survival advantages when compared with conventional techniques, but later studies questioned the significance of early vessel occlusion, as no correlation has been found between the presence of circulating tumour cells and survival. It was also suggested that the good results were attributable to the complete lymphatic resection rather than the isolation technique.

Implantation on to raw surfaces or suture lines   Tumours are easily induced at the site of colonic anastomosis in animal models. It seems that the healing process may promote tumour growth. Spillage of exfoliated malignant cells may be a cause of local recurrence at the time of surgery. There have recently been some data showing an increased incidence of implantation metastases at port sites after resection by laparoscopic methods.

Stapled versus hand sewn anastomosis   There is still some discussion about the use of stapled versus hand sewn anastomosis. However, data from a large, randomised trial in the west of Scotland has shown a decreased local recurrence with stapled anastomosis.[14]

Local recurrence[15]

Local recurrence after surgery for colorectal procedures is a major problem. Between 50 and 70% of patients are reported to undergo "curative" procedures and, of these, 10–15% will develop local recurrence. The main causes of local recurrence are inadequate resection of the primary tumour or the draining lymph nodes and intraoperative tumour cell implantation. The most significant prognostic factor for local recurrence is Dukes's tumour stage. Specific factors such as tumour penetration, lateral pelvic spread, number of rectal quadrants involved by tumour, poor tumour differentiation and the production of mucin have all been associated with a high recurrence rate. There are wide variations in local recurrence rates, both between and within institutions, almost certainly as the result of differences in surgical technique. The prevention of recurrence by adequate surgery and adjuvant therapy should cause recurrence rates to decrease.

Summary

In summary, radical tumour clearance, adequate distal margins, wide mesenteric dissection, and en bloc resection of adherent tissues are advisable to prevent recurrence. Extended lymphatic and vascular resections and isolation techniques have not improved results significantly. Mesorectal excision may increase survival and decrease recurrence rates in some groups of patients with rectal tumours.

Local excision

Selection criteria

Rectal lesions should be superficial tumours of T1 or T2 stage (Dukes's A lesions that do not penetrate the muscularis mucosa), as assessed by endoluminal ultrasonography or MRI.

The approach is usually by transanal excision under local or regional block. The posterior approach (for example, York–Mason) allows local lymph node assessment, but with an associated increase in morbidity.

Transanal endoscopic microsurgery[16]

A minimally invasive method of rectal tumour resection, transanal endoscopic microsurgery (TEM) utilises a 40 mm operating rectoscope sealed in an airtight facepiece. Carbon dioxide is constantly infused to distend the rectum and maintain visibility. Small, large, or even circumferential adenomas and selected carcinomas up to 20 cm from the anal verge can be removed with TEM instrumentation. The optics provide sixfold magnification, which allows precise excision as well as good closure of the wound.

TEM relies on accurate preoperative assessment of the depth of the tumour and the presence of metastases. Problems with the lesions located just above the dentate line include escape of insufflated carbon dioxide and bleeding during dissection. Conversion is always a possibility and full bowel preparation is required. Complications such as rectal stenosis may occur, especially in circumferential lesions. There is a comparatively high recurrence rate at 12–25%, presumably as a result of less than adequate resections margins. There is a documented 10% major complication rate and low mortality rates. The advantages are the minimal trauma and pain, resulting in a shorter hospital stay.

Laser excision

Laser resection of part of an obstructing tumour mass has been shown to decompress adequately the proximal bowel so that an elective operative procedure can be performed. This potentially decreases in-hospital mortality and morbidity rates.

Palliative therapy

Electrocoagulation

Surgical diathermy was first used in the 1900s; it can be used under local or regional block. Fulguration is usually used as palliative therapy but some claim that it can be a curative procedure.

Alcohol injection

Alcohol injection is used as a palliative therapy for unresectable rectal carcinomas and can cause satisfactory destruction of the protruding tumour. As with any therapy, there is a risk of perforation. This procedure needs to be evaluated against the established alternative of laser photocoagulation before further comment can be made.

Local laser therapy

Interstitial laser photocoagulation offers a good palliative treatment for patients with local recurrence and irresectable tumours. In one study 75% of patients reported good symptomatic relief. There are still questions about the ability of laser resection to relieve some of the more troublesome symptoms (for example, tenesmus, urgency), but bleeding and mucous discharge seem well controlled. The future role of laser may be as a substitute for operative diversion in hopeless clinical situations, such as haemorrhage or obstruction in patients with advanced disease.

Elective operations for rectal cancers

Preoperative preparation

1 Bowel preparation
2 Antibiotic therapy
3 Stoma site if needed
4 Placement of ureteric stents if necessary.

Operative procedures

These can be classified as stoma and non-stoma operations.

Abdominoperineal resection   This is indicated if the tumour involves the anal sphincters.

Hartmann's operation   This is advised when the tumour is resectable but a low pelvic anastomosis is not desirable—for example, in patients with preoperative evidence of sphincter compromise or impairment of healing due to a medical condition. This procedure is especially useful in the elderly patient with a compromised sphincter mechanism in whom a perineal wound is undesirable.

The following sphincter saving options should be discussed: low anterior resection, coloanal anastomosis, pull through procedures, and the colonic J pouch.

Total pelvic exenteration[17]   This procedure involves en bloc resection of rectum, distal colon, bladder, lower ureters, all internal reproductive organs, portions of the perineum, draining lymph nodes, and pelvic peritoneum. The indication for pelvic exenteration is a resectable primary colonic carcinoma without evidence of remote spread or a local recurrence without further evidence of spread. The patient's mental state and ability to remain self sufficient after the procedure must be taken into consideration. Despite the use of standard imaging, 25–30% of tumours thought to be resectable by exenteration preoperatively are found to be inoperable at laparotomy. Exenteration has been shown to provide a 40% five year survival rate when successful, but studies comparing similar patients are needed, as is evaluation of quality of life. Many of the large tumours excised are node negative, and in some circumstances the five year survival rate is as high as 70%.

Low anterior resection   This is defined as the resection of a rectal tumour when it is 10 cm from the anal verge. It involves the complete mobilisation of the descending and sigmoid colon, and complete mobilisation of the splenic flexure from its retroperitoneal attachments and omentum. Once the sigmoid colon is mobilised and the gonadal vessels are swept free, the inferior mesenteric artery and vein are isolated and ligated.

After ligation of the mesenteric vessels the rectum is freed by incising the lateral peritoneal reflection and mobilising the rectum from the sacral hollow. The plane between the fascia propria of the mesorectum and the presacral fascia is entered sharply to prevent inadvertent tearing of the sacral veins, which drain through the sacral promontory and may bleed profusely if damaged. The lateral ligaments are then encountered after dissection of the rectum down to the pelvic floor is achieved. Division of the lateral ligaments close to the pelvic side walls is avoided because of the adjacent nervi erigentes. The dissection is then brought anteriorly, the middle rectal arteries are divided, and the anterior plane is developed to the pelvic floor.

To obtain a more extensive radial margin, some surgeons enter the plane anterior to Denonvilliers's fascia. A large bowel clamp is then placed just below the tumour, a cancericidal rectal washout is performed, and a staple gun is placed below the clamp. A purse string suture or a cross stapling technique can be used to close the rectal stump. The largest stapling device possible should be used.

Anastomotic integrity—the anastomosis should be rigorously checked for leakage by:

- palpation of the ring transanally
- direct observation, usually with a rigid proctoscope
- insufflation of air after filling the pelvis with warm saline.

If there is any question as to the integrity of the anastomosis, this should be attended to and a loop ileostomy considered for defunctioning.

Coloanal anastomosis　The anus is prepared by inserting 6–8 heavy sutures around the anal margin. The mucosa is then incised circumferentially at the dentate line, entering the submucosal layer at 1 cm. The dissection is then extended into the muscularis propria for 1–2 cm and then posteriorly to just above the anorectal ring and into the pelvis. The specimen can then be removed and the proximal colon margin anastomised to 1 cm above the dentate line.

Colonic J pouch　An 8–10 cm pouch can be used when a very low colorectal or coloanal anastomosis is indicated. It is said that the presence of a rectal reservoir improves functional outcome. W and J colonic pouches are most commonly used. Both of these can give patients problems with stool frequency, faecal incontinence, and pouchitis.

Autonomic nerve dysfunction

Defecation disturbance The ability to defer defecation and avoid soiling usually remains unchanged in patients with an anastomosis 6 cm from the dentate line. Below this level, however, anorectal function is significantly worse, with changes in bowel frequency and the ability to distinguish flatus from faeces. Careful preoperative patient selection is therefore necessary.

Urinary dysfunction Retention of urine after a rectal cancer operation occurs in between 17 and 100% of patients. Dysfunction is most common in the elderly male, owing to a combination of benign prostatic hypertrophy and damage to the autonomic plexus. It is, however, unusual for long term urinary retention to be a problem. Other types of urinary dysfunction (for example, change in frequency, hesitancy, dysuria) are described and may occasionally persist. Minor urinary difficulties occur in 20% of patients with high anastomoses and 10% with lower anastomoses.

Sexual dysfunction Impotence and abnormal ejaculation can occur after rectal excision. Impotence occurs in between 30 and 70% of patients after conventional anterior resections. This figure increases to almost 100% when radical pelvic procedures are undertaken. Nerve sparing procedures for less invasive carcinomas can reduce this figure to below 20%. Female sexual dysfunction occurs at a similar rate to male dysfunction, with lack of orgasms, decreased vaginal lubrication, and dyspareunia being the most common symptoms.

Extended iliopelvic lymphadenectomy This technique may reduce local recurrence rates at the price of loss of bladder and sexual function. There is a substantial increase in urinary voiding failure. Loss of bladder filling sensation occurs in 40% of the extended group and in only 9% of the conventional group. The impotency rate is 76 versus 38%. Wide pelvic lymphadenectomy is therefore controversial and at present cannot be routinely recommended.

Nerve sparing pelvic node dissection This technique has been devised to decrease the incidence of urinary and sexual dysfunction. It requires an extensive knowledge of the surgical anatomy of the pelvic autonomic nervous system. The main benefit is in urinary rather than sexual function.

Surgery for metastases

Hepatic resection[18]
(See also Chapter 8)

In the United Kingdom 50% of colorectal cancer patients have hepatic metastases at the time of presentation. The mean survival for patients with detectable hepatic metastases without surgery is 12 months. The five year survival for patients who undergo resection is between 20 and 40%, depending on the selection criteria used for hepatic resection. In resections performed for isolated hepatic metastasis 10 year survival is not uncommon. Overall, however, the evidence indicates that hepatic resection is palliative in the majority of cases. Combinations of hepatic resection, cryotherapy, and chemotherapy may become more common in the future.

Pulmonary resection

Pulmonary resection for isolated metastases from colorectal cancer has survival rates comparable to or better than those for resection of isolated hepatic metastases. Fifty per cent five year survival has been reported in some centres.

Laparoscopic resection

With the recent expansion of laparoscopic surgery, colorectal resections are increasingly being performed by this method. Most studies have shown no increase in mortality or 30 day morbidity and that patients having laparoscopic resections may have less postoperative pain, earlier return to work, and shorter stay in hospital. Many surgeons are, however, seriously concerned that the principles of the operative technique may be sacrificed in order to remove the colon laparoscopically. We are beginning to be able to assess local and distant recurrence rates, and some data suggest an increase in local recurrence rates after laparoscopic resections. The use of laparoscopic techniques in curative colorectal cancer resections cannot be routinely recommended at present and needs to be critically evaluated.

Emergency surgery

The obstructed colon and colorectal carcinoma[19]

Between 8 and 9% of patients with colonic carcinoma present with intestinal obstruction. This accounts for more than 75% of all colonic emergencies. Patients presenting with malignant obstruction of the colon are known to have a worse prognosis stage for stage than those with non-obstructing lesions. This may be due to the more aggressive nature of the tumours, but could reflect inadequate attention to radical surgical technique by a surgeon concentrating on the relief of the obstruction rather than curative resection.

Carcinoma of the right colon

A carcinoma presenting with an obstructing lesion proximal to the splenic flexure is easily resected by performing a right or extended right hemicolectomy.

Obstructed carcinoma of the left colon

Fifty per cent of all splenic flexure carcinomas and 25% of all left colonic tumours present with obstruction. Colocolic and colorectal anastomoses are generally considered more susceptible to leakage than ileocolic or ileorectal anastomoses. Blood supply, faecal bulk, and collagen metabolism are possible contributory factors. Treatment options are:

- proximal stoma formation
- Hartmann's procedure
- single stage resection and anastomosis (with or without a covering ileostomy)
- non-laparotomy treatments.

Proximal stoma formation and Hartmann's procedure necessitate a further one or two procedures to reconstruct bowel continuity.

Proximal stoma formation

1 *Caecostomy* is advocated by some as an easy and safe way of decompressing the bowel. Its advantage is that it can be performed under local anaesthesia, either radiologically or surgically. Its disadvantages are that it is a difficult stoma to look after (tube caecostomies have a reputation for obstructing) and the surgeon has not resected the tumour. Caecostomy should only be used as a last resort measure to buy time to improve patients' general condition if they are extremely high risk.

2 *Loop transverse colostomy* can be performed under local anaesthetic and is an easier stoma to deal with long term. Its best use is when further resection is unlikely in a high risk patient.

3 *Three stage procedure* was the standard for many years. It involves a loop colostomy, resection of tumour and anastomosis, and finally reversal of the loop colostomy. Often the third operation was not performed because the patient was insufficiently fit or was unwilling to undergo a further surgical procedure. The technique has a survival advantage but has the disadvantages of prolonging hospital stay and exposing patients to repeated operations.

Hartmann's procedure The two main advantages of this technique compared with the previous procedures are that the colonic tumour is resected at the first operation and that a terminal left iliac fossa colostomy is much more easily managed than a right upper quadrant loop colostomy.

At present Hartmann's procedure accounts for 4% of all elective colorectal carcinoma procedures and 92% of all emergency procedures. Morbidity from the stoma includes skin erosions, strictures, incisional hernias, abscesses, wound infections, and fistulas. The procedure has acceptable morbidity and mortality rates and is the safest option for trainee surgeons or surgeons with limited exposure to colonic resection. Hospital stay is less than for the three stage procedures. Reversal of Hartmann's procedure, however, carries significant morbidity and mortality rates, and many are never reversed.

Primary resection with anastomosis Traditionally this was a taboo procedure, but more favourable results began to be reported when proximal irrigation was performed. Technical refinements to lavage equipment have made faecal spillage rare. Reported 30 day operative mortality rates vary between 4 and 15%, comparable with both Hartmann's procedure and colostomy alone. Lavage lengthens the operation by at least an hour and a mean operating time of 3–4 hours can not be undertaken lightly in an ill elderly patient. Hospital stay is considerably less than that associated with the staged procedures. Five year survival rates are comparable with elective procedures.

An alternative to intraoperative lavage and segmental colectomy is the complete resection of the proximal colon by subtotal colectomy and ileosigmoid or ileorectal anastomosis. Operative mortality rates are similar to the other resection procedures but subtotal colectomy carries a risk of diarrhoea and/or faecal incontinence, particularly in the elderly patient.

Avoidance of a stoma has to be weighed against the risk of anastomotic leakage. A randomised controlled study comparing segmental resection with subtotal colectomy is currently under way.

Non-laparotomy treatments Deflation of the obstructed colon can on occasion be obtained by the introduction of a rectal stent through a flexible sigmoidoscope.

Hydrostatic balloon dilatation is a recent innovation that is at present under evaluation. The early results show relief of two thirds of obstructing tumours with a single dilatation.

Endoscopic neodymium yttrium aluminium garnet (NdYAG) laser recanalisation has been tried on partially obstructing lesions with reasonable results. The data on completely obstructing lesions are scant.

Summary

In general there is no benefit to be gained by deferring tumour resection as part of a staged procedure. Long term survival may be affected by the delay, and completion of staged procedures often fails to occur. Whether primary anastomosis should be performed after segmental resection or subtotal colectomy is at present incompletely evaluated. Surgeons unfamiliar with immediate resection and primary anastomosis should either consider referral to another colleague with the necessary skills or perform a Hartmann's procedure. The future management of rectal tumours will probably be by transanal decompression followed by a semielective procedure.

References

1 Campbell WJ, Spence RAJ, Parks TG. Familial adenomatous polyposis. *Br J Surg* 1994; **81**:1722–33.
2 Warthin TA. The further study of a cancer family. *J Cancer Res* 1925;**9**:279.
3 Lynch HT, Krush AJ. A cancer family "G" revisited 1895–1970. *Cancer* 1971;**27**: 1895–1900.
4 Lovett E. Family studies in cancer of the colon and rectum. *Br J Surg* 1976;**63**:13–18.
5 Peltomaki PT. Genetic basis of hereditary nonpolyposis colorectal carcinoma (HNPCC). *Ann Med* 1994;**26**:215–9.
6 Kinzler KW, Vogelstein B. Colorectal cancer gene hunt: current findings. *Hosp Pract* 1992: 51–8.
7 Mandel JS, Bond JH, Church TR, *et al.* Reducing mortality from colorectal cancer by screening for faecal occult blood. Minnesota Colon Cancer Control Study. *N Engl J Med* 1993;**328**:1365–71.
8 Winawer SJ, Flehinger BJ, Schottenfeld D, *et al.* Screening for colorectal cancer with faecal occult blood resting and sigmoidoscopy. *J Natl Cancer Inst* 1993;**85**:1311–8.
9 Levin B, Lennard-Jones J, Riddell RH, *et al.* Surveillance of patients with chronic ulcerative colitis. *Bull World Health Organ* 1991;**69**:121–6.
10 Kelvin FM, Maglinte DDT. Colorectal carcinoma: a radiological and clinical review. *Radiology* 1987;**164**:1–8.
11 Wang JY, Tang R, Chiang JM. Value of carcinoembryonic antigen in the management of colorectal cancer. *Dis Colon Rectum* 1994;**37**:272–7.
12 Jass JR, Morson BC. Reporting colorectal cancer. *J Clin Pathol* 1987;**40**:1016–23.
13 Fisher GR, Turnbull RB. The cytologic demonstration and significance of tumour cells in the mesenteric venous blood in patients with colorectal carcinoma. *Surg Gynecol Obstet* 1955;**8**:100–2.
14 Akyol AM, McGregor TR, Galloway DJ, *et al.* Recurrence of colorectal cancer after sutured and stapled large bowel anastomosis. *Br J Surg* 1991;**78**:1297–1300.
15 Abulafi AM, Williams NS. Local recurrence of colorectal cancer: the problem, mechanisms, management and adjuvant therapy. *Br J Surg* 1994;**81**:7–19.
16 Buess G. Review: transanal endoscopic microsurgery. *J R Coll Surg Edinb* 1993;**38**:239–45.
17 Yeung RS, Moffat FL, Falk RE. Pelvic exenteration for recurrent colorectal carcinoma: a review. *Cancer Invest* 1994;**12**:176–88.
18 Shumate CR. Colorectal cancer hepatic metastases: the surgeon's role. *Ala Med* 1994; **63**(8):15–8.
19 Deans GT, Krukowski ZH, Irwin ST. Malignant obstruction of the left colon. *Br J Surg* 1994;**81**:1270–6.

Chemotherapy, radiotherapy, palliative care, and new approaches

NICHOLAS D JAMES and DAVID J KERR

Radiotherapy

Aims of radiotherapy

The role of radiotherapy in colorectal cancer can be subdivided into radical and palliative. Definitive radical therapy for colorectal cancer is centred around surgical resection of the tumour and the adjacent mesentery bearing the draining nodes. There are, however, potential roles for radiotherapy in the radical treatment programme, both in the downstaging of disease preoperatively and in the reduction of the risks of local recurrence postoperatively. In both settings there is a local control benefit, with a trend to improved survival seen in overviews of published trials.[20 21] In addition, in locally advanced inoperable disease, long term survivors have been reported after radical radiotherapy. Radiotherapy also has a significant role in the palliation of both local and metastatic recurrences.

Patient selection

Radiotherapy can be given either preoperatively to downstage disease, increasing the probability of complete resection at surgery, or postoperatively in patients at high risk of local recurrence. Most studies have only examined the role of radiotherapy in tumours below the peritoneal reflection, as the local recurrence rates for colonic carcinomas are less. Furthermore, the radiosensitivity of organs such as liver and kidneys and the difficulties of accurate and consistent localisation render colonic radiotherapy impracticable. The remaining radiotherapy discussion will be restricted to rectal carcinomas. Palliative radiotherapy is dealt with below.

Preoperative radiotherapy

A number of studies have examined the role of radiotherapy as an adjunct to definitive surgery. The aim of preoperative radiotherapy has been to downstage disease, reduce tethering, and thereby render the primary tumour more susceptible to surgical removal. Additionally, where staging suggests that definitive resection may be difficult, preoperative radiotherapy may increase the likelihood that colostomy may be avoided. Most of these studies have shown a decrease in local recurrence rates for rectal cancer. Studies such as MRC1 (reviewed in *The Journal of Cancer Research*[2]) also showed a significant reduction in the size of tumour at operation and also a significant reduction in the number of tethered tumours; however, because of the logistic problems in identifying patients suitable for radiotherapy before surgery, preoperative radiotherapy is probably not used as widely as it could be. When the results of all the preoperative radiotherapy studies are pooled, there is a trend to improved odds of survival of around 9%, which approaches statistical significance.[21]

Postoperative radiotherapy

At least four large randomised studies, including two studies organised by the Medical Research Council (MRC), have looked at the role of postoperative radiotherapy in locally advanced rectal carcinomas. Again, there was a trend to improved local control, which reached statistical significance in the case of MRC3 (reviewed in *The Journal of Cancer Research*[2]). As with the preoperative studies, there was a trend to improved survival of $14 \pm 11\%$, again approaching statistical significance.[20 21]

Who, then, should receive radiotherapy, and should it be preoperative or postoperative? Patients in whom the tumour seems to be fixed in the preoperative assessment, or in whom the imaging suggests removal may be difficult, should be considered for preoperative radiotherapy. In general, it will be difficult to identify these patients preoperatively and consideration should be given when the pathological staging is reviewed. As there is convincing evidence that postoperative radiotherapy reduces local recurrence rates, it should be considered for all rectal carcinoma patients with Dukes's stage B2 or C tumours, particularly if there was a degree of fixity at operation or any suspicion of incomplete excision.

Whether or not there is an improvement in overall survival, the improvement in local control, a particularly distressing problem to control, more than justifies consideration of adjuvant radiotherapy in appropriate cases. The currently ongoing AXIS trial is also addressing the role of radiotherapy in rectal cancer, in addition to examining the effects of locally infused chemotherapy on the subsequent development of metastases.[22] Adjuvant chemotherapy with 5-fluorouracil based chemotherapy has been shown in randomised studies—for example, those of the National Surgical Adjuvant Board Project (NSABP)—to improve overall survival in patients with advanced colonic and rectal carcinomas (see below). Patients with advanced rectal carcinomas should therefore be offered both adjuvant radiotherapy and chemotherapy, and this should be given concurrently, as for example in the currently recruiting Quick and Simple and Reliable (QUASAR) trial.

Colonic carcinomas present a much more difficult problem in terms of radiotherapeutic management. For the portions of the colon that are intraperitoneal, such as the transverse colon, local radiotherapy is generally not possible because of uncertainty about the position of the tumour and also the radiosensitivity of adjacent organs, such as the liver and kidneys. For retroperitoneal tumours, such as those in the sigmoid colon where the bowel is fixed and there are no especially sensitive local organs, radiotherapy can be considered in selected cases.

Targeted radioimmunotherapy

In recent years there has been considerable work in the area of radioimmunotherapy. Monoclonal antibodies against epitopes such as carcinoembryonic antigen (CEA) and HMFG1 have been used. These antibodies can be conjugated to radionuclides such as iodine-131 and yttrium-90. Phase I and II studies in advanced disease have shown disappointing results, despite good tumour to normal tissue ratios. The long term role of such therapies is likely to be as adjuvant treatment in patients with completely excised tumours rather than as treatment for advanced disease.[23 24]

Technical aspects

General

Whole pelvic treatments should be administered on megavoltage radiotherapy machines, preferably linear accelerators rather than cobalt-60 machines because of the superior dose distributions that can be produced, especially in larger patients. Treating the patient in the prone position improves the reproducibility of the set-up, based on our internal audit data, as the bony landmarks of the pelvis overlying the rectum can be directly used for field alignment.

Radiotherapy fields

The clinical target volume should include the original tumour volume, the presacral space, and the adjacent pelvic nodes, as defined by preoperative imaging and operative and other clinical findings. When postoperative radiotherapy is given after an abdominoperineal resection, the perineal scar should be included in the volume and should be marked with wire during simulation. Various field arrangements are possible, including a four field box, a posterior and two lateral wedged fields, or a posterior and two wedged posterior oblique fields (Figure 10.2). The field will include the

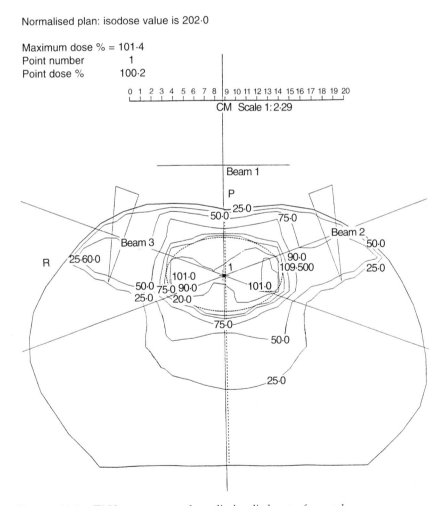

Normalised plan: isodose value is 202·0

Maximum dose % = 101·4
Point number   1
Point dose %   100·2

FIGURE 10.2—*Field arrangements for radical radiotherapy for rectal cancer.*

ovaries in female patients and may include the testes in males; patients should be counselled appropriately for this as the doses given will cause gonadal failure and sterility.

Radiotherapy doses

Various dose schedules are in use worldwide. The schedules used in our centre are 25 Gy in five fractions over one week for preoperative therapy, 45 Gy in 20 fractions over four weeks for postoperative treatment, reduced to 45 Gy in 25 fractions over five weeks when given with concurrent chemotherapy. These are the doses recommended in the QUASAR trial protocol. Doses for palliative treatment are given in the relevant section.

Monitoring

Patients receiving pelvic radiotherapy are prone to the usual side effects of treatment, such as malaise and lethargy. As significant volumes of bone marrow are included in the fields, patients with compromised marrow reserve should be haematologically monitored. This is not usually a problem during radiotherapy but may become one during subsequent chemotherapy. Specific acute side effects include radiation cystitis and proctitis and small bowel irritation, manifesting itself as colic or nausea. Radiation cystitis can be complicated additionally by urinary tract infection, which should be promptly investigated and treated. Some clinicians advocate regular examinations of urine samples during therapy, for occult infection. Radiation proctitis usually manifests itself as diarrhoea, which progressively worsens as the course of radiotherapy progresses. A low residue diet can alleviate the acute symptoms, supplemented with antidiarrhoeals such as loperamide if necessary. Both the cystitis and proctitis gradually settle over the weeks after cessation of treatment. As these side effects can be distressing and debilitating, particularly in older patients, it is essential that patients on treatment are reviewed regularly during therapy.

Mortality and morbidity

Colorectal cancer is the second most common malignant disease in the United Kingdom, with about 26 000 cases and 20 000 deaths each year. Around 70–80% of cases are suitable for "curative" surgery but unfortunately two thirds of these will subsequently relapse and are generally then incurable. Five year survival, as for all cancers, is dependent on stage and is about 80% for Dukes's stage A, 60% for stage B, and 30% for stage C. Local recurrence is uncommon for colonic cancer but occurs in around 30% of patients with rectal tumours.

The acute morbidity of radiotherapy is described in the previous section. Late effects of radiotherapy are dependent on dose given as well as on the nature of the surgery performed. At the dose levels given above, the incidence of late bladder and bowel damage requiring surgical intervention should not exceed a few per cent of treated patients, at most, in the absence of other comorbid conditions.

Outcome

The outcome of treatment with present standard therapies is described above and has changed little in recent years. Ultimately, improved results will depend on the development of new treatment modalities, in particular new drug treatments, and areas such as gene therapy (see below); however, pending the development of new agents, the optimal use of existing technology could still produce substantial saving in terms of both lives and morbidity. Two trials mentioned above, AXIS and QUASAR, are currently recruiting in the United Kingdom and aim to provide important data on the optimal use of adjuvant radiotherapy and chemotherapy.

The AXIS study is examining two questions: the use of postoperative infusional chemotherapy, the rationale for which is discussed below, and adjuvant radiotherapy. The design of the trial is open, in that eligibility criteria are determined by the clinicians entering the patients. The trial, when mature, will thus help to define the area in which there is most clinical uncertainty about the role of radiotherapy, as well as hopefully demonstrating whether radiotherapy, either preoperative or postoperative, can contribute to improved survival.

The QUASAR study, like AXIS, has eligibility criteria that are open, in that clinicians determine which patients should be entered and which randomisation is appropriate (chemotherapy versus no chemotherapy for early tumours, different intensity chemotherapies for patients with more advanced tumours). Again, the aim is both to define the areas in which there is uncertainty and simultaneously to produce a definitive answer as to the optimal therapy.

For both studies, the aim is to detect survival benefits of the order of 10% and to define which patients are most likely to benefit. Although this possible benefit is small numerically, the number of patients affected by colorectal cancer means that potentially large numbers of lives could be saved by optimal use of existing treatments.

Chemotherapy

Aims of chemotherapy

In general terms, chemotherapy may be administered with either curative or palliative intent, and this will be determined by the natural history of the disease and the fitness of the patient. With respect to colorectal cancer, chemotherapy will only be administered with the possibility of cure in an adjuvant setting, whereas advanced or metastatic colorectal cancer is widely held to be incurable and therefore any therapy needs must be palliative. The philosophy of the treatment approach is quite different, in that, if cure is possible, both patient and doctor will strive to achieve this, and consequent side effects are somehow considered less important. If, however, palliation (perhaps without prolongation of life) is the primary objective, then maintenance of quality of life is of paramount importance and may require a trade off between the efficacy and toxicity of the cytotoxic regimen.

Drug selection and rationale

The chemotherapeutic mainstay of colorectal cancer is 5-fluorouracil (5FU), an antimetabolite that has enjoyed over 30 years of clinical use. 5FU is a prodrug that is metabolised inside cells to its active principle, 5-fluorodeoxyuridine monophosphate (5FdUMP), which can inhibit DNA and RNA synthesis (Figure 10.3). An antimetabolite is a drug that is structurally similar to an essential cellular factor and, by virtue of that similarity, is incorporated into a variety of biochemical pathways, which are then inhibited.

5FdUMP inhibits thymidylate synthase, a key enzyme involved in synthesis of thymidine, an essential DNA building block. It can also be further metabolised and incorporated into DNA and RNA, interfering with the synthesis of these macromolecules. Given its mechanism of action, it is not surprising to learn that 5FU is a cycle specific agent—that is, it is particularly effective against cells that are in the DNA synthetic (S) phase of the cell cycle. If the average cell cycle lasts 24 hours and S phase lasts eight hours, then at any given time only one third of the cell population will be in S phase and, therefore, sensitive to 5FU. A clinical prediction stemming from this is that prolonged, continuous or intermittent, frequent exposure would be more active than infrequent, high dose therapy.

The pharmacokinetics of 5FU have been extensively studied and reveal that it has a short half life (10–15 minutes) and saturable cell uptake/ metabolism. Again, this implies that prolonged infusion of the drug would enhance its cellular uptake and, therefore, cytotoxicity.

As a single agent, 5FU has been administered in a wide variety of doses and schedules. In general, in the absence of data from convincing randomised studies, it would appear that intravenous bolus administration daily for five days every month is superior to intermittent high dose weekly or fortnightly and oral 5FU. Being dogmatic, oral 5FU should not be used, given its wide interindividual variation in bioavailability and, therefore, toxicity. Response rates (the percentage of treated patients who show at least a 50% reduction in tumour bulk after therapy) to single agent 5FU are in the range of 10–20% and the duration of these responses is of the order of 6–8 months. The side effects that occur during 5FU therapy depend on the schedule and dose and include nausea, vomiting, myelosuppression, mucositis, and diarrhoea. After prolonged infusion, one unusual side effect is a desquamative erythema of the hands and feet.

There is a dual academic response to this disappointing clinical activity—namely, use currently available drugs optimally, or search for novel therapeutic strategies. By understanding the pharmacokinetics and molecular pharmacology of 5FU, advances have been made in its clinical use.

Pharmacokinetic rationale

The pharmacokinetic and cell cycle hypothesis would suggest that prolonged continuous infusion of 5FU would give superior results compared with intermittent high dose therapy. Lokich *et al* have subjected this hypothesis to a randomised trial in advanced colorectal cancer and have shown that tumour response rates are significantly higher (30%) with the infusion compared with the bolus (7%).[25] Regional chemotherapy with 5FU is similarly predicated on pharmacokinetic principles. In addition to intravenous administration, 5FU has been given by portal venous infusion in an adjuvant setting, and via the hepatic artery and peritoneal cavity for advanced disease. 5FU is an ideal drug for regional chemotherapy as it is readily diffusible, has a high total body clearance, has some efficacy in colorectal cancer, and has a relatively high extraction ratio by the liver. We[26] and others have proven that it is possible to deliver very high drug concentrations to hepatic metastatic colorectal cancer through surgically implanted indwelling arterial catheters. This increases tumour response rates to the order of 50–60% and, although a series of technically flawed randomised studies have not shown a survival benefit for intrahepatic arterial 5FU, the MRC has recently undertaken a pharmacokinetically designed trial of arterial versus systemic chemotherapy in hepatic metastatic disease, which should provide a definitive answer to this question. Postoperative portal venous infusion of 5FU (for a period of one week) has been shown to improve survival significantly in an adjuvant setting. One postulated mechanism of action is through eradication of microscopic tumour metastases, which receive their vascular supply from the portal vein.

Intraperitoneal administration of 5FU through an abdominal Tenckhoff catheter can generate abdominal drug concentrations 1000-fold higher than systemic blood levels. There is a compelling rationale for intraperitoneal therapy in an adjuvant setting as this would allow generation of very high drug concentrations at likely sites of tumour recurrence—for example, locoregional, retroperitoneal lymph nodes, peritoneal carcinomatosis, and the liver—as intraperitoneal 5FU is cleared from the abdominal cavity through the portal vein to the liver (70% of abdominal drug content) and by retroperitoneal lymphatic channels. We are currently conducting a phase I trial of prolonged infusional intraperitoneal 5FU (12 weeks), using a novel dialysate solution, with a view to developing it as an adjuvant therapy.[27]

Pharmacodynamic rationale

Folinic acid is an important cellular cofactor in the synthesis of certain amino acids and nucleotides. It has been shown to stabilise the ternary complex of 5FdUMP and thymidylate synthase and thus increase inhibition of the enzyme, leading to further cellular depletion of thymidine and

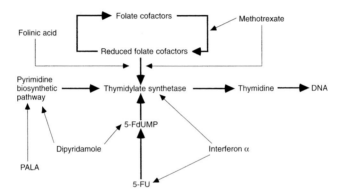

FIGURE 10.3—*Mechanism of action of 5FU and its biochemical modulation (5FU= 5-fluorouracil; 5FdUMP=5-fluorodeoxyuridine monophosphate; PALA=N-phosphonocetyl-L-aspartic acid).*

enhanced cytotoxicity of 5FU (Figure 10.3). These in vitro observations have been translated into a large number of phase II and phase III trials. Recent meta-analysis of nine randomised studies comparing single agent 5FU versus combinations of 5FU and folinic acid, comprising approximately 2000 patients, has shown that the addition of folinic acid significantly increases tumour response rates in advanced colorectal cancer, from 9 to 23%. Although in several individual studies the addition of folinic acid conferred a survival benefit, this was not seen in the meta-analysis. Nevertheless, the combination of 5FU and folinic acid is a step forward and is now regarded by many as the chemotherapy of choice for palliation of advanced colorectal cancer. Although the side effects associated with high dose 5FU and folinic acid can be severe, with debilitating mucositis and diarrhoea, this may be offset by its significantly higher response rate, as symptomatic improvement in patients usually correlates with reduction in tumour mass.

Most other conventional cytotoxic drugs have been assessed in the treatment of advanced colorectal cancer and, apart perhaps from mitomycin C, have been found to be lacking in activity. There was a vogue for combination type chemotherapy, but again with relatively little evidence of worthwhile benefit relative to single agent 5FU. Other drugs have been used in attempts to modulate the bioactivity of 5FU, such as methotrexate (an inhibitor of the enzyme dihydrofolate reductase), dipyridamole (an inhibitor of 5FU metabolism), N-phosphonocetyl-L-aspartic acid (PALA) (an inhibitor of the enzyme aspartate transcarbamylase), and interferon α (an immunomodulatory agent that alters thymidylate synthase expression); however, these combinatorial attempts to improve the therapeutic ratio of 5FU have not met with the same success as folinic acid.

A range of immunomodulatory agents have been tested in the treatment of advanced colorectal cancer. These include the anthelmintic drug, levamisole (which has a postulated immunostimulatory effect), interferon α (which can have a direct cytostatic effect on cancer cells in vitro, in addition to its capacity to alter ratios of helper:suppressor T cells), the T cell growth factor interleukin 2 (which has been infused with lymphokine activated killer cells), and a range of monoclonal antibodies coupled to radionuclides, cell toxins, enzymes, and cytotoxic drugs. These approaches have not proved very rewarding and can be associated with significant toxicity, particularly interleukin 2, which can precipitate a capillary leak syndrome.

Adjuvant chemotherapy for colorectal cancer

Adjuvant chemotherapy has been extensively tested for colorectal cancer but results achieved with the suboptimal chemotherapy regimens used in early studies were generally disappointing. Nevertheless, a meta-analysis of the published data from these studies suggests that six months, or longer, treatment with 5FU containing regimens may reduce the risk of death by around 10–15%, although this difference is of only borderline statistical significance.[22] Such an improvement in survival, if real, would be important, because even a 10% reduction in mortality in a disease as common as colorectal cancer would save tens of thousands of lives worldwide each year.

The early trial with the most striking result was the American intergroup study comparing one year of 5FU and levamisole with levamisole alone and with an untreated control group. This trial reported a one third reduction in the death rate in a subgroup of high risk (Dukes's stage C) patients with colonic cancer who received combination therapy. The contribution of levamisole, an antihelminthic immunomodulatory drug, to the strikingly improved outcome can, however, be questioned. The 5FU–levamisole combination appears no more effective than 5FU alone in advanced disease, and a clear understanding of the biological mechanism of the hypothesised synergy between these drugs has proved elusive. The large survival benefit seen in this study may therefore not be due to synergy between 5FU and levamisole but be simply a "random high"—that is, a 5FU effect that by chance turned out larger in the stage C patients in this study than in previous studies of 5FU on its own.

A second smaller study by the American National Cancer Clinical Trials Group (NCCTG) group has also reported a large reduction in mortality, this time achieved by adding systemic 5FU to radiotherapy in rectal cancer. Again, radiotherapy alone has at best a very moderate influence on survival and so it is unclear whether the benefit seen in this study was inflated by chance or was due to synergy between 5FU and radiotherapy.

Three recent studies, which recruited 2886 patients, of six months adjuvant 5FU coupled with its biomodulator folinic acid (FU/FA) provide more convincing evidence of a worthwhile survival benefit for adjuvant chemotherapy. Firstly, an overview of three randomised studies—from Italy, France, and Canada—that had tested six months of 5FU with high doses $(250 \, mg/m^2)$ of folinic acid has reported a significant benefit of this combination in terms of recurrence free survival, but not, to date, in survival. Secondly, an American intergroup study of 5FU with much lower doses $(20 \, mg/m^2)$ of folinic acid has reported a significant reduction in recurrence free survival, but again not in survival. Finally, an NSABP study comparing 5FU and very high dose $(500 \, mg/m^2)$ folinic acid with MOF (methyl-CCNU, vincristine, 5FU) chemotherapy has shown a significant improvement in recurrence free survival and also a survival benefit for the 5FU and folinic acid combination. These apparent benefits from adjuvant FU/FA are made more plausible by an understanding of the pharmacological rationale for this 5FU potentiation, coupled with definite evidence that folinic acid enhances the activity of 5FU in advanced disease.

Special aspects of palliative care

Patients with locally advanced rectal tumours that are inoperable by virtue of fixity may derive significant benefit from palliative radiotherapy, depending on the age of the patient and whether or not the tumour has metastasised. Patients with locally advanced non-metastatic tumours have achieved long term remissions with radical radiotherapy without surgery and this option should always be considered in such cases. Doses of the order of 55–65 Gy in 20–30 fractions should be used and will provide good symptomatic palliation in 80–90% of patients, although long term control or cure is sadly rare.

Pelvic recurrence in patients previously operated on presents a particularly unpleasant situation to deal with as patients often have great pain from infiltration of the sacral nerve plexus. Short palliative courses of radiotherapy (for example, 21 Gy in three fractions over one week) may produce considerable benefits in terms of pain and other symptom control.

Up to 30–40% of patients with solitary liver metastases from primary colorectal tumours can be cured by resection; however, most patients are unsuitable for curative resection and alternative therapies need to be explored. The usefulness of radiotherapy in the palliation of liver metastases is limited by the radiosensitivity of the liver. External beam irradiation of 20–30 Gy in 10–15 fractions to the whole liver, with or without concurrent chemotherapy, may be used for palliation of metastatic disease to the liver,[28][29] although this is below the desirable dose level for maximum tumour kill. A combination of brachytherapy applied to the tumour bed and external beam irradiation may improve local control and survival rates in patients with unresectable metastases. Techniques examined include implantation of iodine-125 seeds[29] and afterloading of iridium-192 wires into catheters implanted at the time of surgery.[30]

Laser palliation of locally advanced rectal or rectosigmoid cancer can provide good palliation of bowel symptoms such as obstruction, bleeding, and mucous discharge. It is, however, probably less effective with symptoms such as tenesmus, and is thus probably best combined with other palliative therapies for optimal benefit and possibly more prolonged palliative effect. Treatments need to be repeated every 4–6 weeks and this can be extended by the addition of palliative radiotherapy to the laser therapy, the combination being well tolerated.[31][32]

Future developments in treatment

New molecular targets for anticancer drug development

The predominant target for the majority of conventional antineoplastic drugs is inhibition of DNA synthesis. Historically, the screening systems developed to identify new anticancer drugs were mechanistically biased towards DNA synthesis inhibitors, as they were based on rapidly proliferating murine leukaemic cells with a high proportion of cells in the DNA synthetic (S) phase of the cell cycle. There has been an extraordinary increase in our understanding of the molecular process of carcinogenesis, and many of the genes (so called oncogenes and tumour suppressor genes) responsible for initiating and maintaining the transformed cell phenotype have been identified. This implies that there are novel targets that, if inhibited or modulated, might alter the biological behaviour of the cancer cell. The following scientific areas could be fruitful sources of new treatments over the next decade.

Growth factor–receptor–signal transduction pathways

Many cancer cells are genetically programmed, by mutation, constitutively to produce peptide growth factors to which they respond via receptors of the cell membrane. Put simply, the cancer cell can feed itself, and one would imagine that such a cell would have a proliferative advantage relative to the growth regulated normal counterparts and that clonal expansion would soon occur. It is possible to take a reductionist approach to this growth factor loop, dissect out the components of the pathway, and then devise therapeutic interventions. Antisense oligomers are modified nucleotide sequences that can recognise and bind to unique mRNA molecules and therefore prevent expression of key oncogenic proteins. There are immense pharmaceutical problems about delivering these nucleotides to the cancer cell in sufficient quantity, but at least in vitro this approach has been shown to inhibit selectively mutant oncogene activity and reduce the growth of cancer cells. Many growth factors need to be "processed", usually by proteolytic cleavage, to active species and there are some low molecular weight inhibitors of these enzymes available. Monoclonal antibodies have been used in vitro to prevent binding and activation of growth factor receptors, inducing cytostasis in vitro. After activation of growth factor receptors, conformational change initiates a cascade of events, many mediated by kinases, which alter levels of transcription factors and ultimately commit the cell to dividing.

Colorectal cancer cells express high levels of the oncogenic src kinase. We have recently completed a phase I clinical trial of a novel inhibitor of this kinase and found some evidence of antitumour activity.

Metastasis and angiogenesis

The biological features that differentiate cancer cells from normal host cells include incoordinated growth, the ability to invade locally, and the capacity to metastasise to distant organs. Understanding the sequence of events leading to metastasis suggests a series of possible interventions. Subpopulations of cancer cells from within the primary tumour can secrete a range of proteases that can degrade basement membranes and other components of the peritumoral stroma (for example, collagen, gelatin, elastin). Tssue degradation is followed by a movement of tumour cells and invasion into small lymphatic or blood vessels. The cells are then disseminated into the systemic circulation and establish themselves in distant tissue compartments. The specificity of organ metastasis depends on a series of cell surface proteins, addressing, which recognise and bind to specific components on the endothelium of discrete organ systems. The tumour cells then proteolytically break down the endothelial barrier and invade and establish themselves in the tissue's interstitium. The micrometastasis requires a blood supply from the surrounding host tissue if it is to advance beyond about 1 mm in size, therefore the process of angiogenesis is crucial to the establishment of any cancer nodule.

A number of biochemical pathways involved in the metastatic and angiogenic process have been characterised and are being actively investigated as potential therapeutic targets; for example, the matrix metalloproteinases, which include collagenase, elastase, and gelatinase, are believed to be responsible for the breakdown of extracellular matrix and the disruption of tissue architecture that accompany malignant progression. Inhibitors of these enzymes have been developed and preclinical studies have shown that, in animal models of malignancy, these drugs can:

- restrict the growth and regional spread of solid tumours
- inhibit metastatic spread
- block the process of tumour neovascularisation.

Several of these agents have entered clinical trial and the results are awaited with interest.

Gene therapy

The discovery, since the late 1970s, of a large number of cellular oncogenes and a growing number of tumour suppressor genes has identified many important targets for the genetic mutations that characterise multistage carcinogenesis; however, the accumulation of multiple mutations within cancer cells makes it unlikely that transfer of one or a few normal homologues will permanently restore controlled cell growth. Furthermore, with existing technology it appears unlikely that a gene therapy vector could feasibly be delivered to 100% of tumour cells, and thus tumour cells that escape gene delivery or that secondarily lose or inactivate the transduced gene will continue to grow. Virally directed enzyme prodrug therapy (VDEPT) may offer such potential; for example, gene constructs linking the CEA promoter sequence to the structural gene for the enzyme cytosine deaminase (CD) have been packaged into adenoviruses and retroviruses.[33] The fungal enzyme (CD) (Figure 10.4) is not expressed in mammalian cells and has the capacity to convert the inactive prodrug, 5-flucytosine, to the cytotoxic drug, 5FU, which is then capable of killing the cancer cell infected by the virus and surrounding cells—the so called bystander effect. The reasoning underlying the use of the CEA promoter is to impart an

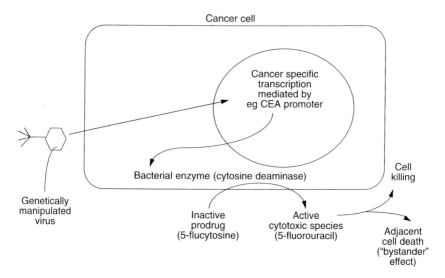

FIGURE 10.4—*Virus directed enzyme prodrug therapy for colorectal cancer. Tumour specificity is provided by carcinoembryonic antigen promoter (CEA = carcinoembryonic antigen).*

element of tumour specific expression of the gene therapy and therefore introduce a degree of tumour selectivity.

The turn of the century will see an extraordinary increase in the range of novel therapeutic strategies being brought to the clinic and will require close cooperation between basic and clinical scientists.

References

20 Cummings BJ. Adjuvant radiation therapy for colorectal cancer. *Cancer* 1992;**70**(suppl 5): 1372–83.

21 James RD. AXIS—a new kind of cancer trial [editorial]. *Clin Oncol* 1990;**2**:125–9.

22 Gray R, James R, Mossman J, *et al.* AXIS a suitable case for treatment. *Br J Cancer* 1991; **63**:841–50.

23 Williams LE, Beatty BG, Beatty JD, *et al.* Estimation of monoclonal antibody-associated ^{90}Yt activity needed to achieve certain tumour radiation doses in colorectal cancer patients. *Cancer* 1990;**50**:1029–30.

24 Boxer GM, Begent RH, Kelly AM, *et al.* Factors influencing variability of localisation of antibodies to carcinoembryonic antigen in patients with colorectal cancer—implications for radioimmunotherapy. *Br J Cancer* 1992;**65**:825–31.

25 Lokich JJ, Ahlgren JD, Gullo JJ, *et al.* A prospective randomised comparison of continuous infusion fluorouracil with a conventional bolus schedule in metastatic colorectal cancer. *J Clin Oncol* 1989;**7**:425–32.

26 de Takats PG, Kerr DJ, Poole CJ, *et al.* Hepatic arterial chemotherapy for colorectal carcinoma [review]. *Br J Cancer* 1994;**69**:372–8.

27 McArdle CS, Kerr DJ, O'Gorman P, *et al.* Pharmacokinetic study of 5-FU in a novel dialysate solution: a long term intraperitoneal approach for advanced colorectal cancer. *Br J Cancer* 1994;**6a**:768–73.

28 James RD, Schofield PF. The value of radiotherapy for rectal cancer. *Baillières Clin Gastroenterol* 1989;**3**:647–69.

29 Donath D, Nori D, Turnbull A, *et al*. Brachytherapy in the treatment of solitary colorectal metastases to the liver. *J Surg Oncol* 1990;**44**:55–61.

30 Thomas DS, Nauta RJ, Rodgers JE, *et al*. Intraoperative high-dose rate interstitial irradiation of hepatic metastases from colorectal carcinoma. Results of a phase I–II trial. *Cancer* 1993;**71**:1977–81.

31 Kashtan H, Stern H. The use of lasers in colorectal cancer. *Cancer Invest* 1993;**11**:33–5.

32 Sargeant IR, Tobias JS, Blackman G, *et al*. Radiation enhancement of laser palliation for advanced rectal and rectosigmoid cancer: a pilot study. *Gut* 1993;**34**:958–62.

33 Huber BE, Richards CA, Krenitsby TA. Retroviral mediated gene therapy for the treatment of hepatocellular cancer: an innovative approach for cancer therapy. *Proc Natl Acad Sci USA* 1991;**88**:8039–43.

11: Lymphomas

HUGH M GILMOUR, ANDREW S KRAJEWSKI, and
ALISTAIR C PARKER

It is estimated that 20–40% of non-Hodgkin's lymphomas present with
extranodal disease, which may reflect either primary or secondary
involvement, and the gastrointestinal tract is the most common site of
primary disease. Extranodal Hodgkin's disease is rare and in the
gastrointestinal tract virtually all cases are secondary to nodal disease arising
at other sites. Over the years, strict criteria have been laid down for the
diagnosis of primary gastrointestinal lymphomas, the best recognised being

---

**Criteria for diagnosis of primary gastrointestinal
lymphoma**

- Patients have no evidence of superficial lymphadenopathy on presentation
- Chest radiograph (scans) shows no enlargement of intrathoracic lymph
  nodes
- Normal total and differential white cell counts (normal bone marrow)
- The tumour lies mainly in the bowel with only local lymph node involvement
- Liver and spleen free of disease

Adapted from Dawson *et al.*[1] Should now include investigations indicated in
parentheses.

---

those of Dawson *et al* (see box)[1]. Unfortunately in many of the series
reported such criteria are either not applied or left unstated. This, along
with the reporting of groups of cases based on anatomical site, histological
features, immunohistochemical characteristics, or clinical behaviour, has
made for difficulties in identifying and comparing incidence and prevalence
rates, diagnostic features, and in particular the effectiveness of therapy.
The last has also been compounded by the lack of standardisation of
treatments and the different modes of therapy applied—often, it would
appear—in a somewhat arbitrary and inconsistent manner. Many of the
series reported are retrospective, the classification and nomenclature have

366

changed over the years. The distinction both between early lymphoma and reactive lymphoid hyperplasias and between primary and secondary involvement of the gastrointestinal tract has posed problems in obtaining a clear picture of how best to diagnose and manage what is, in most Western countries, a relatively rare but none the less important tumour affecting the gastrointestinal tract.

Epidemiology

Notwithstanding the above comments, it is estimated that in developed Western countries primary gastrointestinal lymphomas account for some 30% of all extranodal lymphomas. This tumour forms 1–4% of primary gastrointestinal malignant tumours with an incidence in the United Kingdom and North America of 1–2 per 100 000 of the population. There is a male preponderance in most series of about 2:1, with a wide age range, although the majority of patients are older than 50 years at the time of diagnosis. In childhood the ileocaecal site and Burkitt's histological pattern are more frequent. There are geographical variations in the incidence, anatomical site, and histological pattern, with small intestine being a relatively frequent site in the Mediterranean and Middle East regions and an increased incidence of T cell lymphomas affecting the gastrointestinal tract in parts of Japan. The incidence of lymphomas including gastrointestinal sites is increased in immunocompromised patients and in developed countries this is seen in transplant recipients,[2] whereas it might be expected that in countries where HIV infection is common this would be associated with an increased incidence of gastrointestinal lymphomas.[3] A majority of the lymphomas arising in the gastrointestinal tract are of B cell origin and, while usually of diffuse, large cell type, small B cell lymphomas are relatively common. Many of the latter are derived from mucosal associated lymphoid tissue (MALT) and had previously been classified as pseudolymphomas.

In Western developed countries the most common site of gastrointestinal lymphoma is the stomach, where over half the tumours arise, followed by the small intestine, which accounts for about one third of cases. There is some overlap with the colon in the ileocaecal region, with about 10% involving the colorectum. In many series there is some variation of the distribution within the intestines but Table 11.1 shows the distribution of cases diagnosed in the department of pathology at the University of Edinburgh over the decade 1985–1994. This confirms the stomach as the most common site but shows a reversal of the expected sex distribution at this site. The small intestinal tumours are almost equally divided between the sexes and only in the colorectum is there the expected male preponderance. This illustrates that a small number of cases may present

TABLE 11.1—*Gastrointestinal lymphomas 1985–1994—Department of Pathology, University of Edinburgh*

Site	1985–1989	1990–1994	1985–1994
Stomach	25 (15:10)	18 (12:6)[+3]	43 (27:16)
Small intestine	13 (7:6)*	6 (4:2)[+]	19 (11:8)
Colorectum	6 (3:3)*	6 (1:5)[+]	12 (4:8)
Oesophagus	1	1[+]	2 (1:1)

Values in parentheses are male:female ratios.
* One case involving two gastrointestinal sites.
[+] Three cases involving two gastrointestinal sites.

with tumours at more than one anatomical site, although multiple tumours within a single site are not infrequent, particularly within the small intestine and in early gastric lymphoma. When lymphoma is found in the colorectum there is the increased likelihood of other sites in the gastrointestinal tract being involved, or an association with chronic lymphocytic leukaemia or previously known lymphoma outside the gastrointestinal tract. Indeed, three of the six colorectal cases in the Edinburgh figures for 1990–1994 would not fulfil the criteria for primary gastrointestinal lymphoma because of the above relationship.

In addition to the increased incidence of lymphomas related to immunosuppression, lymphomas may also be seen in relation to coeliac disease, where it is suggested that a gluten free diet may protect against the development of lymphoma,[4] and inflammatory bowel disease, and rare familial cases have also been reported.

Despite this association with a number of diseases in which there is an abnormality of the immune system, due either to suppression or to chronic stimulation, the aetiology of most gastrointestinal lymphomas is unknown. Great interest has, however, been generated in the discovery of the association between *Helicobacter pylori* colonisation of the gastric mucosa and gastric lymphoma. What is even more intriguing is the apparent regression of early gastric lymphomas after the eradication of helicobacter from the stomach.[5] Infection with this organism leads to the accumulation of lymphoid tissue, which is not found in the normal stomach and may become hyperplastic under the influence of chronic infection and other autoimmune phenomena. Mutagens in the diet may also affect proliferating B cells, and there appears to be a stimulatory role for *H. pylori* responsive non-neoplastic T cells in this process. This T cell effect only seems to influence the cells of low grade gastric MALT lymphomas, which may explain the regression of early tumours of this type after treatment of *H. pylori* infection.[6]

Clinical features

Unfortunately there are no specific symptoms or signs that herald the development of a gastrointestinal lymphoma but the most common symptom is abdominal pain, which may or may not be associated with weight loss, malaise, fatigue, nausea, and vomiting, while other less common features are gastrointestinal bleeding, intestinal obstruction, altered bowel habit, or perforation. A presentation with anaemia is relatively rare. While the majority of patients present with chronic symptoms, the mean duration of symptoms in a large series from Saudi Arabia[7] was only about six months for both gastric and intestinal sites of origin, although a longer duration was seen in cases developing in immunoproliferative small intestinal disease (IPSID). A relatively small proportion of patients present acutely, usually as a result of intestinal obstruction or perforation and these features are almost exclusively seen in patients with small intestinal lymphomas. As expected, the symptoms tend to reflect the site of the disease and the pattern of involvement but on clinical examination it is only possible to palpate a mass lesion in perhaps 10% of cases.

When lymphoma is a complication of a pre-existing disease, such as coeliac disease, the development of symptoms such as abdominal pain and weight loss (without dietary alteration) in a previously well patient often indicates the development of gastrointestinal lymphoma; in this situation the high suspicion of such a development should lead to appropriate investigation.[8]

Investigation and diagnosis

Histology is usually required for definitive diagnosis because even with scanning radiology and endoscopy the best diagnosis that can be reached is that of a tumour and, as most primary tumours in the gastrointestinal tract are of epithelial origin, clinical suspicion usually falls on the side of carcinoma for most detected lesions. While scanning modalities may be valuable in diagnosis, their major role is perhaps in staging of lymphomas once diagnosed, as in the large Saudi Arabian series[7] abdominal ultrasound examinations were negative in 40 of the 84 cases examined, as were 50 of 152 cases examined by computed tomography (CT). Contrast gastrointestinal radiology failed to demonstrate tumours in 22 of 125 cases, and there were 12 negative endoscopies out of 101 examinations. The most difficult tumours to identify, both by contrast radiology and by endoscopy, are those within the distal jejunum and ileum, and superficial lesions—even if multifocal—would be difficult to identify by either ultrasonography or CT. Intracavitary ultrasonography, if available, is particularly useful in identifying lesions and assessing the degree of infiltration of the wall of the

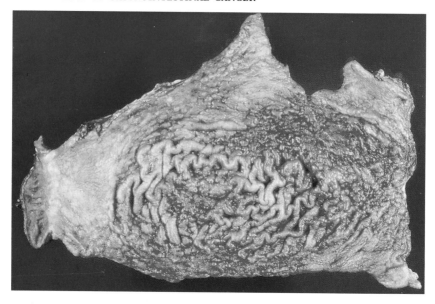

FIGURE 11.1—*This is a low grade B cell gastric lymphoma. An extensive area of hyperaemia affects much of the body and proximal antrum of the stomach, where in areas the rugal folds are exaggerated and thickened and elsewhere are effaced, resulting in a somewhat mamillated appearance.*

gut preoperatively. Double contrast barium meal or enema examinations may be valuable in detecting small mucosal lesions or abnormalities of mucosal pattern (Figure 11.1), but endoscopy has the advantage of allowing biopsies to be taken from the lesions to ascertain the true nature of the neoplastic process.

Pathology

Disease patterns

Before dealing in detail with the histological classification of the gastrointestinal lymphomas, which is still evolving, it is valuable to consider the different patterns that can be related to anatomical sites of origin.

Stomach

A wide variation of tumour patterns may be seen in the stomach, ranging from subtle changes in mucosal architecture barely discernible by endoscopy or contrast radiology to large lesions, which may take the form of giant

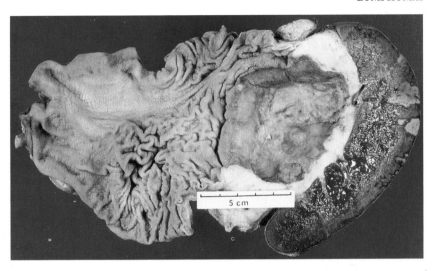

FIGURE 11.2—*A large ulcerated high grade B cell lymphoma on the greater curvature of the stomach that extends to and invades the hilum of the spleen. The remainder of the gastric mucosa appears unremarkable. Small splenic infarcts are noted at the periphery of the spleen; these are caused by invasion of hilar vessels.*

gastric ulcers (Figure 11.2) or multiple tumours often of bizarre appearance. Biopsy diagnosis may be difficult in either case because of the subtlety of early gastric lymphomas or because of necrosis and secondary inflammation on the surface of larger lesions if multiple biopsies are not taken from non-ulcerated areas.

Small intestine

Here the tumours often form stricturing lesions, with or without ulceration (Figure 11.3), but exophytic masses or tumour plaques are not uncommon and the tumours may lead to perforation or intussusception, the latter seemingly more common in Burkitt's lymphomas of the ileocaecal region. In one series of 119 small intestinal lymphomas from London the impression was gained that B cell tumours were more likely to form masses or be annular, whereas T cell tumours more often formed plaques or ulcerated strictures and were more likely to be multifocal.[9] T cell tumours are more likely to develop in association with coeliac disease and there has been a degree of controversy about those tumours that present without a previous history of coeliac disease but where the small intestinal mucosa shows evidence of villous atrophy. The terminology is of an enteropathy associated lymphoma and there is still debate as to whether these patients had "silent coeliac disease" or whether the villous atrophy developed in association with the tumour without there being hypersensitivity to dietary gluten.

371

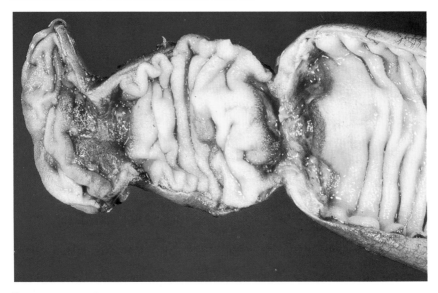

FIGURE 11.3—*An enteropathy associated T cell lymphoma in the ileum. Two circumferential superficial ulcers have caused stricturing of the lumen; there is a third area of mucosal nodularity and superficial erosion midway between the two strictures.*

Lymphomas developing in IPSID are common in the Middle East and account for about a third of gastrointestinal lymphomas in Iraq, Kuwait, and Lebanon. These tumours are extremely rare in Western experience. While the macroscopic tumours within the small intestine may be similar to those described above, there is often the pattern of IPSID in the small intestine, manifest by a diffuse lymphoplasmacytic infiltrate within the mucosa, and it is often within the mesenteric lymph nodes that evidence of a lymphoma is identified at surgery.[10]

Colon

The ileocaecal region is a relatively common site of involvement by lymphoma, which may lead to the presentation of intestinal obstruction due to intussusception; this, as indicated, may be seen in association with a tumour of Burkitt's type occurring in the younger age group. In one series of 45 cases which formed 0·2% of all colonic malignancies the most common clinical presentations were rectal bleeding, diarrhoea, abdominal pain, and alteration in bowel habit.[11] About a quarter were multiple and just under half involved the rectum, but this series excluded ileocaecal tumours in children. A particularly distinctive pattern of lymphomatous involvement of the gut is described as multiple lymphomatous polyposis; although this may be seen throughout the gastrointestinal tract, it is most commonly seen within the colon. The polypoid lesions may vary from a few millimetres to several centimetres in size and may have a similar appearance to the adenomas of familial adenomatous polyposis coli. In lymphomatous polyposis, however, the polyps generally tend to be smoother and more uniform in appearance and size, and later in the disease tend to be larger than the usual adenomas in familial adenomatous polyposis coli. In the colon and rectum lymphomas commonly appear as exophytic ulcerated masses that are difficult to distinguish from adenocarcinomas.

Classification

Although the gastrointestinal tract may be secondarily involved in as many as 25% of cases of nodal lymphoma, the majority of cases of lymphoma presenting with gastrointestinal involvement are believed to arise primarily from intestinal MALT. It is now accepted that these MALT derived lymphomas have quite distinct morphological, immunological, and clinical features that differentiate them from nodal lymphomas.[12] In particular, it is now known that most of these tumours remain localised to the gastrointestinal tract and show prolonged survival compared with nodal lymphomas. When relapses occur these are nearly always within the gastrointestinal tract. Because of these distinctive clinicopathological features it is now generally accepted that commonly used classifications of nodal lymphoma, such as Kiel or Working formulation, are inadequate for classification of intestinal lymphoma,[13] and instead the classification proposed by Isaacson et al should be adopted (see box).[14 15] It should be noted that the categories defined in Isaacson's classification are incorporated as part of the new revised European American Classification of Lymphoma.[16]

Low grade MALT lymphomas

MALT type lymphomas may occur anywhere in the gastrointestinal tract but are most common in the stomach. Low grade tumours account for about 40% of gastric lymphomas and 20% of intestinal lymphomas.

Morphologically low grade tumours show diffuse infiltration of the lamina propria by cells of small to medium size with irregular nuclear contours resembling centrocytes (centrocyte-like cells). A small number of blast cells may be present. In some cases the infiltrating cells may be more like lymphocytes or show more abundant cytoplasm resembling monocytoid B cells. In some cases plasmacytic differentiation may be present and may be sufficiently marked to cause confusion with lymphoplasmacytic lymphoma. A distinctive feature of low grade MALT lymphoma is the formation of lymphoepithelial lesions. These are characterised by infiltration and destruction of gland epithelium by centrocyte-like cells, often associated

---

Classification of gastrointestinal lymphomas

B cell
- Mucosa associated lymphoid tissue (MALT) type
    Low grade
    High grade with or without a low grade component
    Immunoproliferative small intestinal disease
        Low grade
        High grade with or without a low grade component
- Mantle cell (lymphomatous polyposis)
- Burkitt's and Burkitt-like
- Other types of low and high grade lymphoma corresponding to peripheral lymph node equivalents

T cell
- Enteropathy associated T cell lymphoma (EATL)
- Other types unassociated with enteropathy

Rare types (including conditions that may simulate lymphoma)

---

with eosinophilia of glandular epithelium. In mucosa infiltrated by low grade MALT lymphoma reactive lymphoid follicles are almost invariably present. These follicles may appear relatively normal with well defined light and dark zones in the germinal centre or may become progressively colonised by neoplastic centrocyte-like cells. The presence of follicles and follicular colonisation has in the past been misinterpreted as follicular lymphoma or pseudolymphoma.

Immunophenotypically low grade MALT lymphomas resemble splenic marginal zone and Peyer's patch dome cells (expressing pan B cell markers such as CD20 and surface IgM or less commonly IgA plus monotypic κ or λ light chain and also showing immunoglobulin gene rearrangements). In contrast to node based follicle centre cell tumours (follicular lymphomas, centroblastic lymphomas) and lymphocytic or centrocytic lymphomas, MALT lymphomas do not express CD10 or CD5 and do not show bcl-2 (t14;18) or bcl-1 (t11;14) translocations, but may show trisomies, especially trisomy 3 in a high proportion of cases.

High grade MALT lymphomas

High grade MALT lymphomas are more common than low grade tumours.

Morphologically these tumours show diffuse mucosal infiltration by blast cells, somewhat resembling centroblasts, or may have more abundant cytoplasm and resemble plasmablasts. In some cases a low grade component may be present. Lymphoepithelial lesions are rare in high grade MALT lymphoma. Immunophenotypically these tumours are similar to low grade tumours but may show strong cytoplasmic immunoglobulin staining. It is perhaps worth noting that the lack of distinctive morphological characteristics of high grade MALT lymphomas (without concomitant low grade) does raise the problem of whether these are truly distinct from nodal high grade large B cell lymphomas; however, evidence is accumulating that these tumours are immunophenotypically and genetically distinct, resembling low grade MALT lymphomas, and several reports also suggest that the clinical behaviour of these tumours is better than nodal high grade tumours.

Immunoproliferative small intestinal disease

IPSID is a small intestinal variant of MALT lymphoma showing marked plasma cell differentiation with production of IgA heavy chain (with no light chains) by tumour cells. This disease is extremely rare outside the Middle East. The usual clinical presentation is with malabsorption in young adults, which in early cases may respond to antibiotic therapy. The jejunum is the most commonly involved site. This usually shows diffuse thickening but tumour masses may be present in some cases.

Histologically these cases may closely resemble other low grade MALT lymphomas but show marked plasmacytic differentiation of cells in the lamina propria, which is diffusely infiltrated, causing broadening of villi. Lymphoepithelial lesions with crypt epithelium infiltrated by centrocyte-like cells are usually present. Reactive follicles may be present. In the later stages of the disease increased numbers of blast cells may accumulate to form frankly invasive tumour masses.

Mantle cell lymphoma (lymphomatous polyposis)

Lymphomatous polyposis accounts for about 10% of cases of intestinal lymphoma. Most patients are over 50 and present with abdominal pain or bleeding. Multiple polypoid tumours are present in these patients, most commonly in the ileocaecal region but they may be found anywhere in the gastrointestinal tract.

These tumours are distinct from MALT lymphomas and are equivalent to nodal centrocytic (diffuse small cleaved cell) lymphomas. In contrast to those with MALT lymphomas, these patients almost invariably show nodal involvement, which may be localised to the gastrointestinal tract in the early stages but usually involves peripheral nodes early in the course of disease. Bone marrow involvement is common in lymphomatous polyposis, in contrast to MALT lymphoma where bone marrow involvement is extremely rare.

Histologically these tumours cause mucosal nodules or polyps of varying size as the result of mucosal infiltration by a uniform population of small to medium sized lymphoid cells, without nucleoli, showing nuclear irregularity, and resembling centrocytes. Blast cells and lymphoepithelial lesions are not present. In many cases the tumour cells may infiltrate around reactive lymphoid follicles with germinal centres, giving a histological appearance similar to that of low grade MALT lymphomas, but the absence of blast cells and lymphoepithelial lesions helps distinguish these tumours from MALT lymphoma. Immunohistochemistry may also be useful in distinguishing lymphomatous polyposis from MALT lymphoma because in lymphomatous polyposis tumour cells consistently express CD5 antigen (absent in MALT lymphoma) and express IgM with IgD in most cases (IgM alone in MALT lymphoma).

Burkitt's and Burkitt-like lymphoma

This type of tumour is common in some African populations but is rare in European patients, accounting for around 5% of cases of intestinal lymphoma. In Europe the tumour usually occurs in children and involves the ileocaecal region. Histologically these tumours either show a homogeneous infiltrate of monomorphic blasts typical of Burkitt's lymphoma or, in European cases, show slightly more cytological atypia of blast cells (Burkitt-like).

Enteropathy associated T cell lymphoma

Formerly known as malignant histiocytosis, enteropathy associated T cell lymphoma (EATL) accounts for 20–30% of small intestinal lymphomas. These tumours usually occur in the jejunum of patients over 50 years of age, who present either with haemorrhage, obstruction, or perforation. Macroscopically these tumours usually show multiple discrete areas of ulceration associated with thickening of the bowel wall and luminal narrowing. Diagnosis is usually made on resected specimens after an acute surgical episode, although cases may occasionally be diagnosed by endoscopic biopsy. Although the great majority of cases involve the jejunum, a minority of cases may show lesions in the ileum and rarely in the stomach.

EATL has a well known association with coeliac disease. About two thirds of patients give a history of coeliac disease and the remaining third show evidence of enteropathy, often with a recent history of malabsorption, at the time of presentation of the tumour.[8]

Histologically these tumours are high grade lymphomas, containing large blast cells showing variable pleomorphism, with diffuse infiltration of the mucosa, mucosal ulceration, and infiltration of tumour into submucosa and muscularis propria. Variable numbers of small lymphocytes, histiocytes, and eosinophils may be present. Because of this admixture of cell types this is the tumour that has been most commonly misdiagnosed as primary Hodgkin's disease of the intestine in the past.

The mucosa adjacent to the tumour usually shows crypt hyperplastic villous atrophy, with increased lymphocytes and plasma cells in the lamina propria and increased intraepithelial lymphocytes. Cases lacking evidence of enteropathy have been reported but are rare.

EATL can be differentiated from other bowel lymphomas by immunohistochemistry, which shows expression of T cell antigens by tumour cells (CD3 and CD7, without CD4 or CD8).[17] Genetic studies have shown that these tumours show clonal T cell receptor gene rearrangements.[18]

Staging of primary gastrointestinal lymphomas

Staging may be primarily clinical, relying on endoscopy and radiology once a pathological diagnosis has been reached, or combined with the pathological information obtained from resection specimens or lymph node and bone marrow biopsy.

Staging of primary gastrointestinal lymphomas

I_E — Lymphoma confined to one or more gastrointestinal site, on one side of diaphragm, without lymph node infiltration

$\quad I_{E1}$ — Lymphoma confined to mucosa and submucosa

$\quad I_{E2}$ — Lymphoma extending beyond submucosa

II_E — Lymphoma confined to one or more gastrointestinal site with lymph node infiltration on one side of diaphragm (any depth of lymphoma infiltration in gut wall)

$\quad II_{E1}$ — Infiltration of regional lymph nodes contiguous to tumour

$\quad II_{E2}$ — Infiltration of non-contiguous lymph nodes (for example, para-aortic or paracaval)

III_E — Gastrointestinal tract involvement and involvement of lymph nodes on both sides of the diaphragm or the spleen (III_S)

IV_E — Gastrointestinal lymphoma with dissemination to bone marrow or other non-lymphoid tissues

---

The current staging is shown in the box, but at a recent European workshop a modification of the above classification was proposed.[13] This is almost identical to the above classification but the E subscript is not used unless there is penetration of serosa to involve adjacent organs (for example, II_E pancreas) and stages III and IV are combined into stage IV with no stage III. It is obvious that if Dawson's criteria are used to define primary gastrointestinal tumours then any tumour above stage II should be excluded!

Treatment

As the incidence of gastrointestinal lymphomas is relatively low, experience of management outwith large oncology centres is limited. What follows is an outline of the available treatment. At the present time evaluation of the individual patient by staging, histology, and surgical and medical observation is essential for determining the most appropriate therapeutic approach. This includes surgery, chemotherapy, or radiotherapy, either alone or in combination.

Role of surgery

Surgical intervention will be required when patients present acutely with obstruction or perforation. Surgical excision at this time may attempt cure or may be used to debulk tumour or remove tumour from sites where a rapid response to chemotherapy or radiotherapy could lead to perforation—for example, in the small intestine.

Radiotherapy

This can be used to follow up local resection and when limited nodal disease adjacent to the primary tumour is identified, but careful follow up is required. When "bulk" disease is present then radiotherapy can be used as additional treatment after chemotherapy.

Gastric MALT lymphoma

At present, many authorities are convinced that an attempt should be made to eradicate *H. pylori* in cases of low grade MALT lymphoma of the stomach. Cases of early gastric MALT lymphomas have regressed after eradication of this organism, and this present stance is supported by in vitro results showing that proliferation of low grade MALT lymphomas depends on *H. pylori* induced, T cell mediated stimulation.[6]

The picture is not, however, absolutely clear because it is not known whether the initial encouraging results apply only to "early" tumours or can be extrapolated and indeed shown to occur in more advanced disease. Most commonly, omeprazole and ampicillin given for 10–14 days are prescribed, although many other combinations are available. To date, follow up is obviously very short. As some studies have shown persistent molecular evidence of a monoclonal B cell population after such treatment, long term results are uncertain. Endoscopic mucosal resection has been suggested as an alternative method of treatment, after endoscopic ultrasonography to confirm the superficial location of the lesions, but careful follow up is warranted because these early lesions have often proved to be multifocal.

Many high grade primary gastric lymphomas evolve from low grade MALT lymphomas and they have a more favourable clinical behaviour when compared with nodal lymphoma. Despite this apparent evolution there is as yet no clinical evidence to suggest that *H. pylori* eradication is of benefit in high grade MALT lymphoma. In the case of high grade lymphoma of the stomach the practice of our centre is to stage the tumour, but relatively few will prove to be localised to the stomach and even in these cases surgery is probably not the treatment of choice as the tumour is chemotherapy and radiotherapy sensitive. A standard chemotherapeutic regimen, such as CHOP (cyclophosphamide, doxorubicin, vincristine, prednisolone), with the potential of adjunctive radiotherapy to the site of disease is an appropriate approach.

High grade lymphomas at other sites

After appropriate staging procedures the decision on management can be made; however, as stated previously, some localised lesions present as acute surgical emergencies and appropriate resection at laparotomy could potentially be curative. In other cases the disorder is found to be more widely disseminated at laparotomy or on clinical and radiological investigation. In such cases chemotherapy is the appropriate therapy and additional radiotherapy can be considered.

Enteropathy associated T cell lymphoma

This disorder of the small intestine complicating coeliac disease has been shown to be of T cell origin on the basis of T cell receptor gene rearrangement studies. As this disorder often involves the bowel at multiple sites and metastatic disease is common, chemotherapy is the therapy of choice in most cases. The general principles of chemotherapy are outlined below.

Lymphoma arising in IPSID

This rare lymphoma, occurring in young adults from low socioeconomic groups in North Africa and the Middle East, is associated with abnormalities in immunoglobulin production, particularly IgA. Chemotherapy is used together with antibiotics but the outlook is poor.

Chemotherapy

Hodgkin's disease affecting the gastrointestinal tract as a primary tumour is a rarity. If it is encountered chemotherapy should be used as a first line treatment.

Low grade lymphoma

As far as the management of so called low grade lymphomas is concerned the exciting new development in gastrointestinal disease has been the treatment of low grade MALT lymphomas in the stomach; this has already been outlined.

If initial attempts with eradication therapy fail, and there is some discussion as to how long the interval may be between eradication and regression of the lymphoma, then regimens such as CVP (cyclophosphamide 400 mg/m² orally days 1–5, vincristine 1·4 mg/m² i.v. infusion day 1, and prednisolone 40 mg orally days 1–5) repeated every 21 days for approximately six cycles are acceptable. Radiotherapy should be considered. Advances in the therapy of low grade disease in general have not been as good as in high grade. Survival is, however, often prolonged, with or without therapy.

High grade lymphomas

At present, when chemotherapy is chosen as the optimum treatment for these tumours, no regimen has been shown to be superior to that of CHOP (cyclophosphamide 750 mg/m², i.v. infusion day 1, doxorubicin 50 mg/m² i.v. infusion day 1, vincristine 1·4 mg/m² i.v. infusion but no more than 2 mg day 1, prednisolone 25 mg QDS orally days 1–5). The regimen results overall in a complete remission rate of about 60%, and 30–40% long term survival.

At present, younger patients (below age 60 years) with features indicating high risk disease—for example, high serum lactate dehydrogenase and poor performance status—can be selected for high dose chemotherapy with progenitor cell rescue after initial cytoreductive treatment to bring them into remission. Preliminary results are encouraging and the use of progenitor cells from the peripheral blood has significantly reduced the mortality, morbidity, and expense of this approach.

The quality of life of most patients actively receiving chemotherapy is relatively good. This is because of the support given by the specialised units concerned and the use of more effective antiemetics. Major improvements still require to be made in this area, however, in terms of the recognition of many social and other problems, often not revealed by patients undergoing such treatment.

There are few studies that indicate the incidence of secondary tumours arising as a result of therapy in patients with non-Hodgkin's lymphoma. Other side effects and toxicity using the CHOP regimen are myelosuppression, sterility, peripheral neuropathy, and cardiotoxicity. Of these, myelosuppression is the most common and is usually self limiting.

Prognosis and survival in gastrointestinal non-Hodgkin's lymphoma

Because of the rarity of gastrointestinal lymphoma there are few prospective studies of clinical outcome[19] and almost all large series reported in the recent literature depend upon retrospective analyses.[9 20–22] Comparison of data from these different studies is difficult because of differences in the method of patient selection, differences in therapy, and lack of standardisation in histopathological classification. Nevertheless, from these studies it is possible to draw some important conclusions regarding prognosis in gastrointestinal lymphoma. Statistically significant prognostic variables include the site of tumour, stage, and histopathological subtype, and whether radical (complete) tumour resection is carried out.

Patients with gastric lymphomas have a better overall prognosis than those with intestinal lymphoma, with a 70–90% five years survival for low grade gastric lymphomas and around a 40% five years survival for patients with high grade gastric tumours. Patients with early stage (I_E) gastric lymphoma show an 80–90% five years survival, with over 50% 10 year survival.[19 22]

The prognosis for patients with intestinal lymphoma is usually considered to be worse than for those with gastric lymphoma, but simple comparisons are misleading because patients with intestinal lymphoma constitute a more heterogeneous group with more high grade and non-MALT lymphomas, which are likely to present at a later stage. Patients with low grade B cell, MALT lymphomas and high grade B cell lymphomas probably show a similar survival to patients with gastric lymphoma at the same stage. Possibly the most important prognostic factor in these cases is the tumour stage and whether the tumour is resectable, with several studies showing five year survivals for stage I tumours of around 70%. In contrast, patients with non-MALT lymphomas, such as lymphomatous polyposis, have been reported to show a median survival of 15 months, with none surviving beyond three years.[19] Similarly, the great majority of patients with intestinal T cell lymphomas die within a year of diagnosis, with few reported long term survivals.[18]

No doubt further refinements of classification will result from advances in molecular pathology but in order for better survivals to be achieved advances in therapy are required. This has to be accompanied by standardisation of staging, pathological classification, and therapy so that valid comparisons can be made between centres in order to identify the most effective methods of management for this relatively uncommon but important gastrointestinal neoplasm.

References

1 Dawson IMP, Cornes JS, Morson BC. Primary malignant lymphoid tumours of the intestinal tract. Report of 37 cases with a study of the factors influencing prognosis. *Br J Surg* 1961;**49**:80–9.
2 Guettier C, Hamilton-Dutoit S, Guillemain R, *et al.* Primary gastrointestinal malignant lymphomas associated with Epstein–Barr virus after heart transplantation. *Histopathology* 1992;**20**:21–8.
3 Parente F, Rizzardini G, Cernuschi M, *et al.* Non-Hodgkin's lymphoma and AIDS: frequency of gastrointestinal involvement in a large Italian series. *Scand J Gastroenterol* 1993;**28**:315–8.
4 Holmes GKT, Prior P, Lane MR, *et al.* Malignancy in coeliac disease—effect of a gluten free diet. *Gut* 1989;**30**:333–8.
5 Wotherspoon AC, Doglioni C, Diss TC, *et al.* Regression of primary low grade B-cell gastric lymphoma of mucosa-associated lymphoid tissue type after eradication of *Helicobacter pylori*. *Lancet* 1993;**342**:575–7.
6 Isaacson PG. Gastric lymphoma and *Helicobacter pylori*. *N Engl J Med* 1994;**330**:1310–1.
7 Amer MH, El-Akkad S. Gastrointestinal lymphoma in adults: clinical features and management of 300 cases. *Gastroenterology* 1994;**106**:846–58.
8 Swinson CM, Coles EC, Booth CC. Coeliac disease and malignancy. *Lancet* 1983;**i**:111–5.
9 Domizio P, Owen RA, Shepherd NA, *et al.* Primary lymphoma of the small intestine. A clinicopathological study of 119 cases. *Am J Surg Pathol* 1993;**17**:429–42.
10 Galian A, Lecestre M-J, Scotto J, *et al.* Pathological study of alpha-chain disease, with special emphasis on evolution. *Cancer* 1977;**39**:2080–101.
11 Shepherd NA, Hall PA, Coates PJ, *et al.* Primary malignant lymphoma of the colon and rectum. A histopathological and immunohistochemical analysis of 45 cases with clinicopathological correlations. *Histopathology* 1988;**12**:235–52.
12 Isaacson PG, Norton AJ. Malignant lymphoma of the gastrointestinal tract. In: *Extranodal Lymphomas*. Edinburgh: Churchill Livingstone, 1994: chap. 3.
13 Rohatiner A, d'Amore F, Coiffier B, *et al.* Report on a workshop convened to discuss the pathological and staging classifications of gastrointestinal tract lymphoma. *Ann Oncol* 1994;**5**:397–400.
14 Isaacson PG, Spencer J, Wright DH. Classifying primary gut lymphomas. *Lancet* 1988;**ii**:1148–9.
15 Isaacson PG. Gastrointestinal lymphoma. *Hum Pathol* 1994;**25**:1020–9.
16 Chan JKC, Banks PM, Cleary ML, *et al.* A proposal for classification of lymphoid neoplasms (by the International Lymphoma Study Group). *Histopathology* 1994;**25**:517–36.
17 Salter DM, Krajewski AS, Dewar AE. Immunophenotype analysis of malignant histocytosis of the intestine. *J Clin Pathol* 186;**39**:8–15.
18 Murray A, Cuevas EC, Jones DB, *et al.* Study of the immunohistochemistry and T cell clonality of enteropathy-associated T cell lymphoma. *Am J Pathol* 1995;**146**:509–19.
19 Ruskone-Fourmestraux A, Aegerter P, Delmer A, *et al.* Primary digestive tract lymphoma: a prospective multicentric study of 91 patients. *Gastroenterology* 1993;**105**:1662–71.
20 Cogliatti SB, Schmid U, Schumacher U, *et al.* Primary B-cell gastric lymphoma: a clinicopathological study of 145 patients. *Gastroenterology* 1991;**101**:1159–70.

21 Radaszkiewicz T, Dragosics B, Bauer P. Gastrointestinal malignant lymphomas of the mucosa-associated lymphoid tissue: factors relevant to prognosis. *Gastroenterology* 1992; **102**:1628–38.
22 Morton JE, Leyland MJ, Vaughan Hudson G, *et al.* Primary gastrointestinal non-Hodgkin's lymphoma: a review of 175 British National Lymphoma Investigation cases. *Br J Cancer* 1993;**67**:776–82.

Index

α-catenin 38, 39, 95
α heavy chain disease 54
α_1 antitrypsin deficiency 70
abdominoperineal resection (of
    rectum) 343
acetylator status 84
achlorhydria 304
addressins 363
adenoma-carcinoma
    sequence 57–8, 59, 67, 68,
    324–5
adherens junctions 38
adhesion molecules 38–41
adrenocorticotrophic hormone
    (ACTH), ectopic 308
Adriamycin *see* doxorubicin
aflatoxin 21, 63, 69, 283
    B1 (AFB1) 69, 70
AFP *see* alphafetoprotein
agricultural chemicals 52
alcohol consumption 53
    colorectal cancer and 17
    hepatocellular carcinoma
        and 21, 69, 283
    oesophageal cancer and 5–6
    pancreatic cancer and 26, 71
alcohol injection
    in liver metastases 278
    in oesophageal cancer 121
    in rectal cancer 342
alcoholism
    hepatocellular carcinoma
        and 21, 283
    oesophageal cancer and 5
alkaline phosphatase, serum 203,
    244
alkylating agents
    carcinogenicity 63
    in pancreatic cancer 226–7

allele loss *see* heterozygosity, loss
    of
alphafetoprotein (AFP)
    serum 284
    in viral constructs 294–5
aminoimidazoazarenes (AIAs) 16
amphiregulin 85–6, 88, 93
ampullary carcinoma
    investigations 203, 205
    surgery 216, 218–19
ampullectomy, endoscopic 219
anabolic steroids 283
anaemia
    in colorectal cancer 331
    in glucagonoma 305
    pernicious 54, 158
analgesia
    in pancreatic cancer 238–9
    in radiation oesophagitis 130
anastomosis
    integrity 344
    stapled *v* hand sewn 340
    tumour implantation at 340
angiogenesis 362–3
angiography
    in bile duct cancer 245
    in endocrine tumours 309,
        313
    in hepatocellular
        carcinoma 284–5
    in liver metastases 273–4
    in pancreatic cancer 205–7,
        208
angiosarcoma, liver 22
ankylosing spondylitis 10, 26,
    322
anorectal manometry 338
antacid mixtures 130
anthracyclines *see also*
    doxorubicin; epirubicin

385

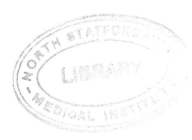